INTRODUCTORY
CLINICAL
PHARMACOLOGY

INTRODUCTORY CLINICAL PHARMACOLOGY

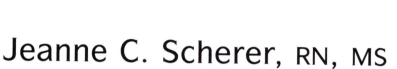

Jeanne C. Scherer, RN, MS

Former Assistant Director, Medical-Surgical Coordinator, and Instructor
Sisters of Charity Hospital School of Nursing
Buffalo, New York

FOURTH EDITION

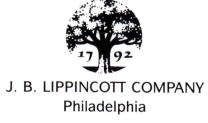

J. B. LIPPINCOTT COMPANY
Philadelphia

New York   London   Hagerstown

Acquisitions Editor: Ellen M. Campbell
Project Editor: Grace R. Caputo
Indexer: Anne Cope
Designer: Doug Smock
Production Manager: Helen Ewan
Production Coordinator: Kathryn Rule
Compositor: Circle Graphics
Printer/Binder: Courier Companies, Inc.

4th Edition

6   5   4   3   2

Library of Congress Cataloging-in-Publication Data

Scherer, Jeanne C.
    Introductory clinical pharmacology / Jeanne C. Scherer. —4th ed.
      p.   cm.
    Includes index.
    ISBN 0-397-54843-5
    1. Clinical pharmacology.   2. Nursing.   I. Title.
    [DNLM: 1. Drug Therapy-nurses' instruction.   2. Pharmacology,
Clinical-nurses' instruction.   QV 38 S3261]
RM301.28.S34 1992
615.5′8-dc20
DNLM/DLC
for Library of Congress   91-21768
                                                            CIP

PREFACE

The fourth edition of *Introductory Clinical Pharmacology* reflects the ever-changing science of pharmacology. The information contained in this textbook has been revised and updated according to the latest available information.

This text is designed for those wishing a clear, concise introduction to pharmacology. However, the basic explanations presented in this textbook are not intended to suggest that pharmacology is an easy subject. Drug therapy is one of the most important and complicated treatment modalities in modern health care. Because of its importance and complexity and the frequent additions and changes in the field of pharmacology, it is imperative that all health professionals constantly review and update their knowledge.

Arithmetic and the calculation of drug dosages are reviewed in chapter 1. Material on the nursing process as it applies to the administration of pharmacologic agents follows. Chapters on patient teaching and the administration of medications have been retained.

As in previous editions, drugs are discussed primarily according to their classification rather than according to the disorders they are used to treat. This approach is implemented because many drugs may be used to treat disorders in more than one body system, resulting in extensive cross referencing or repetition of information.

The headings divide the chapter into drug reactions, drug uses, and adverse reactions associated with the administration of a particular pharmacologic agent. In this edition, the nursing process applicable to the administration of a specific class or type of drug is presented after the discussion of a particular class or type of drug. The nursing diagnoses identify patient problems applicable to the drug being administered. Additional nursing diagnoses pertaining to the patient's identified needs and related specifically to the patient's disease or disorder are not included, since this information can be retrieved from other sources, such as a medical-surgical nursing textbook. Patient teaching, which in previous editions was placed at the end of most chapters, has been incorporated into the nursing process under the nursing diagnosis of Knowledge Deficit.

The summary drug tables are representative of the type or class of drugs covered in the chapter. The trade names listed for each generic name are representative of the drugs discussed in the chapter.

In most instances, the adult dose *ranges* are given in the summary drug tables because space does not permit the inclusion of all the possible dosages for various types of disorders. Pediatric dose ranges usually have been omitted because of the increasing complexity of determining the pediatric dose of many pharmacologic agents. Citing pediatric dose ranges could be misleading because many of the drugs given to children are determined on the basis of weight or body surface area (square meters) and have a variety of dosage schedules. Space would not permit an *accurate* presentation of pediatric dosages. When drugs are given to the pediatric patient, the practitioner is encouraged to consult references that give *complete* pediatric dosages.

For current drug information and dosages, the practitioner is advised to consult references such as the *Physician's Desk Reference, Facts and Comparisons*, and *The Hospital Formulary*, as well as the package inserts that accompany most drugs. If reliable references are not available, the hospital pharmacist should be contacted for information concerning a specific pharmacologic agent. If there is a question about the dosage, adverse reactions, or the administration of a particular drug, the physician and pharmacist are appropriate and reliable sources of information.

I wish to thank those involved in the fourth edition of this textbook. The guidelines offered by Ellen Campbell, Acquisitions Editor, assisted in the inclusion of the nursing process throughout the text. The skillful editing of Maria Quici, the production supervision of Kathy Rule, and the design work of Doug Smock improved readability and the presentation of material. I am especially grateful to Grace Caputo, Project Editor, who helped me develop and finalize the changes in this edition.

Jeanne C. Scherer, RN, MS

CONTENTS

► ANTIARRHYTHMIC DRUGS
Actions of the Antiarrhythmic Drugs
Uses of the Antiarrhythmic Drugs
Adverse Reactions Associated with the
Administration of Antiarrhythmic Drugs
Nursing Process: The Patient Receiving an
Antiarrhythmic Drug

Contents

INTRODUCTORY CLINICAL PHARMACOLOGY

Review of Arithmetic and Calculation of Drug Dosages

On completion of this chapter the student will:

► *Accurately perform mathematical calculations when they are necessary to compute drug dosages*

► REVIEW OF ARITHMETIC

▷ Fractions

The two parts of a fraction are the numerator and the denominator.

$$\frac{2}{3} \quad \begin{array}{l} \longleftarrow \text{numerator} \\ \longleftarrow \text{denominator} \end{array}$$

A **proper fraction** may be defined as a part of a whole or any number less than a whole number. An **improper fraction** is a fraction having a numerator the same as or larger than the denominator.

Parts of a Fraction

Proper Fraction $\quad \dfrac{1}{2} \quad \begin{array}{l} \longleftarrow \text{numerator} \\ \longleftarrow \text{denominator} \end{array}$

Improper Fraction $\quad \dfrac{7}{5} \quad \begin{array}{l} \longleftarrow \text{numerator} \\ \longleftarrow \text{denominator} \end{array}$

The numerator and the denominator *must be of like entities or terms,* that is:

Correct (like terms)	Incorrect (unlike terms)
$\dfrac{2 \text{ grams}}{3 \text{ grams}}$	$\dfrac{3 \text{ grams}}{5 \text{ milliliters}}$
or	or
$\dfrac{30 \text{ milligrams}}{60 \text{ milligrams}}$	$\dfrac{60 \text{ milligrams}}{15 \text{ grains}}$

Mixed Numbers and Improper Fractions

A **mixed number** is a whole number and a proper fraction. These are mixed numbers

$$2 \tfrac{2}{3} \qquad 3 \tfrac{1}{4} \qquad 5 \tfrac{4}{5} \qquad 2 \tfrac{1}{8}$$

When doing certain calculations, it is sometimes necessary to change a mixed number to an improper fraction or change an improper fraction to a mixed number.

To change a mixed number to an improper fraction, multiply the denominator of the fraction by the whole number, add the numerator, and place the sum over the denominator.

EXAMPLE: mixed number $3\tfrac{3}{5}$

1. Multiply the denominator of the fraction (5) by the whole number (3) or ($5 \times 3 = 15$):

$$3 \diagdown \tfrac{3}{5} \times$$

2. Add this number (15) to the numerator (3) ($15 + 3 = 18$):

$$3 \diagdown \tfrac{+3}{5} \times$$

3. And place the sum (18) over the denominator of the fraction:

$$\frac{18}{5}$$

To change an improper fraction to a mixed number, divide the denominator into the numerator. The quotient (the result of the division of these two numbers) is the whole number. Then place the remainder over the denominator of the improper fraction.

EXAMPLE: improper fraction

$$\frac{15}{4} \quad \begin{array}{l} \longleftarrow \text{numerator} \\ \longleftarrow \text{denominator} \end{array}$$

1. Divide the denominator into the numerator. The quotient is the whole number.

$$\begin{array}{r} 3 \quad \longleftarrow \text{quotient} \\ 4\overline{)15} \\ \underline{12} \\ 3 \quad \longleftarrow \text{remainder} \end{array}$$

2. Place the remainder over the denominator of the improper fraction.

$$3\tfrac{3}{4}$$

Adding Fractions with Like Denominators

When the denominators are the *same*, fractions are added by adding the numerators and placing the sum of the numerators over the denominator. If the

answer is an improper fraction, it may then be changed to a mixed number. In the second example, the answer is 4/8, which is reduced to 1/2. When giving a final answer, fractions are *always* reduced to the lowest possible terms.

EXAMPLES

$$\begin{array}{c} \frac{2}{3} \\ \frac{1}{3} \\ \frac{1}{3} \\ \hline \frac{4}{3} \text{ or } 1\tfrac{1}{3} \end{array} \qquad \begin{array}{c} \frac{1}{8} \\ \frac{3}{8} \\ \hline \frac{4}{8} \text{ or } \tfrac{1}{2} \end{array}$$

Adding Fractions with Unlike Denominators

Fractions with *unlike denominators* cannot be added until the denominators are changed to like numbers. The first step is to find the *lowest common denominator*, which is the lowest number divisible by (or that can be divided by) all the denominators.

EXAMPLE: add 2/3 and 1/4

$$\begin{array}{l} \frac{2}{3} \longleftarrow \\ \frac{1}{4} \longleftarrow \end{array}$$ The lowest number that can be divided by these two numbers is 12; therefore, 12 is the lowest common denominator.

1. Divide the lowest common denominator by each of the denominators ($12 \div 3$ and $12 \div 4$):

$$\frac{2}{3} = \frac{}{12}$$
$$\frac{1}{4} = \frac{}{12}$$

2. Multiply the quotient by the numerators (4×2 and 3×1) and place the result over the denominator:

$$\frac{2}{3} = \frac{8}{12} \quad \longleftarrow$$
$$\frac{1}{4} = \frac{3}{12} \quad \longleftarrow$$

3. Add the numerators:

$$\begin{array}{l} \frac{2}{3} = \frac{8}{12} \\ \frac{1}{4} = \frac{3}{12} \\ \hline \frac{11}{12} \end{array}$$

Adding Mixed Numbers or Fractions with Mixed Numbers

When adding two or more mixed numbers or adding fractions and mixed numbers, the mixed number is first changed to an improper fraction.

EXAMPLES

Add $3\frac{3}{4}$ and $3\frac{3}{4}$

$3\frac{3}{4}$	changed to an improper fraction	$\frac{15}{4}$
$3\frac{3}{4}$	changed to an improper fraction	$\frac{15}{4}$

$$\frac{30}{4} = 7\frac{2}{4} = 7\frac{1}{2}$$

Add $2\frac{1}{2}$ and $3\frac{1}{4}$

$2\frac{1}{2}$	changed to an improper fraction	$\frac{5}{2} = \frac{10}{4}$
$3\frac{1}{4}$	changed to an improper fraction	$\frac{13}{4} = \frac{13}{4}$

$$\frac{23}{4} = 5\frac{3}{4}$$

In the example above, 5/2 and 13/4 cannot be added because the denominators are not the same; it was necessary therefore to find the lowest common denominator before these fractions could be added.

Add $1\frac{1}{2}$ and $\frac{2}{3}$

$$1\frac{1}{2} = \frac{3}{2} = \frac{9}{6}$$
$$\frac{2}{3} = \frac{2}{3} = \frac{4}{6}$$
$$\frac{13}{6} = 2\frac{1}{6}$$

In the example above, 3/2 and 2/3 cannot be added because the denominators are not the same; it was therefore necessary to find the lowest common denominator before these fractions could be added.

Comparison of Fractions

When fractions with *like* denominators are compared, the fraction with the *largest numerator* is the *largest* fraction.

EXAMPLES

Compare 5/8 and 3/8   Answer: 5/8 is larger than 3/8

Compare 1/4 and 3/4   Answer: 3/4 is larger than 1/4

When the denominators are *not* the same, for example comparing 2/3 and 1/10, the lowest common denominator must first be determined. The same procedure is followed as in the addition of fractions with unlike denominators.

EXAMPLE

Compare 2/3 and 1/10

$$\frac{2}{3} = \frac{20}{30}$$
$$\frac{1}{10} = \frac{3}{30}$$

The largest numerator in these two fractions is 20; therefore 2/3 is larger than 1/10.

Multiplying Fractions

When fractions are multiplied, the numerators are multiplied *and* the denominators are multiplied.

EXAMPLES

$$\frac{1}{8} \times \frac{1}{4} = \frac{1}{32} \qquad \frac{1}{2} \times \frac{2}{3} = \frac{2}{6} = \frac{1}{3} \qquad \frac{4}{5} \times \frac{3}{6} = \frac{12}{30} = \frac{2}{5}$$

In the above examples, it was necessary to reduce two of the three answers to their lowest possible terms.

Multiplying Whole Numbers and Fractions

When whole numbers are multiplied with fractions, the numerator is multiplied by the whole number and the product is placed over the denominator. If the answer is an improper fraction, it may be changed to a mixed number.

EXAMPLES

$$2 \times \frac{1}{2} = \frac{2}{2} = 1$$
$$4 \times \frac{2}{3} = \frac{8}{3} = 2\frac{2}{3}$$
$$2 \times \frac{3}{8} = \frac{6}{8} = \frac{3}{4}$$

Multiplying Mixed Numbers

To multiply mixed numbers, the mixed numbers are changed to *improper fractions* and then multiplied.

EXAMPLES

$$2\frac{1}{2} \times 3\frac{1}{4} = \frac{5}{2} \times \frac{13}{4} = \frac{65}{8} = 8\frac{1}{8}$$
$$3\frac{1}{3} \times 4\frac{1}{2} = \frac{10}{3} \times \frac{9}{2} = \frac{90}{6} = 15$$

Multiplying a Whole Number and a Mixed Number

To multiply a whole number and a mixed number, *both* numbers must be changed to improper fractions.

EXAMPLES

$$3 \times 2\frac{1}{2} = \frac{3}{1} \times \frac{5}{2} = \frac{15}{2} = 7\frac{1}{2}$$
$$2 \times 4\frac{1}{2} = \frac{2}{1} \times \frac{9}{2} = \frac{18}{2} = 9$$

A whole number is converted to an improper fraction by placing the whole number over 1. In the above examples, 3 becomes 3/1 and 2 becomes 2/1.

Dividing Fractions

When fractions are divided, the *second* fraction (the divisor) is inverted (turned upside down) and then the fractions are multiplied.

EXAMPLES

$$\frac{1}{8} \div \frac{1}{4} = \frac{1}{8} \times \frac{4}{1} = \frac{4}{8} = \frac{1}{2}$$

$$\frac{2}{3} \div \frac{5}{6} = \frac{2}{3} \times \frac{6}{5} = \frac{12}{15} = \frac{4}{5}$$

$$\frac{3}{4} \div \frac{1}{2} = \frac{3}{4} \times \frac{2}{1} = \frac{6}{4} = 1\frac{2}{4} = 1\frac{1}{2}$$

In the above examples, answers were reduced to their lowest possible terms.

Dividing Fractions and Mixed Numbers

Some problems of division may be expressed as (1) fractions and mixed numbers, (2) two mixed numbers, (3) whole numbers and fractions, or (4) whole numbers and mixed numbers.

Mixed Numbers and Fractions
When a mixed number is divided by a fraction, the whole number is changed to a fraction.

EXAMPLES

$$2\frac{1}{3} \div \frac{1}{4} = \frac{7}{3} \div \frac{1}{4} = \frac{7}{3} \times \frac{4}{1} = \frac{28}{3} = 9\frac{1}{3}$$

$$2\frac{1}{2} \div \frac{1}{2} = \frac{5}{2} \div \frac{1}{2} = \frac{5}{2} \times \frac{2}{1} = \frac{10}{2} = 5$$

Mixed Numbers
When two mixed numbers are divided, they are both changed to improper fractions.

EXAMPLE

$$3\frac{3}{4} \div 1\frac{1}{2} = \frac{15}{4} \div \frac{3}{2} = \frac{15}{4} \times \frac{2}{3} = \frac{30}{12} = 2\frac{6}{12} = 2\frac{1}{2}$$

Whole Numbers and Fractions
When a whole number is divided by a fraction, the whole number is changed to an improper fraction by placing the whole number over 1.

EXAMPLE

$$2 \div \frac{2}{3} = \frac{2}{1} \div \frac{2}{3} = \frac{2}{1} \times \frac{3}{2} = \frac{6}{2} = 3$$

Whole Numbers and Mixed Numbers
When whole numbers and mixed numbers are divided, the whole number is changed to an improper fraction and the mixed number is changed to an improper fraction.

EXAMPLE

$$4 \div 2\frac{2}{3} = \frac{4}{1} \div \frac{8}{3} = \frac{4}{1} \times \frac{3}{8} = \frac{12}{8} = 1\frac{4}{8} = 1\frac{1}{2}$$

▷ Ratios

A ratio is a way of expressing *a part of a whole* or *the relation of one number to another*. For example, a ratio written as 1 : 10 means 1 in 10 parts, or 1 to 10. A ratio may also be written as a fraction; thus 1 : 10 can also be expressed as 1/10.

EXAMPLES

1 : 1000 is 1 part in 1000 parts, or 1 to 1000, or 1/1000
1 : 250 is 1 part in 250 parts, or 1 to 250, or 1/250

Some drug solutions are expressed in ratios, for example 1 : 100 or 1 : 500. These ratios mean that there is 1 part of a drug in 100 parts of solution or 1 part of the drug in 500 parts of solution.

▷ Percentages

The term *percentage (%)* means *parts per hundred*.

EXAMPLES

25% is 25 parts per hundred
50% is 50 parts per hundred

A percentage may also be expressed as a fraction.

EXAMPLES

25% is 25 parts per hundred or 25/100
50% is 50 parts per hundred or 50/100
30% is 30 parts per hundred or 30/100

The above fractions may also be reduced to their lowest possible terms: 25/100 = 1/4, 50/100 = 1/2, 30/100 = 3/10.

Changing a Fraction to a Percentage

To change a fraction to a percentage, divide the denominator by the numerator and multiply the results (quotient) by 100 and then add a percent sign (%).

EXAMPLES

Change 4/5 to a percentage
$4 \div 5 = 0.8$
$0.8 \times 100 = 80\%$

Change 2/3 to a percentage
$2 \div 3 = 0.666$
$0.666 \times 100 = 66.6\%$

Changing a Ratio to a Percentage

To change a ratio to a percentage, the ratio is first expressed as a fraction with the first number or term of the ratio becoming the numerator and the second number or term becoming the denominator. For example, the ratio $1:500$ when changed to a fraction becomes 1/500. This fraction is then changed to a percentage by the same method shown in the preceding section.

EXAMPLE

Change $1:125$ to a percentage
$1:125$ written as a fraction is 1/125
$1 \div 125 = 0.008$
$0.008 \times 100 = 0.8$
adding the percent sign $= 0.8\%$

Changing a Percentage to a Ratio

To change a percentage to a ratio, the percentage becomes the numerator and is placed over a denominator of 100.

EXAMPLES

Change 5% and 10% to ratios

5% is $\dfrac{5}{100} = \dfrac{1}{20}$ or $1:20$

10% is $\dfrac{10}{100} = \dfrac{1}{10}$ or $1:10$

▷ Proportion

A proportion is a method of expressing equality between two ratios. An example of two ratios expressed as a proportion is

3 is to 4 as 9 is to 12

This may also be written as

$3:4$ as $9:12$
or
$3:4::9:12$
or
$\dfrac{3}{4} = \dfrac{9}{12}$

Proportions may be used to find an unknown quantity. The unknown quantity is assigned a letter, usually X. An example of a proportion with an unknown quantity is

$$5:10::15:X$$

The first and last terms of the proportion are called the *extremes*. In the above expression 5 and X are the extremes. The second and third terms of the proportion are called the *means*. In the above proportion 10 and 15 are the means.

means
$$5:10::15:X$$
extremes

extreme $\dfrac{5}{10} = \dfrac{15}{X}$ mean
mean   extreme

To solve for X:

1. Multiply the extremes and place the product (result) to the left of the equal sign.

$5:10::15:X$
$5X =$

2. Multiply the means and place the product to the right of the equal sign.

$5:10::15:X$
$5X = 150$

3. Now solve for X by dividing the number to the right of the equal sign by the number to the left of the equal sign ($150 \div 5$).

$5X = 150$
$X = 30$

4. To prove the answer is correct, substitute the answer for X in the equation.

$5:10::15:X$
$5:10::15:30$

Then multiply the means and place the product to the left of the equal sign. Then multiply the extremes and place the product to the right of the equal sign.

$5:10::15:30$
$150 = 150$

If the numbers are the same on both sides of the equal sign, the equation has been solved correctly.
If the proportion has been set up as a fraction, cross multiply and solve for X.

$\dfrac{5}{10} = \dfrac{15}{X}$
5 times X = 5X and 10 times 15 = 150
$5X = 150$
$X = 30$

To set up a proportion, remember that a *sequence must be followed*. If a sequence is not followed, the proportion will be stated incorrectly.

EXAMPLES

If a man can walk 6 **miles** in 2 **hours**, how many **miles** can he walk in 3 **hours**?

MILES is to HOURS as MILES is to HOURS

or

MILES : HOURS : : MILES : HOURS

or

$$\frac{MILES}{HOURS} = \frac{MILES}{HOURS}$$

6 miles : 2 hours : : X miles : 3 hours

2X = 18

X = 9 miles (he can walk 9 miles in 3 hours)

If there are 15 **grains** in 1 **gram**, 30 **grains** equals how many **grams**?

15 grains : 1 gram : : 30 grains : X grams

15X = 30

X = 2 grams (30 grains = 2 grams)

▷ Decimals

Decimals are used in the metric system. A **decimal** is a fraction in which the denominator is 10 or some power of 10. For example, 2/10 (read as two tenths) is a fraction with a denominator of 10; 1/100 (one one-hundredth) is an example of a fraction with a denominator that is a power of ten (ie, 100).

A power (or multiple) of 10 is the *number 1 followed by one or more zeros*. Therefore, 100, 1000, 10,000 and so on are powers of 10 because the number 1 is followed by two, three, and four zeros, respectively. Fractions whose denominators are 10 or a power of 10 are often expressed in decimal form.

Parts of a Decimal

There are three parts to a decimal:

| | 1 | . | 25 |

number (s) to the left of the decimal point

d e c i m a l

number(s) to the right of the decimal point

Types of Decimals

✱ A decimal may consist only of numbers to the right of the decimal point. This is called a **decimal fraction**. Examples of decimal fractions are 0.05, 0.6, and 0.002.

A decimal may also have numbers to the *left* and *right* of the decimal point. This is called a **mixed decimal fraction**. Examples of mixed decimal fractions are 1.25, 2.5, and 7.5.

Both decimal fractions and mixed decimal fractions are commonly referred to as decimals. When there is no number to the left of the decimal, a zero may be written, for example, 0.25. Although in general mathematics the zero may not be required, it should be used in the writing of drug doses in the metric system. *Use of the zero lessens the chance of medication errors*, especially when the dose of a drug is hurriedly written and the decimal point is indistinct. For example, a drug order for dexamethasone is written as dexamethasone .25 mg by one physician and written as dexamethasone 0.25 by another. If the decimal point in the first written order is indistinct, the order might be interpreted as 25 mg, which is 100 times the prescribed dose!

Reading Decimals

To read a decimal, the position of the number to the left or right of the decimal point indicates how the decimal is to be expressed.

hundred thousands	ten thousands	thousands	hundreds	tens	units	DECIMAL POINT	tenths	hundredths	thousandths	ten thousandths	hundred thousandths
0	0	0	0	0	0	.	0	0	0	0	0

Adding Decimals

When adding decimals, place the numbers in a column so that the whole numbers are aligned to the left of the decimal and the decimal fractions are aligned to the right of the decimal.

EXAMPLE

20.45 + 2.56 is written as:

20.45
2.56
23.01

2 + 0.25 is written as:

2.00
0.25
2.25

Subtracting Decimals

When subtracting decimals, the numbers are aligned to the left and right of the decimal in the same manner as for the addition of decimals.

EXAMPLE

20.45 − 2.56 is written as:

20.45
2.56
17.89

Multiplying a Whole Number by a Decimal

To multiply a whole number by a decimal, move the decimal point of the product as many places to the left as there are places to the right of the decimal point.

EXAMPLES

500
.05 ← there are two places to the right of the decimal
2500. ← the decimal point is moved two places to the left

The answer now reads 25.

250
.3 ← there is one place to the right of the decimal
750. ← the decimal point is moved one place to the left

The answer now reads 75.

Multiplying a Decimal by a Decimal

To multiply a decimal by a decimal, move the decimal point of the product as many places to the left as there are places to the right in *both* decimals.

EXAMPLE

2.75 ← there are two places to the right of the decimal
0.5 ← plus one place to the right of the decimal equals three
1375. ← move the decimal point three places to the left

The answer now reads 1.375.

Dividing Decimals

The **divisor** is a number that is divided into the dividend.

EXAMPLE

$$0.69 \div 0.3 \qquad 0.3)\overline{0.69}$$

DIVIDEND   DIVISOR   DIVISOR   DIVIDEND

This may be written or spoken as 0.69 divided by 0.3. To divide decimals:

1. The *divisor* is changed to a whole number. In this example, the decimal point is moved one place to the right so that 0.3 now becomes 3, which is a whole number.

$$0.3)\overline{0.69}$$

2. The decimal point in the *dividend* is now moved the *same number of places* to the right. In this example, the decimal point is moved one place to the right, the same number of places the decimal point in the divisor was moved.

$$3)\overline{0.69}$$

3. The numbers are now divided.

$$\frac{2.3}{3)\overline{6.9}}$$

When only the dividend is a decimal, the decimal point is carried to the quotient (answer) in the same position.

EXAMPLES

$$\frac{.375}{2)\overline{0.750}} \qquad \frac{1.736}{2)\overline{3.472}}$$

To divide when only the divisor is a decimal, for example, $.3)\overline{66}$:

1. The divisor is changed to a whole number. In this example the decimal point is moved one place to the right.

$$.3)\overline{66}$$

2. The decimal point in the dividend must also be moved one place to the right.

$$3)\overline{66.0}$$

3. The numbers are now divided.

$$\frac{220}{3)\overline{660}}$$

Whenever the decimal point is moved in the dividend *it must also be moved* in the divisor, and whenever the decimal point in the divisor is moved *it must be moved* in the dividend.

Changing a Fraction to a Decimal

To change a fraction to a decimal, divide the numerator by the denominator.

EXAMPLES

$$\frac{1}{5} = 5)\overline{1.0} \quad .2 \qquad \frac{3}{4} = 4)\overline{3.00} \quad .75 \qquad \frac{1}{6} = 6)\overline{1.000} \quad .166$$

"thousands"

Changing a Decimal to a Fraction

To change a decimal to a fraction:

1. Remove the decimal point and make the resulting whole number the numerator

0.2 = 2

2. The denominator is stated as 10 or a power of 10. In this example, 0.2 is read as two *tenths*, and therefore the denominator is 10.

$$0.2 = \frac{2}{10} \text{ (which is reduced to the lowest possible number)} = \frac{1}{5}$$

ADDITIONAL EXAMPLES

$$0.75 = \frac{75}{100} = \frac{3}{4} \qquad 0.025 = \frac{25}{1000} = \frac{1}{40}$$

► CALCULATION OF DRUG DOSAGES

▷ Systems of Measurement

There are three systems of measurement of drug dosages: the **metric system, the apothecaries' system,** and **household measurements.** The metric system is the most commonly used system of measurement in medicine. A physician may prescribe a drug dosage in the apothecaries' system, but for the most part this ancient system of measurements is rarely used. The household system is rarely used in the hospital, but may be used to measure drug dosages in the home.

The Metric System

The metric system uses decimals (or the decimal system). In the metric system the **gram** is the unit of weight, the **liter** the unit of volume, and the **meter** the unit of length.

Table 1-1 lists the measurements used in the metric system. The abbreviations for the measurements are given in parenthesis.

TABLE 1–1
Metric Measurements

WEIGHT

The unit of weight is the gram
1 kilogram (kg) = 1000 grams (g)
1 milligram (mg) = 0.001 gram (g)
1 microgram (mcg) = 0.000001 gram (g) *hundred thousand*
1 nanogram (ng) = 0.000000001 gram (g)

VOLUME

The unit of volume is the liter
1 decaliter (dL) = 10 liters (L)
1 liter (L) = 1000 milliliters (mL)
1 milliliter (mL) = 0.001 liter (L)

LENGTH

The unit of length is the meter
1 meter (m) = 1000 centimeters (cm)
1 centimeter (cm) = 0.01 meter (m)
1 millimeter (mm) = 0.001 meter (m)

TABLE 1–2
Apothecaries' Measurements

WEIGHT

The units of weight are grains, drams, and ounces
60 grains (gr) = 1 dram (3)
1 ounce (3) = 480 grains (gr)

VOLUME

The units of volume are minims, fluid drams, and fluid ounces
1 fluid dram (fl 3) = 60 minims (m)
1 fluid ounce = (fl 3) = 8 fluid drams

The Apothecaries' System

The apothecaries' system uses whole numbers and fractions. Decimals are *not* used in this system. The whole numbers are written as lowercase roman numerals, for example x instead of 10, or v instead of 5.

The units of weight in the apothecaries' system are **grains, drams,** and **ounces.** The units of volume are **minims, fluid drams,** and **fluid ounces.**

Table 1-2 lists the measurements used in the apothecaries' system. The abbreviations (or symbols) for the measurements are given in parenthesis.

Household Measurements

When used, household measurements are for volume only. In the hospital, household measurements are rarely used, because they are inaccurate when used to measure drug dosages. On occasion, the nurse may use the pint, quart, or gallon when ordering irrigating or sterilizing solutions or stock solutions.

Table 1-3 lists the more common household measurements.

Conversion Between Systems

To convert between systems, it is necessary to know the equivalents, or what is equal to what in each

---

TABLE 1–3
Household Measurements

3 teaspoons (tsp) = 1 tablespoon (tbsp)
2 tablespoons (tbsp) = 1 ounce (oz)
2 pints (pt) = 1 quart (qt)
4 quarts (qt) = 1 gallon

TABLE 1—4
Approximate Equivalents

METRIC	APOTHECARIES'	HOUSEHOLD
WEIGHT		
0.01 mg	gr 1/600	
0.15 mg	gr 1/400	
0.2 mg	gr 1/300	
0.3 mg	gr 1/200	
0.4 mg	gr 1/150	
0.6 mg	gr 1/100	
1 mg	gr 1/60	
2 mg	gr 1/30	
4 mg	gr 1/15	
6 mg	gr 1/10	
8 mg	gr 1/8	
10 mg	gr 1/6	
15 mg	gr 1/4	
20 mg	gr 1/3	
30 mg	gr ss (1/2)	
60 mg	gr 1	
100 mg	gr i ss (1 1/2)	
120 mg	gr ii	
1 g (1000 mg)	gr xv	
VOLUME		
0.06 mL	min (♏) i	
1 mL	min (♏) xv or xvi	
4 mL	fluidram (fl ℨ) i	1 teaspoon (tsp)
15 mL	fluidrams (fl ℨ) iv	1/2 ounce (oz)
30 mL	fluid ounce (fl ℨ) i	1 ounce (oz)
500 mL	1 pint (pt)	1 pint (pt)
1000 mL (1 liter)	1 quart (qt)	1 quart (qt)

system. Table 1-4 lists the more common equivalents. These equivalents are only *approximate* because the three systems are different and are not truly equal to each other.

Several methods may be used to convert from one system to another using an equivalent, but most conversions can be done by using proportion.

EXAMPLES

Convert 120 mg (metric) to grains (apothecaries')
Using proportion and a known equivalent:
60 mg = gr i
1 gr: 60 mg :: X gr : 120 mg

$$60 X = 120$$
$$X = 2$$

or

$$\frac{1 \text{ gr}}{60 \text{ mg}} = \frac{X \text{ gr}}{120 \text{ mg}}$$
$$X = 2$$

Therefore, 120 mg = 2 grains (gr ii). Note the use of gr and mg when setting up the proportion. This shows that the proportion was stated correctly and helps in identifying the answer as 2 *grains*.

Convert gr 1/100 (apothecaries') to mg (metric).
Using proportion and a known equivalent:
60 mg = 1 gr
60 mg : 1 gr :: X mg : 1/100 gr

$$X = 60 \times \frac{1}{100} = \frac{60}{100} = \frac{3}{5}$$
$$X = \frac{3}{5} \text{ mg}$$

or

$$\frac{60 \text{ mg}}{1 \text{ qr}} = \frac{X \text{ mg}}{1/100 \text{ gr}}$$
$$X = 60 \times \frac{1}{100} = \frac{60}{100} = \frac{3}{5}$$
$$X = \frac{3}{5} \text{ mg}$$

Because fractions are *not* used in the metric system, the fraction must be converted to a decimal by dividing the denominator into the numerator, or $3.0 \div 5 = 0.6$. Therefore, gr 1/100 is equal to 0.6 mg.

When setting up the proportion, the apothecaries' system was written in arabic numbers instead of roman numerals, and their order was reversed (1 gr instead of gr i) so that all numbers and abbreviations are uniform in presentation.

Convert 0.3 milligrams (mg) [metric] to grains (gr) [apothecaries'].

Using proportion and a known equivalent:
1 mg = gr 1/60

1/60 gr : 1 mg :: X gr : 0.3 mg

$$X = \frac{1}{60} \times 0.3 = \frac{0.3}{60} = \frac{3}{600} = \frac{1}{200}$$
$$X = \frac{1}{200} \text{ gr}$$

or

$$\frac{1/60 \text{ gr}}{1 \text{ mg}} = \frac{X \text{ gr}}{0.3 \text{ mg}}$$
$$X = \frac{1}{60} \times 0.3 = \frac{0.3}{60} = \frac{3}{600} = \frac{1}{200}$$
$$X = \frac{1}{200} \text{ gr}$$

Therefore, 0.3 mg equals gr 1/200.

There is no rule stating which equivalent must be used. In the above problem, another equivalent (60 mg = 1 grain) could have been used. If this equivalent is used, the proportion would be

$$60 \text{ mg} : 1 \text{ gr} :: 0.3 \text{ mg} : X \text{ gr}$$
$$60 X = 0.3$$
$$X = 0.005$$

or

$$\frac{60 \text{ mg}}{1 \text{ gr}} = \frac{0.3 \text{ mg}}{X \text{ gr}}$$
$$60 X = 0.3$$
$$X = 0.005$$

Therefore, 0.3 mg = 0.005 grains.

Because decimals are not used in the apothecaries' system, this decimal answer must be converted to a fraction. 0.005 is 5/1000, which, when reduced to its lowest terms, is 1/200. The final answer is now 0.3 mg = gr 1/200.

Converting Within a System

Sometimes it is necessary to convert within the same system, for example, changing grams (g) to milligrams (mg) or milligrams to grams. Proportion and a known equivalent may be used for this type of conversion.

EXAMPLE

Convert 0.1 gram (g) to milligrams (mg).
Using proportion and a known equivalent:

1000 mg = 1 g

$$1000 \text{ mg} : 1 \text{ g} : : X \text{ mg} : 0.1 \text{ g}$$
$$X = 1000 \times 0.1$$
$$X = 100 \text{ mg}$$

or

$$\frac{1000 \text{ mg}}{1 \text{ g}} = \frac{X \text{ mg}}{0.1 \text{ g}}$$
$$X = 1000 \times 0.1$$
$$X = 100 \text{ mg}$$

Therefore, 0.1 gram (g) is 100 milligrams (mg).

▷ Oral Dosages of Drugs

It is sometimes necessary to compute an oral drug dosage, because the dosage ordered by the physician may not be available, or the dosage may have been written in the apothecaries' system and the drug or container label is in metric.

Tablets and Capsules

To find the correct dosage of a solid oral preparation, the following formula may be used:

$$\frac{\text{dose desired}}{\text{dose on hand}} = \text{dose administered (the unknown)}$$

This formula may be abbreviated as

$$\frac{D}{H} = X$$

When the dose ordered by the physician (dose desired) is written in the *same system* as the dose on the drug container (dose on hand), these two figures may be inserted into the formula.

EXAMPLE
The physician orders ascorbic acid 100 mg ←—— metric
The dose on hand is ascorbic acid 50 mg ←—— metric

$$\frac{D}{H} = X$$

$$\frac{100 \text{ mg}}{50 \text{ mg}} = \begin{array}{l}\text{2 tablets of ascorbic acid 50 mg to}\\ \text{give the prescribed dose of 100 mg}\end{array}$$

The fraction in the above example denotes $\frac{\text{milligrams}}{\text{milligrams}}$.
If the physician had ordered ascorbic acid 0.5 g and the drug container was labeled ascorbic acid 250 mg, a *conversion of grams to milligrams* (because the drug container is labeled in milligrams) would be necessary before this formula can be used. If the 0.5 g were *not* converted to milligrams the fraction of the formula would look like this:

$$\frac{0.5 \text{ grams}}{250 \text{ milligrams}}$$

A fraction must be stated in *like* terms; therefore, proportion may be used to convert grams to milligrams.

$$1000 \text{ mg} : 1 \text{ g} : : X \text{ mg} : 0.5 \text{ g}$$
$$X = 1000 \times 0.5$$
$$X = 500 \text{ mg}$$
$$\frac{D}{H} = X$$
$$\frac{500 \text{ mg}}{250 \text{ mg}} = \text{2 tablets of 250 mg of ascorbic acid}$$

As with all fractions, the numerator and the denominator must be of like terms, for example, milligrams over milligrams or grams over grams. Errors in using this and other drug formulas, as well as proportions, will be reduced if the entire dose is written rather than just the numbers.

$$\frac{100 \text{ mg}}{50 \text{ mg}} \text{ rather than } \frac{100}{50}$$

This will eliminate the possibility of using *unlike* terms in the fraction.

Even if the physician's order was written in the apothecaries' system, the drug container will most likely be labeled in the metric system. A conversion of *apothecaries' to metric* will now be necessary because the drug label is written in the metric system.

EXAMPLE
The physician's order reads:
codeine sulfate gr 1/4 ←—— apothecaries'
The drug container is labeled:
codeine sulfate 15 mg ←—— metric
Grains must be converted to milligrams or milligrams must be converted to grains.

Grains to milligrams
60 mg : 1 gr : : X mg : 1/4 gr

$$X = 60 \times \frac{1}{4}$$

X = 15 mg (gr 1/4 is approximately equivalent to 15 mg)

or

$$\frac{60 \text{ mg}}{1 \text{ gr}} = \frac{X \text{ mg}}{1/4 \text{ gr}}$$

$$X = 60 \times \frac{1}{4}$$

$$X = 15 \text{ mg}$$

Milligrams to grains
60 mg : 1 gr : : 15 mg : X gr
60 X = 15
X = 1/4 gr (15 mg is approximately equivalent to gr 1/4)

or

$$\frac{60 \text{ mg}}{1 \text{ gr}} = \frac{15 \text{ mg}}{X \text{ gr}}$$
60 X = 15
X = 1/4 gr

The formula $\frac{D}{H} = X$ can now be used.

$$\frac{D}{H} = X$$

$$\frac{15 \text{ mg}}{15 \text{ mg}} = 1 \text{ tablet}$$

or

$$\frac{1/4 \text{ gr}}{1/4 \text{ gr}} = 1 \text{ tablet}$$

Liquids

In liquid drugs there is a specific amount of drug in a given volume of solution. For example, if a container is labeled as 10 mg per 5 mL (or 10 mg/5 mL), this means that for every 5 mL of solution there is 10 mg of drug.

As with tablets and capsules, the prescribed dose of the drug may not be the same as what is on hand (or available). For example, the physician may order 20 mg of an oral liquid preparation and the bottle is labeled as 10 mg/5 mL.

The formula for computing the dosage of oral liquids is

$$\frac{\text{dose desired}}{\text{dose on hand}} \times \text{quantity} = \text{volume administered}$$

This may be abbreviated as

$$\frac{D}{H} \times Q = X$$

The quantity (or Q) in this formula is the amount of liquid in which the available drug is contained. For example, if the label states that there is 15 mg/5 mL, 5 mL is the *quantity* (or volume) in which there is 15 mg of this drug.

EXAMPLE
The physician orders cephradine 250 mg PO oral suspension. The drug container is labeled cephradine 125 mg/5 mL. The 5 mL is the amount (quantity or Q) that contains 125 mg of the drug.

$$\frac{D}{H} \times Q = X \text{ (the amount or volume to be given)}$$

$$\frac{250 \text{ mg}}{125 \text{ mg}} \times 5 \text{ mL} = X$$

$$2 \times 5 \text{ mL} = 10 \text{ mL (the volume to be given)}$$

Therefore, 10 mL contains 250 mg (the desired dose).

Liquid drugs may also be ordered in drops (gtt) or minims. With the former, a medicine dropper is usually supplied with the drug and is always used to measure the ordered dosage. Eye droppers are not standardized, and therefore the size of a drop from one eye dropper may be different than one from another eye dropper.

To measure an oral liquid drug in minims, a measuring glass *calibrated in minims* must be used.

▷ Parenteral Dosages of Drugs

Drugs for parenteral use must be in liquid form before they are administered. Parenteral drugs may be available in the following forms:

1. As liquids in disposable cartridges or disposable syringes that contain a specific amount of a drug in a specific volume, for example, meperidine 50 mg/mL. After administration, the cartridge or syringe is discarded.

2. In ampules or vials that contain a specific amount of the liquid form of the drug in a specific volume. The vials may be single-dose vials or multidose vials. A multidose vial contains more than one dose of the drug.

3. In ampules or vials that contain powder or crystals, to which a liquid (called a **diluent**) must be added before the drug can be removed from the vial and administered. Vials may be single-dose or multidose vials.

4. As small tablets that are manufactured for parenteral use. These are called hypo tablets and are rarely used today. The tablet is placed in a syringe, and the syringe is filled with a diluent and gently rotated until the tablet dissolves.

Parenteral Drugs in Disposable Syringes or Cartridges

There may be instances when a specific dosage strength is not available and it will be necessary to administer less than the amount contained in the syringe.

EXAMPLE

The physician orders Valium 5 mg IM. The drug on hand is Valium Tel-E-Ject 2 mL = 10 mg.

$$\frac{D}{H} \times Q = X$$

$$\frac{5 \text{ mg}}{10 \text{ mg}} \times 2 \text{ ml} = X$$

$$X = \frac{1}{2} \times 2 = 1 \text{ mL (volume administered)}$$

Because the syringe contained 2 mL (and 10 mg), 1 mL is discarded and 1 mL is administered to give the prescribed dose of 5 mg.

Parenteral Drugs in Ampules and Vials

If the drug is in liquid form in the ampule or vial, the desired amount is withdrawn from the ampule or vial. In some instances the entire amount is used; in others only part of the total amount is withdrawn from the ampule or vial and administered.

Whenever the dose to be administered is different from the label, the volume to be administered must be calculated. To determine the volume to be administered, the formula for liquid preparations is used. The calculations are the same as for parenteral drugs in disposable syringes or cartridges given in the preceding section.

EXAMPLE

The physician orders hydroxyzine 12.5 mg.
The dosage available is hydroxyzine 25 mg/mL
(in a 10-mL multidose vial labeled as 25 mg/mL).

$$\frac{D}{H} \times Q = X$$

$$\frac{12.5 \text{ mg}}{25 \text{ mg}} \times 1 \text{ mL} = X$$

$$\frac{1}{2} \times 1 \text{ mL} = \frac{1}{2} \text{ mL (or 0.5 mL) volume to be administered}$$

When the dose is less than 1 mL, it may be necessary, in some instances, to convert the answer to minims. A conversion factor of 15 or 16 minims/mL may be used.

EXAMPLES

Physician orders chlorpromazine 10 mg.
The dosage available is 25 mg/mL.

$$\frac{D}{H} \times Q = X$$

$$\frac{10 \text{ mg}}{25 \text{ mg}} \times 1 \text{ mL} = X$$

$$\frac{2}{5} \times 1 \text{ mL} = \frac{2}{5} \text{ ml which is now converted to minims}$$

$$\frac{2}{5} \times 15 \text{ minims} = 6 \text{ minims}$$

Because 15 can be divided by 5, the conversion factor of 15 minims/mL is used.

The physician's order reads: methadone 2.5 mg IM.
The dosage available is 10 mg/mL.

$$\frac{D}{H} \times Q = X$$

$$\frac{2.5 \text{ mg}}{10 \text{ mg}} \times 1 \text{ mL} = X$$

$$\frac{1}{4} \times 1 \text{ mL} = X$$

$$\frac{1}{4} \times 16 \text{ minims} = 4 \text{ mimims}$$

Because 16 (and not 15) minims can be divided by 4, the conversion factor of 16 is used.

WARNING: ALWAYS CHECK DRUG LABELS CAREFULLY. Some may be labeled in a manner different from others.

EXAMPLES

a 2-mL ampule labeled: 2 mL = 0.25 mg

a 2-mL ampule labeled: 1 mL = 5 mg

In these two examples, one manufacturer states the entire dose contained in the ampule: 2 mL = 0.25 mg. The other manufacturer gives the dose per milliliter: 1 mL = 5 mg. In this 2-mL ampule, there is a total of 10 mg.

Parenteral Drugs in Dry Form

Some parenteral drugs are available as a crystal or a powder. Because these drugs have a short life in liquid form, they are available in ampules or vials in dry form and must be made a liquid (reconstituted) before they are removed and administered. Some of these products have directions for reconstitution on the label or on the enclosed package insert. The manufacturer may give either of the following information for reconstitution:

▷ the diluent(s) that must be used with the drug

▷ the amount(s) of diluent to be added

In some instances, the manufacturer supplies a diluent with the drug. If a diluent is supplied, no other stock diluent should be used. Before a drug is reconstituted, the label should be carefully checked for instructions.

EXAMPLES

Add 4 mL of sterile distilled water to vial (final volume is 4.4 mL) 2.2 mL = 0.5 g.

Directions for dilution of 1-g vial: add 2 mL of diluent, 2.2 mL = 1 g; add 2.5 mL of diluent, 3 mL = 1 g; add 3.6 mL of diluent, 4 mL = 1 g.

In each case there is *more liquid in the vial than what was added.* This is because the dry form, once dissolved, sometimes adds to the total volume. This is not always the case, however, and the final volume of some reconstituted solutions is the same as the amount of diluent added to the vial or ampule.

In the second example, the manufacturer has given three possible dilutions: the addition of 2, 2.5, or 3.6 mL to a vial that is large enough to hold 4 mL, when necessary. The reason for the three choices for dilution is the possibility of using a dosage of 1 gram or less. If the patient is to receive 1 gram of the drug, the vial is diluted with the smallest amount (2 mL). But if the patient is to receive 350 mg (0.35 g), the dilution of 2.5 mL (to equal a final volume of 3 mL) would be the best selection. If the patient is to receive 250 mg (0.25 g), the best selection is dilution with 3.6 mL to equal 4 mL.

There is another reason for the manufacturer recommending more than one amount of diluent. For example, when a vial contains 1 gram and there is the possibility that a patient may receive only 250 mg of the amount (or one fourth the amount), adding a small amount of diluent would mean the 250 mg would be contained in a small volume (in this case 0.55 mL). When *some* drugs available in dry form are reconstituted with a small amount of diluent, and then only a fraction of the final amount is withdrawn for administration, there is a problem with accuracy. Thus, the larger amount of diluent (when so specified by the manufacturer) is used for reconstitution when less than the total dosage is given.

When no directions for reconstitution are given, 1 to 1.5 mL may be added to the single-dose vial. In multiple-dose vials, 10 to 20 mL or more (depending on the size of the vial) is added to the dry form of the drug. If there is any doubt about the reconstitution of the dry form of a drug and there are no manufacturer's directions, the hospital pharmacist should be consulted.

Once a diluent is added, the volume to be administered is determined. In some cases, the entire amount is given; in others, a part (or fraction) of the total amount contained in the vial or ampule is given.

EXAMPLE

Penicillin G aqueous 5,000,000 units per vial; physician orders 500,000 units IM.

Directions for dilution: add 23 L, 18 mL, 8 mL, or 3 mL to provide 200,000 U, 250,000 U, 500,000 U, or 1 million U per mL, respectively.

Solution: add 8 mL of diluent to vial, which will give 500,000 U/mL, and 1 mL (500,000 U) is given.

Following reconstitution of this or any multi-dose vial, the following information *must* be added to the label:

▷ amount of diluent added
▷ dose of drug in mL (500 mg/mL, 10 mg/2 mL, etc.)
▷ the date of reconstitution

Hypo Tablets

This solid form of a drug is rarely used today. *Only* drugs labeled as **hypo tablets** may be used in this manner.

If the drug is available in the dose prescribed, the tablet is placed in the syringe and sterile diluent is drawn into the syringe, usually in the amount of 1 mL or 1.5 mL. The syringe is gently rotated until the tablet has fully dissolved. If the dose desired is not available, the formula $\frac{D}{H} = X$ may be used. The X (unknown quantity) is the number of hypo tablets required to give the prescribed dose.

These tablets cannot be cut in half. The whole tablet must be dissolved and either all or part of the solution in the syringe is given.

▷ Temperatures

Two scales used in the measuring of temperatures are **Fahrenheit (F)** and **Celsius (C)** (also known as **centigrade**). On the Fahrenheit scale, the freezing point of water is 32°F and the boiling point of water is 212°F. On the Celsius scale, 0°C is the freezing point of water and 100°C is the boiling point of water.

To convert from one scale to the other, the following formula used:

$$C : F - 32 :: 5 : 9$$

EXAMPLES

Convert 30° Celsius to Fahrenheit.	Convert 50° Fahrenheit to Celsius.
$C : F - 32 :: 5 : 9$	$C : F - 32 :: 5 : 9$
$30 : F - 32 :: 5 : 9$	$C : 50 - 32 :: 5 : 9$
$270 = 5 F - 160$	$9 C = 5 (50 - 32)$
$5 F = 270 + 160$	$9 C = 5 \times 18$
$5 F = 430$	$9 C = 90$
$F = 86°$	$C = 10°$

▷ Pediatric Dosages

The dosages of drugs given to children are usually less than those given to adults. The dosage may be based on age, weight, or body surface area (BSA).

Body Surface Area

Charts are used to determine the BSA in square meters according to the child's height and weight. Once the BSA is determined, the following formula is used:

$$\frac{\text{surface area of the child in square meters}}{\text{surface area of an adult in square meters}} \times \text{usual adult dose} = \text{child dose}$$

The figure for the average BSA of an adult in square meters is 1.7.

Pediatric dosages may also be based on the child's weight in pounds or kilograms.

EXAMPLES

$$5 \text{ mg/kg}$$
$$0.5 \text{ mg/lb}$$

Today, most pediatric dosages are clearly given by the manufacturer, thus eliminating the need for formulas except for determining the dose based on the child's weight or BSA.

▷ Solutions

A **solute** is a substance dissolved in a **solvent.** A solvent may be water or some other liquid. Usually water is used for preparing a solution unless another liquid is specified.

Solutions are prepared by using a solid (powder, tablet) and a liquid, or a liquid and a liquid. Today, most solutions are prepared by a pharmacist and not by a nurse.

Types of Solutions

Weight to Weight—A given weight of solute is dissolved in a given weight of solvent. These are almost always prepared by a pharmacist, because scales are needed to measure the weight of the solute and solvent.

Volume to Volume—A given volume of solute is added to a given volume of solvent.

Weight to Volume—A given weight of solute is dissolved in the amount of solvent necessary to make the required amount of solution. The weight is usually expressed in grams, grains, or ounces.

Solutions from Liquid Drugs (Volume to Volume)

Several facts must be known before a solution can be prepared from a liquid drug:

1. The amount of solution finally required; for example, 500 mL, 1 liter
2. The strength of the solution desired; for example, 10%, 5%
3. The strength of the drug available; for example, 100%, 50%

A proportion can be set up to determine the amount of drug (solute) to be used:

strength desired : strength on hand : : amount of solute : amount of solution desired

EXAMPLE

Strength of drug on hand: 100%
Strength desired: 10%
Amount of solution desired: 1000 mL (1 liter)
Unknown: amount of solute needed

Using the above formula:

$$10\% : 100\% : : X : 1000 \text{ mL}$$
$$100 X = 10,000$$
$$X = 100 \text{ mL}$$

Therefore, 100 mL of the 100% drug is needed to make 1000 mL of a 10% solution.

There is another formula that also may be used:

$$\frac{\text{strength desired}}{\text{strength on hand}} \times \text{quantity of solution desired} = \text{amount of solute}$$

Using this formula and the same example given above:

$$\frac{10\%}{100\%} \times 1000 \text{ mL} = X$$

$$\frac{1}{10} \times 1000 = X$$

$$X = 100 \text{ mL}$$

Solutions from Solid Drugs (Weight to Volume)

Some solutions are made from tablets or powders. The number of grams of (solid) solute per 100 mL of solution can be read as a percentage.

EXAMPLES

100 mL of solution containing 4 grams of solute is a 4% solution $\left(\frac{4}{100} \times 100 = 4\%\right)$; or, said another way, 4 grams of solute is necessary to make 100 mL of a 4% solution. 1000 mL of solution containing 100 grams of solute is a 10% solution $\left(\frac{10}{1000} \times 100 = 10\%\right)$; or, said another way, 100 grams of solute is necessary to make 1000 mL of a 10% solution.

2

The Administration of Medication

On completion of this chapter the reader will:

▶ *Name the five rights of drug administration*

▶ *List the various routes by which a drug may be given*

▶ *Discuss the administration of oral and parenteral medications*

▶ *Calculate IV flow rates*

▶ *Discuss nursing responsibilities before, during, and after a drug is administered*

▷ The Five Rights of Drug Administration

The nurse preparing and administering a drug to a patient assumes responsibility for this professional activity. Responsibility entails preparing and administering the prescribed drug. There are five "rights" in the administration of drugs:

Right patient
Right drug
Right dose
Right route
Right time

Many medication errors occur because one or more of these "rights" has become a "wrong." Each time a drug is prepared and administered, the five rights *must* be a part of the procedure. In addition to these rights, the nurse must have factual knowledge of *each* drug given—the reasons for use of the drug, the drug's general action, the more common adverse reactions associated with the drug, special precautions in administration (if any), and the normal dose ranges.

Some drugs may be given frequently, and the nurse becomes familiar with pharmacologic information about a specific drug. Other drugs may be given less frequently, or a new drug may be introduced, requiring the nurse to obtain information from reliable sources such as the drug package insert or the hospital department of pharmacy. *It is always good practice to check current and approved references for all drug information.*

After the administration of any drug, it is most important that the process be recorded. When medications are given on an as-needed basis (prn medications), recording should be done immediately after the drug is administered. For example, most analgesics require 20 to 30 minutes before the medication begins to relieve pain. The patient may have forgotten that he or she received a medication for pain, may have not been told that the administered medication was for pain, or may not have known that pain relief would not be immediate and may ask another nurse for medication. If the administration of the analgesic was not recorded, the patient may receive a second dose of the analgesic shortly after the first dose was administered. This situation could be extremely serious, especially when narcotics or other central nervous system depressants are administered. Immediate documentation prevents accidental administration of a drug by another individual.

▷ Preparing a Drug for Administration

Whenever any drug is prepared for administration, certain rules must be followed:

1. *A physician's written order is necessary for the administration of all drugs.* The exception to this rule is an emergency, when the nurse may administer a drug with a verbal order from the physician. However, the physician must write the order as soon as the emergency is over.

2. *Any order that is unclear must be questioned.* This includes unclear directions for the administration of the drug, illegible handwriting on the physician's order sheet, or a drug dose that is higher or lower than the dosages given in approved references.

3. *The physician's written orders must be checked.*

4. *Medications are prepared for administration in a quiet, well-lit area.*

5. *The label of the drug is checked three times:* (1) when the drug is taken from its storage area, (2) immediately before removing the drug from the container, and (3) before returning the drug to its storage area.

6. *A drug is never removed from an unlabeled container or from a container whose label is illegible.*

7. *The hands are washed immediately before preparing a drug for administration.*

8. *The hands must not touch capsules or tablets.* To remove an oral drug from the container, the correct number of tablets or capsules is shaken into the cap of the container and from there into the medicine cup.

9. *Aseptic technique is observed when handling syringes and needles.*

10. *Once the drug is removed from the container, the medicine cup, medicine glass, or needle and syringe is placed on or next to the medication card.* Medicine trays with sections for medicine cups, unit dose drugs, and containers for liquid medications, along with clips or slots for the medicine cards, are commonly used in hospitals. This type of tray prevents accidental mixing of the medicine cards and containers.

11. *The caps of drug containers are replaced immediately after the drug is removed.*

12. *Drugs requiring special storage are returned to the storage area immediately after they are prepared for administration.* This rule applies mainly to the refrigeration of drugs but may also apply to those drugs that must be protected from exposure to light or heat.

13. *Tablets should not be crushed or capsules opened without first checking with the pharmacist.* Some tablets can be crushed or capsules can be opened and the contents added to water or a tube feeding when the patient cannot swallow a whole tablet or capsule. Some tablets have a special coating that delays the absorption of the drug. Crushing the tablet may destroy this drug property and result in problems such as improper absorption of the drug or gastric irritation. Capsules are gelatin and dissolve on contact with a liquid. The contents of some capsules do not mix well with water and therefore are best left in the capsule. If the patient cannot take an oral tablet or capsule, the physician is consulted because the drug may be available in liquid form.

14. *Never give a drug that someone else has prepared.* Except in an emergency situation, the individual preparing the drug **must** administer the drug.

15. Many drugs are packaged by their manufacturers in unit doses. That is, each package is labeled by the manufacturer and contains one tablet or capsule, a premeasured amount of a liquid medication, a prefilled syringe, or one suppository. Hospital pharmacists may also prepare unit doses. *With a unit-dose system, the wrappings of the unit dose are not removed until the drug reaches the bedside of the patient who is to receive it.*

▷ General Points of Drug Administration

Immediately before administering any drug to a patient, the patient's identity must be verified. An identification band is attached to the patient's wrist and the band is checked against the medication card. On occasion, identification bands become illegible or have been removed. If the medication must be given immediately, the patient is asked his or her name, and the response is checked against the medication card. The patient's identification band is then replaced as soon as possible.

If the patient makes any statement about the medication or if there is any change in the patient, these must be carefully considered *before* the medication is given. Examples of situations that require consideration before a drug is given include the following:

1. Problems that may be associated with the drug such as nausea, dizziness, ringing in the ears, and difficulty walking. Comments made by the patient *may* indicate the occurrence of an adverse reaction. The drug should be withheld until references are consulted and the physician is contacted. The decision to withhold the drug must have a sound rationale and must be based on a knowledge of pharmacology.
2. Comments stating that the medication looks different from the one previously received, that the medication was just given by another nurse, or that the patient thought the physician discontinued the medication.
3. A change in the patient's condition, a change in one or more vital signs, or the appearance of new symptoms. Depending on the drug being administered and the patient's diagnosis, these changes *may* indicate that the drug should be withheld and the physician contacted.

▷ Administration of Drugs by the Oral Route

The oral route is the most frequent route of drug administration. Oral administration is relatively easy for most patients and rarely causes physical discomfort.

The following points are considered when giving an oral drug:

1. The patient is placed in an upright position. It is difficult, as well as dangerous, to swallow a solid or liquid when lying down.

2. A full glass of water is readily available.
3. The patient's need for assistance in removing the tablet or capsule from the container, holding the container, holding a medicine cup, or holding a glass of water is assessed. Some patients with physical disabilities cannot handle or hold these objects and may require assistance.
4. The patient is advised to take a few sips of water before placing a tablet or capsule in the mouth.
5. The patient is instructed to place the pill or capsule on the back of the tongue and tilt the head back to swallow a tablet or slightly forward to swallow a capsule. A few sips of water are then taken to move the drug down the esophagus and into the stomach. The patient is then encouraged to finish drinking the glass of water.
6. The patient is given any special instructions, such as drinking extra fluids or remaining in bed, that are pertinent to the drug being given.
7. A medication is *never* left at the patient's bedside to be taken later unless there is a specific order to do so. There are a few drugs (eg, antacids and nitroglycerin) that may be ordered to be left at the bedside.

▷ Administration of Drugs by the Parenteral Route

Parenteral drug administration means the giving of a drug by the subcutaneous (SC), intramuscular (IM), intravenous (IV), or intradermal route (Fig. 2-1). Other routes of parenteral administration that may be used by the physician are intralesional (into a lesion), intraarterial (into an artery), intracardiac (into the heart), and intraarticular (into a joint). In some instances, intraarterial drugs are administered by a nurse. However, administration is not by direct arterial injection but by means of a catheter that has been placed in an artery.

The following points are considered when giving a drug by the parenteral route:

1. After selecting the site for injection, the skin is cleansed. Most hospitals have a policy regarding the type of skin antiseptic used for cleansing the skin before parenteral drug administration. The skin is cleansed with a circular motion, starting at an inner point and moving outward.
2. After insertion of the needle for SC and IM administration, the syringe barrel is pulled back (eg, the needle is aspirated). Puncture of a blood vessel is not likely to occur with SC administra-

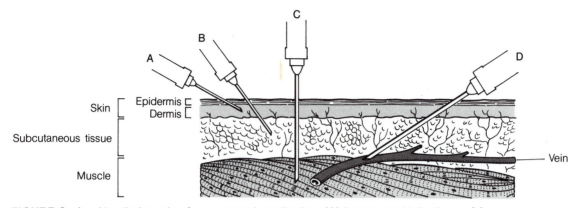

FIGURE 2–1. Needle insertion for parenteral medication. **(A)** Intradermal injection: a 26-gauge, ³/₈-inch long needle is inserted at a 10° to 15° angle. **(B)** Subcutaneous injection: a 25-gauge, ¹/₂-inch long needle is inserted at an angle that depends on the size of the patient. **(C)** Intramuscular injection: a 20-gauge to 23-gauge, 1-inch to 3-inch long needle is inserted into the relaxed muscle with a dart-throwing type of hand movement. **(D)** Intravenous injection: the diameter and length of the needle used depend on the substance to be injected and on the site of injection.

tion, but it may occur with IM administration. If blood does appear in the syringe, the needle is removed and the drug is not injected. The contaminated needle is removed, a new needle is attached, and another injection site is selected.

3. After insertion of a needle into a vein for IV drug administration, the syringe barrel is pulled back. Blood should flow back into the syringe.

4. After removal of the needle from an IM, SC, or IV injection site, pressure is placed on the area. Patients with bleeding tendencies often require prolonged pressure on the area.

5. Depending on hospital policy, gloves may be worn when administering drugs by the parenteral route. Gloves must be worn if the patient has or is suspected of having a disease such as the acquired immunodeficiency syndrome (AIDS), which is transmitted by direct contact with body fluids.

Subcutaneous Injections

An SC injection places the drug into the tissues between the skin and the muscle (Fig. 2-1B). Drugs administered in this manner are absorbed somewhat slowly. A volume of 0.5 to 1 mL is used for SC injection. Larger volumes (eg, more than 1 mL) are best given as IM injections. If a larger volume is ordered by the SC route, the injection is given in two sites with separate needles and syringes.

The sites for SC injection are the upper arms, the upper abdomen, and the upper back (Fig. 2-2). Most SC injections are given in the upper arms. The other areas are used when the drug is given for prolonged periods and injection sites must be rotated.

When giving a drug by the SC, the needle is inserted at a 45-degree angle. Obese patients have excess subcutaneous tissues, and the injection may also be given at a 90-degree angle. If the patient is thin or cachectic, there usually is less SC tissue. For these patients, the skin over the area is picked up between the fingers and the needle is inserted at a 90-degree angle.

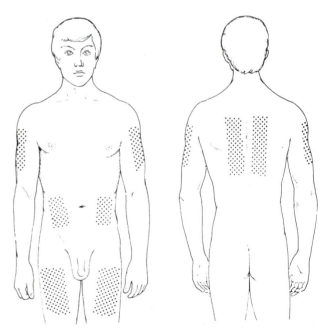

FIGURE 2–2. Sites on the body at which subcutaneous injections can be given.

Intramuscular Injections

An IM injection is the administration of a drug into a muscle (Fig. 2-1C). Drugs given by this route are absorbed more rapidly than drugs given by the SC route. In addition, a larger volume (1–5 mL) can be given at one site.

The sites for IM administration are the deltoid muscle (upper arm), the ventrogluteal or dorsogluteal sites (hip), and the vastus lateralis (thigh; Fig. 2-3). The vastus lateralis site is frequently used for infants and small children because it is often more developed than the gluteal or deltoid sites. This site may also be used for adults.

When giving a drug by the IM route, the needle is inserted at a 90-degree angle. When injecting a drug into the ventrogluteal or dorsogluteal muscles, the patient is placed in a comfortable position, pref-erably in a prone position with the toes pointing inward. When injecting the drug into the deltoid, a sitting or lying down position may be used. The patient is placed in a recumbent position for injection of a drug into the vastus lateralis.

Z-TRACK TECHNIQUE

The Z-track method of IM injection is used when a drug is highly irritating to SC tissues or has the ability to permanently stain the skin. The procedure below is followed when using the Z-track technique (Fig. 2-4):

1. The drug is drawn up into the syringe.
2. The needle is discarded and a new needle is placed on the syringe. This prevents any solution that may remain in the needle (that was used to

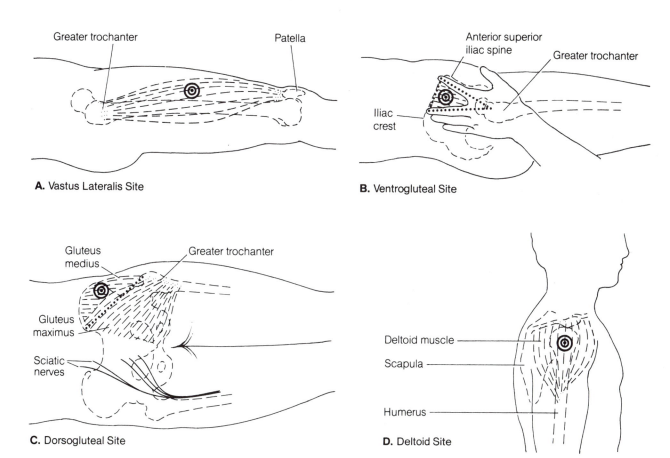

A. Vastus Lateralis Site

B. Ventrogluteal Site

C. Dorsogluteal Site

D. Deltoid Site

FIGURE 2–3. (A) Vastus lateralis site: the patient is supine or sitting. **(B)** Ventrogluteal site: the nurse's palm is placed on the greater trochanter and the index finger is placed on the anterior superior iliac spine; the injection is made into the middle of the triangle formed by the nurse's fingers and the iliac crest. **(C)** Dorsogluteal site: to avoid the sciatic nerve and accompanying blood vessels, an injection site is chosen above and lateral to a line drawn from the greater trochanter to the posterior superior iliac spine. **(D)** Deltoid site: the mid-deltoid area is located by forming a rectangle, the top of which is at the level of the lower ede of the acromion, and the bottom of which is at the level of the axilla; the sides are one third and two thirds of the way around the outer aspect of the patients arm.

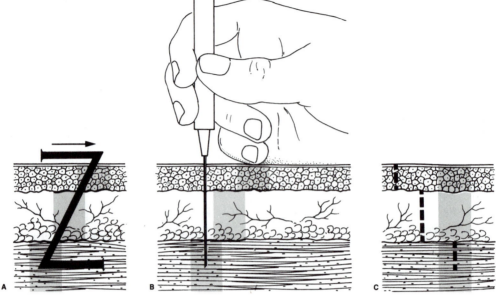

FIGURE 2—4. Z-track injection. **(A)** The tissue is tensed laterally at the injection site before the needle is inserted. This pulls the skin, subcutaneous tissue, and fat planes into a Z formation. **(B)** After the tissue has been displaced, the needle is thrust straight into the muscular tissue. **(C)** After injection, tissues are released while the needle is withdrawn. As each tissue plane slides by the other, the track is sealed.

draw the drug into the syringe) from contacting tissues as the needle is put into the muscle.

3. The plunger is pulled down to draw approximately 0.1 to 0.2 mL of air into the syringe. The air bubble in the syringe follows the drug into the tissues and seals off the area where the drug was injected, thereby preventing oozing of the drug up through the extremely small pathway created by the needle.

4. The patient is placed in the usual position for an IM injection.

5. The skin is cleansed.

6. The skin, subcutaneous tissues, and fat (that are over the injection site) are pulled laterally.

7. While the tissues are still held in the lateral position, the needle is inserted and the drug injected.

8. As soon as the drug is injected, the tissues are released and then the needle is withdrawn.

Intravenous Administration

A drug administered by the IV route is given directly into the blood by a needle inserted into a vein. Drug action occurs almost immediately.

Drugs administered IV may be given:

▷ Slowly, over 1 or more minutes

▷ Rapidly (IV push)

▷ Diluted or undiluted (according to specific instructions in the enclosed package insert and the physician's written order)

▷ Into an existing IV line (the IV port)

▷ Into a heparin lock (a small IV needle with a small fluid reservoir and a rubber cap through which the needle is inserted)

▷ By being added to an IV solution and allowed to infuse into the vein over a longer period.

When administering a drug into a vein by a venipuncture, a tourniquet is place *above* the selected vein. The tourniquet is tightened so that venous blood flow is blocked but there is arterial blood flow. The veins are allowed to fill (distend). The skin is then pulled taut (to anchor the vein and the skin) and the needle is inserted into the vein, bevel up, and at a short angle to the skin (Fig. 2-5). Blood should immediately flow into the syringe if the needle is properly inserted into the vein.

Performing a venipuncture requires practice. Some veins are difficult to enter, and a suitable vein for venipuncture may be hard to find. At no time should the nurse repeatedly and unsuccessfully attempt a venipuncture. Depending on clinical judgment, three unsuccessful attempts on the same patient warrant having a more skilled individual attempt the venipuncture.

Some drugs are added to an IV solution such as

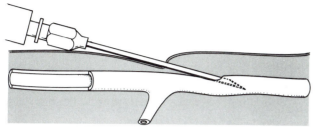

FIGURE 2–5. Needle-bevel position for venipuncture. (Courtesy of Pfizer Laboratories, New York, NY)

1000 mL of dextrose 5% and water. The drug is usually added to the IV fluid container immediately before adding the fluid to the IV line. Whenever a drug is added to an IV fluid, the bottle *must* have a label attached indicating the drug and drug dose added to the IV fluid. In some hospitals, a pharmacist is responsible for adding specific drugs to IV fluids.

CALCULATING IV FLOW RATES

When the physician orders a drug added to an IV fluid, he or she may also indicate the amount of fluid to be administered over a specified period, such as 125 mL/h or 1000 mL over 8 hours. If no infusion rate had been ordered, 1 L (1000 mL) of IV fluid should infuse over 6 to 8 hours.

To allow the IV fluid to infuse over a specified period, the IV flow rate must be determined. Before using one of the methods below, the drop factor must be known. Drip chambers on the various types of IV fluid administration sets vary. Some deliver 12 drops/mL and others deliver more. This is called the *drop factor*. The drop factor (number of drops/mL) is given on the package containing the drip chamber and IV tubing. Two of several methods for determining the IV infusion rate follow.

Method 1

Step 1. Total amount of solution ÷ number of hours = number of mL/h

Step 2. mL/h ÷ 60 = number of mL/min

Step 3. mL/min × drop factor = number of drops/min

EXAMPLE

1000 mL of an IV solution is to infuse over a period of 8 hours. The drop factor is 14.

Step 1. 1000 mL ÷ 8 hours = 125 mL/h

Step 2. 125 ÷ 60 = 2.08 mL/min

Step 3. 2.08 × 14 = 29 drops/min

Method 2

Step 1. Total amount of solution ÷ number of hours = number of mL/h

Step 2. mL/h × drop factor ÷ 60 = number of drops per minute

EXAMPLE

1000 mL of an IV solution is to infuse over a period of 6 hours. The drop factor is 12.

Step 1. 1000 mL ÷ 6 = 166.6 mL/h

Step 2. 166.6 × 12 ÷ 60 = 33 to 34 drops/min

NURSING RESPONSIBILITIES

After the start of an IV infusion, the type of IV fluid and, when applicable, the drug added to the IV solution are entered on the patient's chart. The nurse must check the infusion rate every 15 to 30 minutes. At this time, the needle site is also inspected for signs of redness, swelling, or other problems. Swelling around the needle may indicate that the needle is no longer in the vein and the IV fluid is being deposited in SC tissue. Two events may have occurred: extravasation and infiltration. *Extravasation* refers to the escape of fluid from a blood vessel into surrounding tissues while the needle or catheter is in the vein. *Infiltration* is the collection of fluid into tissues (usually SC tissue) when the needle or catheter is out of the vein. Both events necessitate discontinuation of the infusion and insertion of an IV line in another vein. Some drugs are capable of causing severe tissue damage if extravasation or infiltration occurs.

If extravasation or infiltration should occur, the IV must be stopped and restarted in another vein. The physician should be contacted if a drug, for example, norepinephrine (Levophed), capable of causing tissue damage has escaped into the tissues surrounding the needle insertion site.

INTRAVENOUS INFUSION PUMPS

An infusion pump may be used to deliver the desired number of drops per minute accurately. An alarm is set to sound if the IV is more than or less than the preset rate. Use of an infusion pump still requires nursing supervision and frequent monitoring of the IV infusion.

Intradermal Administration

Drugs given by the IM route are usually agents for sensitivity tests, for example, the tuberculin test or allergy skin testing (see Fig. 2-1A). The inner part of the forearm and the upper back may be used for IM sensitivity testing. The area should be hairless; areas near moles, scars, or pigmented skin areas should be avoided. The area is cleansed in the same manner as for SC and IM injections. The results of the IM injection are read after the prescribed period.

Other Parenteral Routes

The physician may administer a drug by the intracardial, intralesional, intraarterial, or intraarticular routes. The nurse may be responsible for preparing the drug for administration. The physician should be asked what special materials will be required for administration.

▷ Topical Application of Drugs

Drugs may be applied to the skin and mucous membranes. This is called topical application of a drug. Most topical drugs are not absorbed through the skin, and their action is to the skin, not the structures lying below the skin surface. A few topical drugs (eg, nitroglycerin) are absorbed through the skin. These drugs are applied topically for their systemic effects.

Topical drugs may be in the form of ointments, lotions, liquids, solids, or creams. When applied to the skin for their local effect, they are usually used to soften, disinfect, or lubricate the skin. A few topical drugs are enzymes that have the ability to remove superficial debris, such as the dead skin and purulent matter present in skin ulcerations. Other topical agents are used to treat minor, superficial skin infections.

The various forms of topical applications include the following:

▷ Creams, lotions, or ointments applied to the skin with a tongue blade, gloved fingers, or gauze

▷ Sprays applied to the skin or into the nose or oral cavity

▷ Liquids inserted into body cavities such as fistulas

▷ Liquids inserted into the bladder or urethra

▷ Solids (eg, suppositories) or jellies inserted into the urethra

▷ Liquids dropped into the eyes, ears, or nose

▷ Ophthalmic ointments applied to the eyelids or dropped into the lower conjunctival sac

▷ Solids (eg, suppositories, tablets), foams, liquids, and creams inserted into the vagina

▷ Continuous or intermittent wet dressings applied to skin surfaces

▷ Solids (eg, tablets, lozenges) dissolved in the mouth

▷ Sprays or mists inhaled into the lungs

▷ Liquids, creams, or ointments applied to the scalp

▷ Solids (eg, suppositories), liquids, or foams inserted into the rectum

The physician may write special instructions for the application of a topical drug, for example, to apply the drug in a thin, even layer or to cover the area following application of the drug to the skin. Other drugs may have special instructions provided by the manufacturer, such as to apply the drug to a clean, hairless area or to let the drug dissolve slowly in the mouth. All of these instructions are important because drug action may depend on correct administration of the agent.

▷ Nursing Responsibilities After Drug Administration

After the administration of any type of drug, the nurse is responsible for the following:

1. *Recording the administration of the drug.* This task is completed as soon as possible. This is particularly important when prn medications (especially narcotics) are given.

2. *Recording (when necessary) any information concerning the administration of the drug.* This includes information such as the IV flow rate, the site used for parenteral administration, problems with administration (if any), and vital signs taken immediately before administration.

3. *Evaluating and recording the patient's response to the drug* (when applicable). Evaluation may include such facts as relief of pain, decrease in body temperature, relief of itching, decrease in the number of stools passed, and so on.

4. *Observing the adverse reactions.* The frequency of these observations will depend on the drug administered. All suspected adverse reactions are recorded, as well as reported, to the physician. Serious adverse reactions are reported to the physician immediately.

3

General Principles of Pharmacology

On completion of this chapter the student will:

▶ *List the factors that may influence drug action*

▶ *Calculate drug dosages on a weight basis*

▶ *Discuss the types of drug interactions that may be seen with drug administration*

▶ *List and discuss the various types of adverse drug reactions*

▶ *Define drug tolerance and cumulative drug effects*

▶ *Discuss the nursing implications associated with drug actions, interactions, and effects*

▶ *Discuss the laws governing the manufacture, distribution, and sale of drugs*

▷ Drug Actions, Interactions, Reactions, and Effects

Drug Actions

Factors that may influence drug action often must be taken into account when the physician prescribes and the nurse administers a drug.

AGE

The age of the patient may influence the action of a drug. Children almost always require smaller doses of a drug than adults do. Elderly patients may also require smaller doses, although this may depend on the type of drug administered. For example, the el-

derly patient may be given the same dose of an antibiotic as a younger adult, but may require a smaller dose of a drug that depresses the central nervous system, such as a narcotic or a drug to induce sleep (a hypnotic).

WEIGHT

Drug dosages for children are often calculated on a weight basis; however, some drug dosages for adults may also be calculated in this manner. When drug dosages are determined by the patient's weight in kilograms (kg) or pounds (lb), references list the dosage as the amount of drug per kilogram or pound. The following are examples of drug dosages given in this manner:

▷ 20 mg/kg/d (a total of 20 milligrams per kilogram per day)

▷ 100 mg/kg/d in three equally divided doses (a total of 100 milligrams per kilogram per day, which is then divided into three equal doses)

▷ 25 mg/lb/d in four equally divided doses (a total of 25 milligrams per pound per day, which is then divided into four equal doses)

To determine the dose of a drug that is based on weight, the patient is first weighed. If scales that weigh the patient in either kilograms or pounds are available, the patient's weight is obtained on the scale matching the drug dosage. If the drug dosage is stated in kilograms and a scale giving the weight in pounds is the only one available, the patient's weight has to be converted to kilograms. The reverse is also true.

To convert pounds to kilograms, the patient's weight in pounds is divided by 2.2, because there are 2.2 pounds per kilogram. To convert kilograms to pounds, the weight in kilograms is multiplied by 2.2. An example of determining a drug dosage is shown in Table 3-1.

Although the dosages of some drugs administered to adults are based on weight, there are many drugs whose dosages are not based on weight. Instead, these dosages are based on a weight of approximately 150 pounds, which is calculated to be the "average" weight of men and women. In most instances, the individual whose weight varies widely from the 150-pound average will benefit from the drug dose based on this average weight. A drug dose may sometimes be increased or decreased because the patient's weight is significantly higher or lower than the average. An example of this is when narcotics are prescribed. Higher or lower than average dosages may be necessary to produce relief of pain in the patient who weighs significantly more than or less than the average weight.

SEX

The sex of an individual may influence the action of some drugs. Women may require a smaller dose of some drugs than men. This is based on the fact that many women are smaller than men and have a different ratio of body fat and water than men do.

DISEASE

The presence of disease may influence the action of some drugs, and, in some instances, may be an indication for not prescribing a drug or for reducing the dose of a certain drug. In liver disease, for example, the ability to metabolize or detoxify a specific type of drug may be impaired. If the average or normal dose of the drug is given, the liver would be unable to metabolize the drug at a normal rate. Consequently, the drug may be excreted from the body at a much slower rate than normal. The physician may then decide to prescribe a lower dose and lengthen the time between doses because liver function is abnormal.

ROUTE OF ADMINISTRATION

Intravenous (IV) administration of a drug produces the most rapid drug action. Next in order of time of action is the intramuscular (IM) route, followed by the subcutaneous (SC) route. Giving a drug orally usually produces the slowest drug action. Some drugs can be given only by one route, for example, antacids are only given orally. Other drugs are available as oral *and* parenteral drugs. The physician selects the route of administration based on many factors including the desired rate of action. For example, the patient with a severe cardiac problem may require IV administration of a drug that affects the heart, whereas another patient with a mild cardiac problem will respond well to oral administration of the same drug.

Drug Interactions

DRUG–DRUG INTERACTIONS

Some drugs interact with or interfere with the actions of other drugs. An example of one drug interfering with the action of another is the use of certain types of antacids at the same time the antibiotic tetracycline is taken orally. The antacid may chem-

---

TABLE 3–1
Example of Drug Dosage Determination

DRUG DOSAGE

5 mg/kg/d in 3 equally divided doses

WEIGHT OF PATIENT

120 pounds (which, when converted to kilograms, is 54.54 kg)

CALCULATIONS

5 mg/kg is 5 × 54.54 or 272.7 mg/d. The total of 272.7 is divided into 3 equal doses or 272.7 ÷ 3 = 90.9 mg for each dose.

ADMINISTRATION

The drug is available in 50- and 100-mg tablets. The 100-mg tablet is given because it is the closest dose available, and tablets cannot be broken so that nine tenths of the tablet is administered.

ically interact with the tetracycline and impair its absorption into the bloodstream, thus reducing the effectiveness of the tetracycline.

Drug interactions can also be *antagonistic* or *synergistic*. Some drugs may interact with food, chemicals, or other drugs and produce an antagonistic (opposite) effect. Drug synergism may occur when a drug interacts with another drug (or drugs) and produces an effect that is *greater than* the sum of the separate actions of two (or more) drugs.

An example of drug synergism is seen in the person taking more than the prescribed dose of a hypnotic (a drug that induces sleep). If alcohol is also taken at the same time or shortly before or after the hypnotic is taken, the action of the hypnotic is potentiated (increased). The individual is likely to experience a drug effect that is greater than if either of these two agents were taken alone. On occasion, the occurrence of a synergistic drug effect can be serious and even fatal.

DRUG–FOOD INTERACTIONS

Depending on the oral drug given, food may impair or enhance its absorption. Eating certain foods at the same time a specific drug is taken may also influence the action of some drugs. When a drug is taken on an empty stomach, it is absorbed into the bloodstream at a faster rate than when taken with food in the stomach. Some drugs, especially those capable of irritating the stomach, result in nausea or vomiting and epigastric distress and are best given with food or meals.

Some drugs *must* be taken on an empty stomach to achieve an optimal effect. Other drugs should be taken with food. When it is necessary to take a drug on an empty stomach or with food manufacturers give these directions in the package inserts. Approved drug references also give this information. When the drug is dispensed by a pharmacist, this same information is placed on the prescription label. In the hospital, this information may or may not be on the drug label. If this information is not provided, the nurse must check approved references for information regarding the administration of a specific oral drug.

Drug Reactions

ADVERSE DRUG REACTIONS

Patients may experience one or more adverse reactions when they are given a drug. Adverse reactions (side effects) may occur after the first dose, after several doses, or even after many doses. In many instances, an adverse reaction is unpredictable although some drugs are known to cause certain ad-

verse reactions in a large number of patients. For example, drugs used in the treatment of cancer are very toxic and are known to produce adverse effects (reactions) in most of the patients receiving them. Other types of drugs, although capable of producing adverse reactions, do so in a smaller number of patients. Thus, while some adverse reactions to a few drugs are fairly predictable, many adverse drug reactions occur without warning.

DRUG ALLERGY

Drug allergy, or being allergic to a drug, is also called a hypersensitivity reaction. Allergy to a drug begins to occur after more than one dose of the drug is given. When a drug allergy occurs, the individual has become *sensitized* to the drug, that is, the drug has become an *antigen*, which stimulates the body to produce *antibodies*. If the patient takes the drug after the antigen/antibody response has occurred, an allergic reaction results. This can be compared to an allergy produced by ragweed pollen (hay fever). The ragweed pollen is the antigen and the response of the individual to exposure to ragweed is an allergic reaction, which often consists of itching and watering of the eyes, increased nasal discharge, swollen nasal membranes, and sneezing.

Allergic reactions to drugs can range from very mild to extremely serious and even life-threatening. Even a mild reaction can become serious if it goes unnoticed and the drug is given again. This is why even the most mild allergic reaction must be detected early and reported to the physician before the next dose of the drug is given. Serious allergic reactions require contacting the physician immediately because emergency treatment may be necessary.

Some allergic reactions occur within minutes (and even seconds) after the drug is given; others may be delayed for hours or days. In many instances, allergic reactions that occur immediately are the most serious.

Allergic reactions may be manifested by a variety of signs and symptoms that are observed by the nurse or reported by the patient. Examples of some allergic symptoms include itching, various types of skin rashes, hives (urticaria), difficulty breathing, asthmalike symptoms, cyanosis, a sudden loss of consciousness, and swelling of the eyes, lips, or tongue.

Another type of allergic drug reaction is an *anaphylactic* reaction, which usually occurs shortly after the administration of a drug to which the individual is sensitive (or allergic). This type of allergic reaction is extremely serious and requires immediate medical attention. Symptoms of an anaphylactic reaction include bronchospasm, extremely low blood pressure (also called anaphylactic shock), cyanosis, dyspnea (due to the severe bronchospasm), loss of consciousness, convulsions, and cardiac arrest. All or only some of these symptoms may be present. Treatment is aimed at raising the blood pressure, improving breathing, restoring cardiac function, and treating other symptoms as they occur.

Angioedema (angioneurotic edema) is another type of allergic drug reaction. It is manifested by the collection of fluid in SC tissues. The areas that may be affected are the eyelids, lips, mouth, throat, hands, and feet, although other areas may also be affected. Angioedema can be dangerous when the mouth is affected because the swelling may block the airway and asphyxia may occur. Any patient with swelling of any area of the body occurring after a drug is given is closely observed for difficulty in breathing. The physician is contacted immediately if *any* signs of angioedema occur.

DRUG IDIOSYNCRASY

Drug idiosyncrasy is a term used to describe any unusual or abnormal reaction to a drug. It is any reaction that is different from the one normally expected of a specific drug and dose. For example, a patient may be given a drug to help her or him sleep (eg, a hypnotic). Instead of falling asleep, the patient remains wide awake and shows signs of nervousness or excitement. This is a response different from what is expected from this type of drug. Another patient may receive the same drug and dose, fall asleep, and then after 8 hours find it difficult to waken from sleep. This, too, is abnormal and can be described as an overresponse to the drug.

The cause of drug idiosyncrasy is not clear. It is believed to be due to a genetic deficiency wherein the patient is unable to tolerate certain chemicals, including drugs.

Drug Effects

DRUG TOLERANCE

Drug tolerance is a term used to describe a *decreased* response to the dose of a drug, usually requiring an *increase* in dosage to give the desired effect. Drug tolerance may develop when certain drugs, for example, narcotics and tranquilizers, are taken for a long period of time. The individual taking these drugs at home may have a tendency to increase the dose when the expected drug effect does not occur. The development of drug tolerance is one of the signs of drug addiction (see chap 13). Drug tolerance may also occur in the hospitalized patient. Drug tolerance (and possibly drug addiction) is *suspected* when the patient receiving a narcotic for more than 10 to 14 days begins to ask for the drug at more frequent intervals.

CUMULATIVE DRUG EFFECT

A cumulative drug effect may be seen in those with liver or kidney disease because these organs are the major sites for the breakdown and excretion of most drugs.

This drug effect occurs when the body is unable to metabolize and excrete one (normal) dose of a drug before the next dose is given. Thus, if a second dose of this same drug were given, some of the drug from the first dose remains in the body. Because toxicity can occur with some drugs when there is too much of that drug in the body, a cumulative drug effect, which can be serious, may be seen.

Patients with liver or kidney disease are usually given drugs with caution because a cumulative effect may occur. In some instances, the physician lowers the dose of the drug to prevent a toxic drug reaction due to failure to excrete the drug at a normal rate and the accumulation of the drug in the body.

▷ Nursing Implications

Many factors can influence drug action. Appropriate references or the hospital pharmacist should be consulted if there is any question about the dosage of a drug, about whether other drugs the patient is receiving will interfere with the drug being given, or about whether the oral drug should or should not be given with food.

Drug reactions are potentially serious. All patients are observed for adverse drug reactions, drug idiosyncrasy, and evidence of drug tolerance (when applicable). All drug reactions or any unusual drug effect is reported to the physician. The nurse must use judgment as to when adverse drug reactions or unusual drug effects are reported to the physician. Accurate observation and evaluation of the circumstances are essential; all observations are recorded in the patient's record. If there is any question regarding the events that are occurring, the drug can usually be withheld but the physician must be contacted immediately.

▷ Drug Legislation

The *Pure Food and Drug Act*, passed in 1906, was the first attempt by the government to regulate and control the manufacture, distribution, and sale of drugs. Before 1906, any substance could be called a drug, and no testing or research was required before placing the drug on the market. Before this time, drug potency and the purity of many drugs were questionable and some were even dangerous for human use.

The *Harrison Narcotic Act* of 1914 regulated the sale of narcotic drugs. Before the passage of this act, any narcotic could be purchased without a prescription.

In 1938, Congress passed the *Pure Food, Drug, and Cosmetic Act*, which gave the Food and Drug Administration (FDA) control over the manufacture and sale of drugs, as well as food and cosmetics. Before the passage of this act, some drugs, as well as foods and cosmetics, contained chemicals that were often harmful to humans. This law requires that these substances are safe for human use. It also requires pharmaceutical companies to perform toxicology tests before a new drug is submitted to the FDA for approval. Following FDA review of the tests performed on animals, as well as other research data, approval may be given to market the drug.

The *Comprehensive Drug Abuse Prevention and Control Act* was passed by Congress in 1970. This act was written because of the growing problem of drug abuse. It regulates the manufacture, distribution, and dispensation of drugs that have the potential for abuse. Title II of this law, the *Controlled Substances Act*, deals with control and enforcement. The Drug Enforcement Agency (DEA) within the US Department of Justice is the leading federal agency responsible for the enforcement of this act.

Drugs under jurisdiction of the Controlled Substances Act are divided into five schedules based on their potential for abuse and physical and psychological dependence. These schedules are as follows:

Schedule I (C-I)—high abuse potential and no accepted medical use (heroin, marijuana, LSD)

Schedule II (C-II)—high abuse potential with severe dependence liability (narcotics, amphetamines, barbiturates)

Schedule III (C-III)—less abuse potential than schedule II drugs and moderate dependence liability (nonbarbiturate sedatives, nonamphetamine stimulants, limited amounts of certain narcotics)

Schedule IV (C-IV)—less abuse potential than schedule III drugs and limited dependence liability (some sedatives and antianxiety agents, nonnarcotic analgesics)

Schedule V (C-V)—limited abuse potential; primarily small amounts of narcotics (codeine) used as antitussives or antidiarrheals

Prescriptions for controlled substances must include the name and address of the patient and the DEA number of the physician. Prescriptions for these drugs cannot be filled more than 6 months after the prescription was written or be filled more than five times. Under federal law, limited quantities of certain C-V drugs may be purchased without a prescription, with the purchase recorded by the dispensing pharmacist.

▷ Pregnancy Categories

The use of any medication, prescription or nonprescription, carries a risk of causing birth defects in the developing fetus. The FDA has established five categories indicating the potential of a drug for causing birth defects. Information regarding the pregnancy category of a specific drug is found in reliable drug literature such as the inserts accompanying drugs and approved drug references.

Pregnancy category A—Studies have not demonstrated a risk to the fetus in the first trimester of pregnancy and there is no evidence of risk in the second and third trimesters.

Pregnancy category B—This category includes two distinctions. One is that animal studies have not demonstrated a risk to the fetus but there are no adequate studies in pregnant women. The other is that animal studies have demonstrated an adverse effect but adequate studies on pregnant women have not demonstrated a risk to the human fetus during the first, second, or third trimester of pregnancy.

Pregnancy category C—This category includes two distinctions. One is that animal studies have shown an adverse effect on the fetus but there are no adequate studies in humans. The other is that there are no animal reproduction studies and no adequate studies performed in humans.

Pregnancy category D—Evidence indicates a risk to the human fetus.

Pregnancy category X—Studies in animals and humans demonstrate fetal abnormalities or reports indicate evidence of fetal risk.

During pregnancy, no woman should consider taking *any* drug, legal or illegal, prescription or non-prescription, unless the use of the drug is prescribed or recommended by the physician. Smoking or drinking any type of alcoholic beverage also carries risks such as low birthweight, premature birth, and fetal alcohol syndrome. Children born of mothers using addictive drugs such as cocaine or heroin are often born with an addiction to the drug abused by the mother.

The Nursing Process and the Administration of Pharmacologic Agents

On completion of this chapter the student will:

▶ *List the five parts of the nursing process*

▶ *Discuss assessment, planning, implementation, and evaluation as they apply to the administration of pharmacologic agents*

▶ *Differentiate between objective and subjective data*

▶ *Discuss and demonstrate how the nursing process may be used in daily life, as well as when administering pharmacologic agents*

▷ The Five Parts of the Nursing Process

The nursing process is a framework for nursing action. Although there are various ways of describing the nursing process, it is generally considered to consist of five parts: *assessment, nursing diagnosis, planning, implementation,* and *evaluation*. Each part is applicable, with modification, to the administration of drugs.

Assessment

Assessment of the patient receiving a pharmacologic agent is an important aspect of drug administration because data obtained during assessment may influence nursing decisions made during the planning, implementation, and evaluation phases of the nursing process. Patient assessment provides a data base from which decisions can be made. Assessment also provides information that is analyzed to identify problems that can be resolved or alleviated by nursing actions.

Assessment involves the collection of *objective* and *subjective* data. *Objective data* are pieces of information obtained during the physical assessment. Examples of the objective data that may be obtained before administering a drug are blood pressure, pulse, respiratory rate, temperature, weight, examination of the skin, and auscultation of the lungs. Recent laboratory tests and diagnostic studies are also reviewed as part of the physical assessment. Only one or two physical assessments may be necessary for one drug, whereas another drug may require many assessments.

Subjective data are pieces of information supplied by the patient or the patient's family. This type of data is usually collected at the time of admission to the hospital through questions asked by the nurse. In some instances, the patient may offer additional information following the initial collection of data. Examples of subjective data are a family history of disease, allergy history, occupational history, a description (in the patient's words) of the current illness or chief complaint, a medical history, and a drug history. The nurse should also review the physician's initial physical examination record, which often contains objective and subjective data relevant to the drug being administered.

Nursing Diagnosis

After the data collected during assessment are analyzed, the patient's unmethodical needs (the patient's problems) are identified and the nursing diagnosis is formulated. This diagnosis is not a medical diagnosis, but a description of the patient's problems and their probable or actual related causes, based on the subjective and objective data in the data base. The nursing diagnosis identifies those problems that can be solved or prevented by *independent nursing actions*. Independent nursing actions are actions that do not require a physician's order and may be legally performed by a nurse.

The North American Nursing Diagnosis Association (NANDA) has approved a list of diagnostic categories to be used in formulating a nursing diagnosis. Many of the nursing diagnoses developed by NANDA may be used to identify patient's problems associated with drug therapy. In some instances, a nursing diagnoses may apply to a specific group or type of drug, for example, fluid volume deficit related to diuresis secondary to administration of a diuretic.

Planning

After data are collected, they are sorted and analyzed, and a plan of action or patient care plan is developed. For example, during the initial assessment interview to collect subjective data, the patient may state an allergy to penicillin. This information is important, and the nurse must now plan the best method of informing all health team personnel of the patient's allergy to penicillin.

Planning also involves the setting of goals, which should be patient-oriented. For example, a patient may need to apply a skin ointment after discharge from the hospital. The planned goal for this patient is stated as "demonstrates the technique of ointment application."

The planning phase also lays the groundwork or plans the steps for carrying out nursing activities that are specific and that will meet the stated goals. This phase also plans the implementation phase, or the carrying out of nursing actions that are specific for the drug being administered. If, for example, the patient is to receive a medication by the intravenous (IV) route, the nurse must plan the materials needed and the patient instruction for administration of the drug by this route. In this instance, the planning phase occurs immediately before the implementation phase and is necessary to carry out the technique of IV administration correctly. Failing to plan effectively may result in forgetting to obtain all of the materials necessary for drug administration.

Goals that are patient-oriented and planning for nursing actions that are specific for the drug to be administered can result in greater accuracy in drug administration, patient understanding of the drug regimen, improved patient compliance with the prescribed drug therapy after discharge from the hospital, and better results from therapy with a specific drug.

Implementation

Implementation is the carrying out of a plan of action, and is a natural outgrowth of the assessment and planning phases of the nursing process. When related to the administration of pharmacologic agents, implementation refers to the preparation and administration of one or more drugs to a specific patient. Before administering a drug, the nurse reviews the subjective and objective data obtained on admission and considers any additional data, such as blood pressure, pulse, or a statement made by the patient. The decision of whether to administer the drug is based on an analysis of all information. For example, Mr. Greene is hypertensive and is supposed to receive a medication to lower his blood pressure. Objective data obtained at the time of admission included a blood pressure of 188/110. Additional objective data obtained immediately before the administration of the drug included a blood pressure of 182/110. A decision was made by the nurse to administer the drug, because there was minimal change in his blood pressure. If, however, Mr. Greene's blood pressure was 132/88 and this was only the second dose of medication, the nurse could decide to withhold the medication and contact Mr. Greene's physician. Giving or withholding a medication or contacting the patient's physician are nursing activities related to the implementation phase of the nursing process.

Evaluation

Evaluation is a decision-making process. When related to the administration of pharmacologic agents, this part of the nursing process is an evaluation of the patient's response to drug therapy. Depending on the drug administered, the nurse may check the patient's blood pressure in an hour, inquire whether pain has been relieved, or monitor the pulse every 15 minutes. After evaluation, certain other decisions may need to be made and plans of action implemented, for example, notifying the physician of a marked change in the patient's pulse and respiratory rate after a drug was administered or changing the bed linen because sweating occurred after administration of a drug to lower the patient's elevated temperature.

▷ Summary

The nursing process is a plan that is used to identify patient problems, develop and implement a plan of action, and then evaluate the results of nursing activities, including the administration of drugs. The five parts of this process are used not only in nursing but in our daily lives. For example, when buying a television, we may first think about whether we need it and then price it in different stores (assessment). We may have to decide how to pay for the television (planning) and then buy it (implementation). After purchase and use, we evaluate the television set (evaluation).

Using the nursing process requires practice, experience, and a constant updating of knowledge. The nursing process is used in this text only as it applies to drug administration. It is not within the scope of this textbook to list *all* of the assessments, plans, implementations, and evaluations for the medical diagnosis that requires the administration of a specific pharmacologic agent.

5

Patient and Family Teaching

On completion of this chapter the student will:

▶ *Discuss some of the causes of medication failure*

▶ *List the general areas that may be included in a patient and family teaching plan*

▶ *Explain how the nursing process can be used to develop a teaching plan*

"Knowledge deficit"

One of the most important roles of the nurse is educating the patient and family. The patient and the family must be made aware of all relevant information about the prescribed drugs. When using the nursing process, patient and family teaching is identified and explained under the nursing diagnosis of *knowledge deficit.*

Unfortunately, there are times when a prescribed or recommended drug fails to produce the desired effect when patients are discharged from the hospital and assume responsibility for their own care. Some of the causes of medication failure are the following:

● Failure to take the drug at the right time

▷ Taking more or less than the prescribed dose of a drug

● Taking a medication that has lost its potency or has undergone a chemical change EXP date

● Omitting one or more doses

● Taking the drug with fruit juice, milk, or food when this is contraindicated

● Not reading the warnings or directions on the container label

● Breaking or crushing drugs that have a special coating or opening capsules

● Not using the drug as prescribed

● Stopping the drug before the course of therapy is completed

non-Compliance

▷ Areas Included in a Teaching Plan

Teaching plans must be individualized because patients do not have identical needs and may lack knowledge about their prescribed medications. Areas that should be covered in an individualized teaching plan vary depending on the drug prescribed and the physician's preference for including or excluding specific facts about the prescribed drug, and identifying what the patient needs to know to take the drug correctly.

The following are general points of information that apply to almost all drugs. In teaching patients and their families, the nurse must select information relevant to a specific drug. Patient and family teaching is adapted to the individual's level of understanding. Medical terminology is avoided unless terms are explained or defined. When patient or family teaching is detailed, such as teaching the diabetic patient about insulin administration, it is best done in several sessions. In some instances, printed directions or instructions will be necessary for the patient or family.

Keep at level of understanding

The Drug, the Drug Container, and the Storage of Drugs

1. The term *drug* applies to nonprescription as well as prescription drugs.
2. A drug should always remain in the container in which it was dispensed or purchased. Some drugs require special containers, such as light-resistant (brown) bottles to prevent deterioration that may occur on exposure to light. *MOSTURE*
3. If any drug changes color or develops a new odor, a pharmacist should be consulted immediately about continued use of the drug.
4. The original label on the drug container must not be removed while it is used to hold the drug.
5. Two or more different drugs must never be mixed in one container, even for a brief time, because one drug may chemically affect another. Mixing drugs can also lead to mistaking one drug for another, especially when the size and color are similar.
6. The lid or cap of the container is replaced immediately after removing the drug from the container. The lid or cap should be firmly snapped or screwed in place. Exposure to air or moisture shortens the life of most drugs.
7. Drugs requiring refrigeration are so labeled. The container should be returned to the refrigerator immediately after removing the medication.
8. *All* drugs should be kept out of the reach of children.
9. Unless otherwise directed, drugs should be stored in a cool, dry place.
10. No drug should be exposed even for a short time

to excessive sunlight, heat, cold, or moisture because deterioration may occur.
11. The *entire* label of the prescription or nonprescription drug container must be read, including the recommended dosage and warnings.
12. All directions printed on the label (eg, "shake well before using," "keep refrigerated," "take before meals") must be followed to ensure drug effectiveness.
13. In some instances, especially when an ointment or liquid drug is prescribed, some medication may remain after it is used or taken for the prescribed time. Some drugs have a short life (a few weeks to a few months) and may deteriorate or change chemically after a time. A prescription must *never* be saved for later use unless the physician so advises.

avoid medically team & abbreviations.

The Dosage Regimen

1. Water is used to take capsules or tablets unless the physician or pharmacist directs otherwise (eg, take with food, milk, or an antacid). Some liquids such as coffee, tea, fruit juice, and carbonated beverages may interfere with the action of some drugs. *"Enteric Coated" never crush*
2. A full glass of water should be used when taking an oral drug. In some instances, it may be necessary to drink extra fluids during the day while taking certain medications.
3. Capsules should not be chewed before swallowing; they must be swallowed whole. Tablets should not be chewed unless labeled as "chewable." Some tablets have special coatings that are required for events such as proper absorption of the drug or prevention of irritation of the lining of the stomach.
4. The dose of a drug or the time interval between doses is *never* increased or decreased unless directed by a physician. A prescription drug or a physician-recommended nonprescription drug is not stopped or omitted except on the advice of a physician.
5. Unless advised to do so by a physician, a prescribed or recommended drug is *not* discontinued.
6. If the symptoms for which the drug was prescribed do not improve or become worse, the physician is contacted as soon as possible because a change in dosage or a different drug may be necessary.
7. If a dose of a drug is omitted or forgotten, the

[handwritten: - Don't wake pt up for hypnotic.]

next dose must *not* be doubled or the next dose or two taken at more frequent intervals unless advised to do so by a physician.

8. Other physicians, dentists, nurses, and health personnel must *always* be informed of all drugs (prescription and nonprescription) currently being taken on a regular or occasional basis.

9. The exact names of all prescription and nonprescription drugs currently being taken should be kept in a wallet or purse for instant reference when seeing a physician or dentist.

10. When taking a drug for a long period of time, especially drugs such as anticoagulants, steroids, oral hypoglycemic agents, insulin, or digitalis, it is advisable to wear a Medic-Alert bracelet or other type of identification. In case of an emergency, the bracelet ensures that medical personnel are aware of health problems and current drug therapy.

Adverse Drug Effects *[handwritten: Side effects]*

1. Some drugs may cause adverse reactions (side effects). There are a wide variety of these reactions. Examples of some of the more common adverse reactions are nausea, vomiting, diarrhea, constipation, skin rash, dizziness, drowsiness, and dry mouth. Some may be mild and disappear with time or when the physician adjusts the dosage. In some instances, mild reactions such as dry mouth may have to be tolerated. Some adverse reactions are potentially serious and even life-threatening.

2. Adverse effects are *always reported* to the physician as soon as possible.

3. When allergic to any drug, medical personnel must be informed of this fact *before* any treatment or drug is given.

Family Members

1. A drug prescribed for one family member is *never* given to another family member, relative, or friend unless directed to do so by a physician.

2. Family members or relatives should be made aware of all drugs, prescription and nonprescription, that are currently being taken.

▷ Using the Nursing Process to Develop a Teaching Plan

The nursing process can be used when teaching patients about their drug and drug regimen.

Assessment

The nurse must first determine the patient's needs. Needs will stem from two areas: (1) the drug about which information is to be given (or what the patient or family needs to know) and (2) the patient or family member's ability to learn, accept, and use information. *[handwritten: take V/S 1st.]*

Some drugs require relatively little information or teaching, for example, teaching a patient about applying a nonprescription ointment to the skin. Other drugs such as insulin require detailed information that may need to be given over a period of several days. In addition, general points of patient teaching such as those given above should be given to all patients whenever possible.

At times, it may be difficult to assess an individual's ability to learn. However, it must be remembered that although most persons readily understand what is being taught, some cannot. For example, a visually impaired patient may be unable to read a label or printed directions supplied by the physician, pharmacist, or nurse. Giving a printed card with directions for taking the medication is of little value and other means of learning will have to be found. The nurse, by means of assessment, also tries to determine what barriers or obstacles (if any) may prevent the patient or family member from fully understanding the material being presented.

Nursing Diagnosis

A lack of knowledge (knowledge deficit) is the nursing diagnosis used for patient and family teaching. In stating the nursing diagnosis, the specific areas to be covered in the teaching plan depend on several factors such as the individual patient and family members, the type of drug prescribed, the ability of the patient or family members to understand the information, and the physician's orders.

Planning and Implementation *[handwritten: hands on (action)]*

Once the patient or family member's needs and the drug information necessary for the individual patient are determined, the nurse develops a teaching plan. Appropriate references may be consulted for a teaching format for a specific drug, but these sources of information may need to be modified to meet individual patient needs.

Teaching should be done at an appropriate time, which is determined on an individual basis. For example, patient teaching should *not* be done when there are visitors (unless they are to be involved in the administration of the patient's medications), immediately before discharge from the hospital, or if the patient has been sedated. Teaching should be done a day or more before discharge and when the patient is alone and alert. The nurse gears teaching to the patient's level of understanding and, when necessary, provides written, as well as oral, instructions. If much information is given, it is often best to present the material in two or more sessions.

Evaluation

To determine the effectiveness of patient teaching, the nurse must evaluate, as far as possible, the patient's knowledge of the material presented. This can be done in several ways depending on the information. For example, if the patient is being taught to test his or her urine for glucose, several demonstrations can be scheduled. When factual material is being given, the nurse may periodically ask the pa-

tient to list or repeat some of the information that was presented. Questions such as "Do you understand?" or "Is there anything you don't understand?" are usually avoided because they may place the patient in an awkward position.

▷ Summary

Patient teaching is an important aspect of total patient care. There are many possible causes of patient noncompliance and failure of the prescribed medication to produce the desired results. Some, but not all, of these causes may be prevented by thorough patient or family member teaching. The nursing process can be adapted to assess the patient's needs and then plan, implement, and evaluate the teaching program.

assess - BP elevated
planning
Implentation - giving pills
evaulation - BP
nrsg DX

6

Adrenergic Drugs

On completion of this chapter the student will:

▶ *Discuss the types, uses, and general drug actions of the adrenergic drugs*

▶ *List some of the adverse reactions associated with the administration of adrenergic drugs*

▶ *Use the nursing process when administering an adrenergic drug*

▶ *Discuss the nursing implications to be considered when administering adrenergic drugs*

▷ The Nervous System

The nervous system is a complex part of the human body concerned with the regulation and coordination of body activities such as movement, the digestion of food, sleep, and the elimination of waste products.

Divisions of the Nervous System

The nervous system may be divided as follows:

1. Central nervous system (CNS)
   a. Brain
   b. Spinal cord
2. Peripheral nervous system (PNS)
   a. Somatic nervous system
   b. Autonomic nervous system
      i. Sympathetic nervous system
      ii. Parasympathetic nervous system

The *peripheral nervous system* is the term used to describe all nerves outside of the brain and spinal cord. The *somatic* part (branch) of the PNS is concerned with sensation and voluntary movement. The sensory part of the somatic nervous system sends messages to the brain concerning the internal and external environment, for example, sensations of heat, pain, cold, and pressure. The voluntary part of the somatic nervous system is concerned with (voluntary) movement of skeletal muscles, for example, walking, chewing food, or writing a letter. The *autonomic nervous system* is concerned with those functions essential to the survival of the organism. The sympathetic nervous system (sympathetic branch of the autonomic nervous system) tends to regulate the expenditure of energy and is operative when the organism is confronted with stressful situations such as danger, intense emotion, or severe illness. The parasympathetic nervous system (parasympathetic branch of the autonomic nervous system) works to help conserve body energy and is partly responsible for such activities as slowing the heart rate, digesting food, and eliminating body wastes.

There are two neurohormones (neurotransmitters) of the sympathetic nervous system: **epinephrine** and **norepinephrine.** Epinephrine is secreted by the adrenal medulla. Norepinephrine is secreted mainly at nerve endings of sympathetic (also called adrenergic) nerve fibers.

▶ ADRENERGIC DRUGS

Adrenergic drugs act like or mimic the activity of the sympathetic nervous system and are also called *sympathomimetic drugs.* Epinephrine and norepinephrine are neurohormones produced naturally by the body. Synthetic preparations of these two neurohormones, which are identical to those naturally produced by the body, are used in medicine. Adrenergic drugs such as metaraminol (Aramine), isoproterenol (Isuprel), and ephedrine are synthetic adrenergic drugs.

▷ Actions of Adrenergic Drugs

Generally, adrenergic drugs produce one or more of the following responses in varying degrees:

Central nervous system—wakefulness; quick reaction to stimuli; quickened reflexes
Peripheral nervous system—relaxation of the smooth muscles of the bronchi; constriction of blood vessels, sphincters of the stomach; dilatation of coronary blood vessels; decrease in gastric motility
Heart—increase in the heart rate
Metabolism—increased use of glucose (sugar) plus liberation of fatty acids from adipose tissue

Adrenergic nerve fibers have either alpha- or beta-receptors. Adrenergic drugs may act on alpha-receptors only, beta-receptors only, or both alpha- and beta-receptors. For example, phenylephrine (Neo-Synephrine) acts chiefly on alpha-receptors, isoproterenol acts chiefly on beta-receptors, and epinephrine acts on both alpha- and beta-receptors. Whether an adrenergic drug acts on alpha-, beta-, or both alpha- and beta-receptors accounts for the variation of responses for this group of drugs. Table 6-1 gives the action of the autonomic nervous system on the body along with the type of adrenergic nerve fiber receptor for each.

▷ Uses of Adrenergic Drugs

Adrenergic drugs have a wide variety of uses and may be given as all or part of the treatment for the following:

▷ Moderately severe to severe episodes of hypotension
▷ Control of superficial bleeding during surgical and dental procedures of the mouth, nose, throat, and skin
▷ Bronchial asthma
▷ Cardiac arrest
▷ Allergic reactions (anaphylactic shock, angioneurotic edema)
▷ Temporary treatment of heart block
▷ Ventricular dysrhythmias (under certain conditions)
▷ Nasal congestion (applied topically)
▷ In conjunction with local anesthetics to prolong anesthetic action in medicine and dentistry

It should be noted that a specific adrenergic agent is selected as all or part of the treatment for any one of the above situations.

▷ Adverse Reactions Associated with the Administration of Adrenergic Drugs

The adverse reactions associated with the administration of adrenergic drugs depend on the drug used, the dose administered, and individualized patient response. Some of the adverse reactions for specific adrenergic agents are listed in Summary Drug Table 6-1. Some of the more common adverse reactions that may be seen with the administration of this group of drugs include cardiac dysrhythmias such as bradycardia and tachycardia, headache, insomnia, nervousness, anorexia, and an increase in blood pressure (which may reach dangerously high levels).

▶ *NURSING PROCESS*
THE PATIENT RECEIVING AN ADRENERGIC DRUG

ASSESSMENT

Assessment of the patient receiving an adrenergic drug depends on the drug, the patient, and the reason for administration. Assessment of the patient in shock who

TABLE 6–1
Action of the Autonomic Nervous System on Body Organs and Structures

ORGANS OR STRUCTURES	SYMPATHETIC (ADRENERGIC) EFFECTS	TYPE OF SYMPATHETIC (ADRENERGIC) RECEPTOR	PARASYMPATHETIC (CHOLINERGIC) EFFECTS
Heart	Increase in heart rate, heart muscle contractility, increase in speed of atrioventricular conduction	Beta	Decrease in heart ralte, decrease in heart muscle contractility
Blood vessels			
1. Skin, mucous membrane	Constriction	Alpha	
2. Skeletal muscle	Usually dilatation	Cholinergic,* beta	
Bronchial muscles	Relaxation	Beta	Contraction
Gastrointestinal			
1. Muscle motility, tone decrease		Beta	Increase
2. Sphincters	Usually contraction	Alpha	Usually relaxation
3. Gallbladder	Relaxation	?	Contraction
Urinary bladder			
1. Detrusor muscle	Relaxation	Beta	Contraction
2. Trigone, sphincter muscles	Contraction	Alpha	Relaxation
Eye			
1. Radial muscle of iris	Contraction (pupil dilates)	Alpha	
2. Sphincter muscle of iris			Contraction (pupil constricts)
3. Ciliary muscle			Contraction
Skin			
1. Sweat glands	Increased activity in localized areas	Cholinergic*	
2. Pilomotor muscles	Contraction (gooseflesh)	Alpha	
Uterus	Relaxation	Beta	
Salivary glands	Thickened secretions	Alpha	Copious, watery secretions
Liver	Glycogenolysis	Beta	
Lacrimal and nasopharyngeal glands			Increased secretion
Male sex organs	Emission	Alpha	Erection

Cholinergic transmission, but nerve cell chain originates in the thoracolumbar part of the spinal cord, and is therefore sympathetic.

is to be treated with norepinephrine is different from that for the patient receiving nose drops containing phenylephrine. Both are receiving adrenergic agents, but the circumstances are different.

For example, if the patient is to receive an adrenergic agent for shock, the nurse obtains the blood pressure, pulse rate and quality, and respiratory rate and rhythm. This information provides an important data base that is used during treatment. A general survey of the patient is also necessary. The nurse should look for additional symptoms of shock such as cool skin, cyanosis, diaphoresis, and a change in the level of consciousness. Other assessments may be necessary if the hypotensive episode is due to trauma, severe infection, or blood loss. When the patient is to have nose drops instilled for nasal congestion, the initial assessment includes an examination of the nasal passages and a description of the type of secretions present in the nose. The blood pressure should be

obtained because nose drops that contain adrenergic agents are not given to those with high blood pressure.

NURSING DIAGNOSIS

Depending on the drug, dose, and reason for administration, one or more of the following nursing diagnoses may apply to a person receiving an adrenergic drug:

▶ Anxiety related to seriousness of disorder (shock, impending or borderline shock), activity of medical personnel in managing the disorder, invasive procedures (insertion of intravenous [IV] or intraarterial lines), actual or perceived threat to biologic integrity, other factors

▶ High risk for altered body temperature: hyperthermia related to infection secondary to invasive procedures

SUMMARY DRUG TABLE 6–1
Adrenergic Drugs

GENERIC NAME	TRADE NAME*	USES	ADVERSE REACTIONS	DOSE RANGES
dopamine	Intropin, *generic*	Severe hypotensive episodes	Ectopic beats, nausea, vomiting, anginal pain	2–50 mcg/kg/min IV
ephedrine sulfate	*Generic*	Acute hypotensive episodes; as systemic bronchodilator and decongestant	Palpitations, tachycardia, headache, insomnia, nausea, vomiting	Hypotension: 25–50 mg IM, SC, slow IV; systemic bronchodilator, decongestant: 25–50 mg IM, SC, IV
epinephrine	Adrenalin, *generic*	Cardiac arrest, anaphylactic shock, angioneurotic edema, acute asthma, topically to control capillary bleeding	Elevation of blood pressure, headache, anxiety, palpitations, cardiac dysrhythmias	Cardiac arrest: 5–10 mL of 1 : 10,000 solution IV; acute asthma: 0.3–0.5 mL of 1 : 1000 SC, IM; anaphylactic shock, angioneurotic edema: same as acute asthma
isoproterenol hydrochloride	Isuprel, *generic*	Cardiac arrest, some cardiac dysrhythmias, Adams-Stokes syndrome, shock; as systemic bronchodilator	Tachycardia, insomnia	2 mg in 500 mL of diluent by IV infusion; 0.1–0.2 mg by IV injection; 0.02–1 mg IM; 0.15–0.2 mg SC; 5–50 mg sublingually; 5–50 mg rectally
metaraminol bitartrate	Aramine, *generic*	Hypotension	Tachycardia or other cardiac dysrhythmias, headache, flushing	2–10 mg IM, SC; 15–100 mg in 500 mL sodium chloride or 5% dextrose by IV infusion; 0.05–5 mg by direct IV injection
norepinephrine (levarterenol)	Levophed	Acute hypotensive states	Bradycardia, headache, hypertension (due to overdose)	Up to 4 mL in 5% dextrose IV *only*
phenylephrine hydrochloride	Neo-Synephrine	Hypotensive episodes; topically as a nasal decongestant	Headache, reflex bradycardia, cardiac dysrhythmias	1–10 mg IM, SC; 0.1–0.5 mg IV; 10 mg in 500 mL dextrose or sodium chloride by IV infusion

* The term generic *indicates that the drug is available in a generic form.*

▶ Potential for infection related to invasive procedures

▶ Knowledge deficit of treatment modalities, drug regimen

PLANNING AND IMPLEMENTATION

The major goals of the patient depend on the reason for administration of an adrenergic agent. Examples of patient goals include a normal body temperature, an absence of infection, a reduction in anxiety, and an understanding of why the drug is being given.

The major goal of nursing management is to perform the appropriate procedures for drug administration and to competently observe the patient for drug response.

Management of the patient receiving an adrenergic agent varies and depends on the drug used, the reason for administration, and the patient's individual response to the drug. In most instances, adrenergic drugs are potent and potentially dangerous drugs. Great care must be exercised in the calculation and preparation of the drug for administration. All adverse effects are reported to the physician as soon as possible, but again, nursing judgment is necessary. Some adverse effects, such as the development of cardiac dysrhythmias, must be reported immediately, regardless of the time of day or night. Other adverse effects, such as anorexia, should be reported but usually are not of an emergency nature.

Any complaint the patient may have (subjective data) also must be reported and recorded, with the nurse using judgment regarding the seriousness of the complaint.

Although adrenergic drugs are potentially dangerous, proper supervision and management before, during, and after administration of the drug aids in minimizing the occurrence of the serious problems associated with administration.

When the patient has marked hypotension and requires administration of a vasopressor (a drug that raises the blood pressure because of its ability to constrict blood vessels), the physician determines the cause of the hypotension and then selects the best method of treatment. Some hypotensive episodes require the use of a less potent vasopressor such as metaraminol, whereas at other times a more potent vasopressor such as dopamine (Intropin) or norepinephrine (Levophed) is necessary.

The following are points regarding the administration of the potent vasopressors, dopamine and norepinephrine:

1. Dopamine cannot be mixed with other drugs, especially sodium bicarbonate or other alkaline IV solutions. Check with the hospital pharmacist before adding a second drug to an IV solution containing this drug.

2. Norepinephrine and dopamine are administered *only* by the IV route. These drugs *must* be diluted in an IV solution before administration. The physician orders the IV solution, the amount of drug added to the solution, and the initial rate of infusion.

3. During administration of these drugs, the blood pressure and pulse rate are monitored at frequent intervals, usually every 3 to 5 minutes.

4. The rate of administration (ie, drops per minute) is adjusted according to the patient's blood pressure.

5. The needle site and surrounding tissues are inspected at frequent intervals for leakage (extravasation, infiltration) of the solution into the subcutaneous [SC] tissues surrounding the needle site.

6. Intravenous solutions containing either of these drugs must not be allowed to extravasate or infiltrate into the SC tissues surrounding the needle site. If either situation occurs, another IV line is established immediately and the IV containing dopamine is discontinued. The physician is notified immediately.

7. The physician will usually order a specific systolic blood pressure to be maintained during administration. The rate of administration of the IV solution is increased or decreased to maintain the patient's blood pressure at the systolic level ordered by the physician.

8. Readjustment of the rate of flow of the IV solution is often necessary during the administration of these drugs. The frequency of adjustment will depend on the patient's response to the vasopressor.

9. At no time must the patient receiving these drugs be left unattended.

The less potent vasopressors, such as metaraminol, also require close supervision during administration. The same procedure as that for norepinephrine and dopamine is followed, but blood pressure and pulse determinations are usually taken at less frequent intervals, usually every 5 to 15 minutes. Sound clinical judgment should always be used because there is no absolute minimum or maximum time limit between determinations.

Other adrenergic agents have specific uses. Isoproterenol may be used in the treatment of some cardiac dysrhythmias, cardiac arrest, shock, Adams-Stokes syndrome, or as a systemic bronchodilator. Epinephrine may be used to treat bronchial asthma, anaphylactic shock, and other allergic reactions. Epinephrine may be used topically to control capillary bleeding, or may be used with a local anesthetic to control bleeding, as well as prolong local anesthetic action. The uses of various adrenergic agents are given in Summary Drug Table 6-1.

The following are points to remember before, during, and after the administration of an adrenergic agent:

1. The patient's symptoms, problems, or needs are assessed before the administration of the drug. Any subjective or objective data are recorded on the patient's chart. In emergency situations assessments must be made quickly and accurately.

2. The patient is observed for the effect of the drug. For example, is the breathing of the asthmatic patient improved? Is the blood pressure responding to the administration of the vasopressor?

3. The effect of the drug is evaluated and recorded. Comparison of assessments made before and after administration may help the physician determine future use of the drug for this patient.

4. The patient is observed for adverse drug reactions and these are reported to the physician as soon as possible. The next dose of the drug is not given until the physician has been contacted.

ANXIETY. Depending on the clinical situation, some anxiety and fear may be experienced by the patient receiving an adrenergic drug for a serious disorder such as shock or bronchial asthma. Invasive procedures (eg, establishing IV or intraarterial lines) also create anxiety.

All treatments and procedures are explained to the patient or family members but the type and length of explanation depend on the clinical situation. The patient and family members are reassured that care is being exercised in performing treatments or procedures and that the patient will be closely observed while the drug is being administered.

ALTERED BODY TEMPERATURE AND INFECTION. When the patient is receiving an adrenergic drug by the IV route, the temperature is monitored every 4 hours or as ordered. A temperature greater than 101°F or any decrease in body temperature less than normal is reported to the physician.

The entrance point of IV or intraarterial line is inspected for signs of infection, namely redness, streaking, or drainage from the site.

KNOWLEDGE DEFICIT. Some adrenergic drugs, such as the vasopressors, are given only by medical personnel. The nurse's responsibility for teaching involves explaining the drug to the patient or family. Depending on the situation, teaching may include facts such as how the drug will be given (eg, the route of administration) and what results are expected from the administration of the drug. The nurse must use judgment regarding some of the information given to the patient or family regarding administration of an adrenergic drug in life-threatening situations because certain facts, such as the seriousness of the patient's condition, are usually best given by the physician.

When a nasal decongestant (drops or spray) containing an adrenergic drug has been recommended or prescribed, the patient or family must be shown the correct method of instillation. Other points to mention are an explanation of possible adverse effects, and an adherence to the dose regimen prescribed or recommended by the physician. Because many nasal decongestants are over-the-counter (OTC) drugs, patients using them should be advised that these drugs are contraindicated in those with high blood pressure and that overuse can *increase* nasal congestion (rebound congestion).

If an adrenergic drug, such as ephedrine or isoproterenol, has been prescribed as a bronchodilator, the patient must have the drug regimen explained. Additional explanation should include the adverse reactions that may occur and the importance of reporting adverse reactions to the physician as soon as possible. If the drug is prescribed in sublingual form, the technique of placing the drug under the tongue is demonstrated. The patient is also warned not to use any nonprescription (OTC) drug unless use has been approved by the physician. Patients receiving a bronchodilator should be encouraged to contact their physician if the drug fails to produce at least partial relief of their symptoms.

EVALUATION

► Anxiety is reduced

► Body temperature is normal

► Localized infection at venipuncture or arterial puncture site is not evidenced

► An understanding of treatment modalities and importance of continued follow-up care is verbalized

7

Adrenergic Blocking Agents

On completion of this chapter the student will:

▶ *Discuss the types, uses, and general drug actions of the adrenergic blocking agents*

▶ *List the general adverse reactions associated with the administration of the various types of adrenergic blocking agents;*

▶ *Describe the nursing actions that may be taken to minimize orthostatic or postural hypotension*

▶ *Use the nursing process when administering an adrenergic blocking agent*

▶ *Discuss the nursing implications to be considered when administering adrenergic blocking agent*

Adrenergic blocking agents, also called sympathomimetic blocking drugs, may be divided into four groups:

Alpha-adrenergic blocking agents—drugs that block alpha-adrenergic receptors

Beta-adrenergic blocking agents—drugs that block beta-adrenergic receptors

Antiadrenergic agents—drugs that block adrenergic nerve fibers

Alpha/beta-adrenergic blocking agents—drugs that block both alpha- and beta-adrenergic receptors

▷ Actions of Adrenergic Blocking Agents

Alpha-Adrenergic Blocking Agents

Alpha-adrenergic blocking agents produce their greatest effect on alpha receptors of adrenergic nerves that control the vascular system. Stimulation of alpha-adrenergic fibers results in vasoconstriction (see Table 6-1 in chap 6). If stimulation of these alpha-adrenergic fibers is interrupted or blocked, the result will be vasodilatation, which is the direct opposite of the effect of an adrenergic drug having mainly alpha activity. Phentolamine (Regitine) is an example of an alpha-adrenergic blocking agent.

Beta-Adrenergic Blocking Agents

Beta-adrenergic blocking agents produce their greatest effect on beta-receptors of adrenergic nerves, primarily the beta-receptors of the heart. Stimulation of beta-receptors of the heart results in an increase in the heart rate. If stimulation of these beta-adrenergic fibers is interrupted or blocked, the heart rate decreases. Examples of beta-adrenergic blocking agents are metoprolol (Lopressor), esmolol (Brevibloc), propranolol (Inderal), and nadolol (Corgard).

Beta-adrenergic blocking agents when used topically as ophthalmic drops appear to reduce the production of aqueous humor in the anterior chamber of the eye.

Antiadrenergic Agents

One group of antiadrenergic drugs inhibits the release of norepinephrine (a neurohormone of the sympathetic nervous system; see chap 6) from certain adrenergic nerve endings in the peripheral nervous system. This group is called a *peripherally acting* (ie, acting on peripheral structures) antiadrenergic drug. An example of a peripherally acting antiadrenergic drug is guanethidine (Ismelin). The other antiadrenergic drugs are called *centrally acting* antiadrenergic drugs because they act on the central nervous system rather than on the peripheral nervous system. This group affects specific central nervous system centers, thereby decreasing some of the activity of the sympathetic nervous system in this part of the nervous system. Although the action of both types of antiadrenergic drugs is somewhat different, the results are basically the same. An example of a centrally acting antiadrenergic drug is clonidine (Catapres-TTS-1).

Alpha/Beta-Adrenergic Blocking Agents

A drug belonging to this group acts on both alpha and beta nerve fibers. Only one drug is in this category: labetalol (Normodyne).

▷ Uses of Adrenergic Blocking Agents

Alpha-Adrenergic Blocking Agents

Phentolamine is used for its vasodilating effect on peripheral blood vessels, and therefore may be beneficial in the treatment of hypertension due to pheochromocytoma, a tumor of the adrenal gland that produces excessive amounts of epinephrine and norepinephrine.

Beta-Adrenergic Blocking Agents

These drugs are primarily used in the treatment of hypertension (Summary Drug Table 7-1; see chap 18) and certain cardiac dysrhythmias. Some of these drugs have additional uses such as the use of propranolol for migraine headaches and naldolol for angina pectoris.

Beta-adrenergic blocking agents as ophthalmic eye drops, for example, timolol (Timoptic) and betaxolol (Betoptic), are used in the treatment of glaucoma. Glaucoma is a narrowing or blockage of the drainage channels (canals of Schlemm) between the anterior and posterior chambers of the eye, which then results in a buildup of pressure (increased intraocular pressure) in the eye. If glaucoma is not treated, blindness may occur.

Antiadrenergic Agents

Antiadrenergic agents are used mainly for the treatment of certain cardiac dysrhythmias and hypertension. The uses of some of the available antiadrenergic agents are given in Summary Drug Table 7-1.

Alpha/Beta-Adrenergic Blocking Agents

Labetalol is the only drug in this category that is available. It is used in the treatment of hypertension, either as a single agent or in combination with another agent such as a diuretic.

▷ Adverse Reactions Associated with the Administration of Adrenergic Blocking Agents

Alpha-Adrenergic Blocking Agents

Administration of an alpha-adrenergic blocking agent may result in cardiac dysrhythmias, hypotension, and tachycardia.

Beta-Adrenergic Blocking Agents

Some of the adverse reactions that may be seen with the administration of beta-adrenergic blocking agents include bradycardia, dizziness, vertigo,

SUMMARY DRUG TABLE 7–1
Adrenergic Blocking Drugs

GENERIC NAME	TRADE NAME*	USES	ADVERSE REACTIONS	DOSE RANGES
ALPHA-ADRENERGIC BLOCKING DRUGS				
phentolamine	Regitine	Hypertension due to pheochromocytoma	Hypotension, tachycardia, cardiac dysrhythmias	5 mg IM, IV
BETA-ADRENERGIC BLOCKING DRUGS				
acebutolol hydrochloride	Sectral	Hypertension, ventricular dysrhythmias	Bradycardia, dizziness, vertigo, rash, hyperglycemia, bronchospasm, hypotension, agranulocytosis	400–1200 mg/d PO in divided doses
atenolol	Tenormin	Hypertension, angina pectoris, acute myocardial infarction	Same as acebutolol	50–200 mg/d PO; 5 mg IV
betaxolol hydrochloride	Kerlone	Hypertension	Same as acebutolol (systemic use)	10 mg/d PO
betaxolol (ophthalmic)	Betoptic	Glaucoma	Brief discomfort, tearing	1–2 drops/d
esmolol hydrochloride	Brevibloc	Supraventricular tachycardia	Same as acebutolol	25–200 mcg/kg/min IV
metoprolol tartrate	Lopressor	Same as atenolol	Same as acebutolol	100–450 mg/d PO in single or divided doses; 5 mg IV
nadolol	Corgard	Angina pectoris, hypertension	Same as acebutolol	Angina: 40–240 mg/d PO; hypertension: 40–320 mg/d PO
pindolol	Visken	Hypertension	See Summary Drug Table 18-2	See Summary Drug Table 18-2
propranolol hydrochloride	Inderal, *generic*	Cardiac dysrhythmias, hypertrophic subaortic stenosis, pheochromocytoma, migraine, angina pectoris, myocardial infarction, hypertension	Same as acebutolol	Dysrhythmias: 10–30 mg PO tid, qid; hypertension: 40–640 mg/d PO in divided doses; angina: 10–320 mg/d PO in divided doses; aortic stenosis: 20–40 mg/d PO in divided doses; pheochromocytoma: preoperatively 60 mg/d PO in divided doses and inoperable tumor 30 mg/d PO in divided doses; life-threatening dysrhythmias: up to 1 mg/min IV; migraine: 160–240 mg/d PO in divided doses
timolol maleate	Blocadren	Hypertension, myocardial infarction	Same as acebutolol (systemic use)	Hypertension: 20–60 mg/d PO in divided doses; myocardial infarction: 10 mg PO bid
timolol (ophthalmic)	Timoptic	Glaucoma	Ocular irritation, headache, dizziness, bradycardia	1–2 drops daily
ANTIADRENERGIC DRUGS				
CENTRALLY ACTING				
clonidine hydrochloride	Catapres TTS-1	Hypertension	See Summary Drug Table 18-2	See Summary Drug Table 18-2
methyldopa	Aldomet	Hypertension	See Summary Drug Table 18-2	See Summary Drug Table 18-2

(continued)

SUMMARY DRUG TABLE 7–1
(continued)

GENERIC NAME	TRADE NAME*	USES	ADVERSE REACTIONS	DOSE RANGES
BETA-ADRENERGIC BLOCKING DRUGS				
PERIPHERALLY ACTING				
guanethidine monosulfate	Ismelin	Hypertension	See Summary Drug Table 18-2	See Summary Drug Table 18-2
ALPHA/BETA-ADRENERGIC BLOCKING AGENTS				
labetolol hydrochloride	Normodyne	Hypertension	See Summary Drug Table 18-2	See Summary Drug Table 18-2

* The term generic *indicates that the drug is available in a generic form.*

bronchospasm (especially in those with a history of asthma), hyperglycemia, nausea, vomiting, and diarrhea. Many of these reactions are mild and may disappear with therapy.

Examples of adverse reactions associated with the use of beta-adrenergic ophthalmic preparations include headache, depression, cardiac dysrhythmias, and bronchospasm.

Antiadrenergic Agents

Some of the adverse reactions associated with administration of a centrally acting antiadrenergic agent include dry mouth, drowsiness, sedation, anorexia, rash, malaise, and weakness. Adverse reactions associated with the administration of the peripherally acting antiadrenergic agents include hypotension, weakness, lightheadedness, and bradycardia.

In some instances, the adverse reaction of an adrenergic blocking agent may be severe and the physician will stop the drug and prescribe a different one.

Alpha/Beta-Adrenergic Blocking Agents

Most adverse effects of labetalol are mild and do not require discontinuation of therapy. Examples of the adverse reactions are fatigue, headache, diarrhea, dyspnea, and skin rash.

▶ NURSING PROCESS
THE PATIENT RECEIVING AN ADRENERGIC BLOCKING AGENT

ASSESSMENT

As with most drugs, assessment depends on the drug, the patient, and the reason for administration. It is important to establish an accurate data base *before* any adrenergic blocking agent is administered for the first time. If, for example, the patient has a peripheral vascular disease, it is important to note the subjective and objective symptoms of the disorder during the initial assessment. Once drug therapy is started, evaluation of the effects of therapy can be made by comparing the patient's present symptoms with the symptoms experienced before therapy was initiated.

Patients with hypertension must have their blood pressure and pulse taken on both arms in sitting, standing, and lying down positions before therapy is begun. If the patient has a cardiac dysrhythmia, the initial assessment includes taking the pulse rate, determining the pulse rhythm, and noting the patient's general appearance. Subjective data (ie, the patient's complaints or description of symptoms) are also obtained at this time. The physician usually orders an electrocardiogram. Additional diagnostic studies and laboratory tests may also be ordered.

NURSING DIAGNOSIS

Depending on the drug, dose, and reason for administration, one or more of the following nursing diagnoses may apply to a person receiving an adrenergic blocking drug:

▶ Anxiety related to symptoms of disorder, diagnosis, other factors (specify)

▶ Diarrhea related to adverse drug reaction

▶ High risk for injury related to vertigo secondary to orthostatic hypotension

▶ Noncompliance related to negative side effects of drug therapy, anxiety, other factors (specify)

► Potential altered health maintenance related to inability to comprehend drug regimen

► Knowledge deficit of treatment regimen

PLANNING AND IMPLEMENTATION

The major goals of the patient depend on the reason for administration of an adrenergic blocking agent but may include an optimal response to drug therapy, a reduction in anxiety, absence of adverse drug reactions, absence of injury, and an understanding of and compliance to the prescribed treatment regimen.

The major goals of nursing management are to observe the patient for the results of drug therapy, to detect adverse drugs reactions, to reduce patient anxiety, and to develop and implement an effective teaching plan.

OBSERVATIONS AND NURSING MANAGEMENT.
Assessment and evaluation are planned, are carried out continuously during drug therapy, and are primarily based on the disease or condition treated, as discussed later. Some patients may experience one or more adverse drug reactions. As with any drug, adverse reactions are reported to the physician and recorded on the patient's chart. The nurse must use judgment in this matter because some adverse reactions are serious or potentially serious in nature; therefore, the next dose of the drug should be withheld and the physician should be contacted immediately. Some adverse reactions pose no serious threat to the patient's well-being. Less serious adverse reactions, such as dry mouth or mild constipation, are reported to the physician but may have to be tolerated by the patient. In some instances, these less serious reactions disappear or lessen in intensity after a time. The nurse should also remember that even minor adverse drug reactions can be distressing to the patient, especially when the reactions persist for a long time.

Whenever possible, the nurse should try to relieve minor adverse reactions with simple nursing measures. For example, a dry mouth can often be relieved by giving frequent sips of water or allowing a piece of hard candy to dissolve in the mouth (provided that the patient is not a diabetic or on a special diet that limits sugar intake). Constipation can often be relieved by increasing the fluid intake, unless extra fluids are contraindicated. The physician may also order a laxative or stool softener. A record of bowel elimination is maintained daily.

THE PATIENT WITH HYPERTENSION. During therapy with an adrenergic blocking agent for hypertension, the blood pressure must be taken before each dose is given. Some patients have an unusual response to the drugs, and some drugs may, in some individuals, decrease the blood pressure at a more rapid rate than other drugs. If there is a significant decrease in the blood pressure since the last dose was given, the drug should be withheld and the physician should be notified immediately. If there is a significant rise in the blood pressure, the drug is given but the physician is still notified immediately because additional drug therapy may be necessary.

It is good practice to monitor the blood pressure on both arms and in the sitting, standing, and lying down positions for the first week or more of therapy. Once the patient's blood pressure has stabilized, the blood pressure can be taken before each drug administration using the *same* arm and position for each reading. A notation should be made on the Kardex about the position and arm used for blood pressure determinations.

THE PATIENT WITH A CARDIAC DYSRHYTHMIA. Some adrenergic blocking agents are used to treat cardiac dysrhythmias. Ongoing assessment and nursing management of these patients depend on the type of dysrhythmia and the method of treatment. Some dysrhythmias, such as ventricular fibrillation, are life-threatening and require immediate attention. Other dysrhythmias are serious and require treatment but are not immediately life-threatening.

The patient with a life-threatening dysrhythmia may receive an adrenergic blocking drug such as propranolol by the intravenous route. When these drugs are given intravenously, cardiac monitoring is necessary. Patients not in a specialized unit, such as a coronary care unit, are usually transferred to one as soon as possible. Administering these drugs for a life-threatening dysrhythmia requires constant patient supervision, frequent monitoring of the blood pressure and respiratory rate, and cardiac monitoring. The nurse needs to be in frequent communication with the physician about the patient's response to the drug. When propranolol is given orally for a less serious cardiac dysrhythmia, cardiac monitoring is usually not necessary. The blood pressure and pulse rate and rhythm are monitored at varying intervals depending on the length of treatment and the patient's response to the drug. If propranolol is given for angina, the patient is asked about the relief of symptoms and responses are recorded on the patient's chart. If the angina worsens or does not appear to be controlled by the drug, the physician is contacted immediately.

THE PATIENT WITH GLAUCOMA. The patient with glaucoma who is using a beta-adrenergic blocking ophthalmic preparation, such as timolol, requires periodic follow-up examination by the ophthalmologist. At the time of the examination, the intraocular pressure is obtained to determine the effectiveness of drug therapy.

ANXIETY. Some patients may experience anxiety because of their diagnosis, treatment regimen, or the appearance of adverse drug reactions. The treatment regimen is thoroughly explained to the patient and the patient is informed of possible adverse drug reactions. It should also be explained that most drug reactions are mild, transient in nature, and may disappear in time.

ADVERSE REACTIONS. The patient is continually observed for the appearance of adverse drug reactions. All drug reactions are reported to the physician and recorded in the patient's record or chart. Whereas some adverse reactions are mild, others such as diarrhea may cause a problem especially if the patient is elderly or debilitated.

HIGH RISK FOR INJURY. On occasion, patients receiving an adrenergic blocking agent may experience orthostatic or postural hypotension. Postural hypotension is characterized by a feeling of lightheadedness and dizziness when *suddenly* changing from a lying to a sitting or standing position or from a sitting to a standing position. Orthostatic hypotension is characterized by principally the same symptoms as postural hypotension when the patient changes or shifts position after standing in one place for a long period. These adverse reactions can be minimized as follows:

1. Patients are instructed to rise slowly from a sitting or lying position.
2. When symptoms of postural hypotension are severe, a patient must receive assistance when getting out of a bed or a chair. The call light should be placed nearby and these patients should be instructed to ask for assistance each time they get in and out of a bed or a chair.
3. If a patient is experiencing postural hypotension, symptoms can be minimized by assisting the bed patient to a sitting position and having the patient sit on the edge of the bed for about 1 minute before standing. Patients sitting in a chair should be helped to a standing position and instructed to stand in one place for about 1 minute before ambulating. The nurse must remain with the patient while he or she is standing in one place, as well as during ambulation.
4. The patient experiencing orthostatic hypotension should be instructed to avoid standing in one place for prolonged periods. This is rarely a problem in the hospital, but should be included in the patient and family teaching plan.

Often, symptoms of postural or orthostatic hypotension lessen with time, and the patient may be allowed to get out of a bed or chair slowly without assistance. The nurse must always exercise good judgment in this matter and allow the patient to rise from a lying or sitting position without help only when it has been determined that the symptoms have lessened and ambulation poses no danger of falling.

NONCOMPLIANCE AND ALTERED HEALTH MAINTENANCE. Some patients do not adhere to the prescribed drug regimen for a variety of reasons such as failure to comprehend the prescribed regimen, cost of drug therapy, and failure to understand the importance of continued and uninterrupted therapy. If the nurse detects failure to adhere to the prescribed drug regimen, it becomes necessary to investigate the possible cause of the problem. In some instances, financial aid may be necessary; in other instances, patients need to know *why* they are taking a drug and *why* therapy must be continuous to attain and maintain an optimal state of health and well-being.

KNOWLEDGE DEFICIT. The drug regimen and the importance of continued and uninterrupted therapy are stressed when teaching the patient who is prescribed an adrenergic blocking drug.

THE PATIENT WITH HYPERTENSION, CARDIAC DYSRHYTHMIA, OR ANGINA. If a beta-adrenergic blocking drug has been prescribed for hypertension, cardiac dysrhythmia, angina, or other cardiac disorders, the patient must have a full understanding of the treatment regimen. In some instances, the physician may advise the hypertensive patient to lose weight or eat a special diet such as a diet low in salt. A special diet may also be recommended for the patient with angina or a cardiac dysrhythmia. When appropriate, the importance of diet and weight loss in the therapy of hypertension or a special diet for other disorders is stressed. The following are additional points that should be included in the teaching plan for the patient with hypertension, angina, or a cardiac dysrhythmia:

▶ Do not not stop abruptly except on the advice of a physician.
▶ Notify the physician promptly if adverse drug reactions occur.
▶ Observe caution while driving or performing other hazardous tasks because these drugs (beta-adrenergic blocking agents) may cause drowsiness, dizziness, or lightheadedness.
▶ Do not use any nonprescription drug unless use of a specific drug has been approved by the physician.

► Inform dentists and other physicians of therapy with this drug.
► Keep all physician appointments, because close monitoring of therapy is essential.
► Check with a physician or pharmacist to determine if the drug is to be taken with food or on a empty stomach.

When an adrenergic blocking drug is prescribed for hypertension, the physician may want the patients to monitor their blood pressure between office visits. If this is recommended, the patient and a family member are taught how to take a blood pressure reading. It is also advisable to supervise the patient and a family member during several trial blood pressure readings to ensure accuracy of their measurements. It should also be suggested that the same arm and body position be used each time the blood pressure is taken. Patients should also understand that the blood pressure can vary slightly with emotion, the time of day, the position of the body, and so on. A slight change in readings is normal, but if a drastic change in either or both the systolic or diastolic readings occurs, the physician should be contacted as soon as possible.

THE PATIENT WITH GLAUCOMA. The technique of eye drop instillation is demonstrated, and the prescribed treatment regimen is explained to the patient. The importance of adhering to the instillation schedule is stressed because omitting or discontinuing the drug without approval of the physician may result in a marked increase in intraocular pressure, which can lead to blindness.

EVALUATION

► Anxiety is reduced
► Adverse reactions are identified and reported to the physician
► No evidence of injury
► Patient complies to the prescribed drug regimen
► Patient and family demonstrate understanding of drug regimen

8

Cholinergic Drugs

On completion of this chapter the student will:

▶ *Discuss the uses and drug actions of the cholinergic drugs*

▶ *List some of the adverse reactions associated with the administration of cholinergic drugs*

▶ *Use the nursing process when administering a cholinergic drug*

▶ *Discuss the nursing implications to be considered when administering cholinergic drugs*

Cholinergic drugs mimic the activity of the parasympathetic nervous system. They are also called *parasympathomimetic drugs.*

The parasympathetic nervous system is a part of the autonomic nervous system; it helps conserve body energy. It is partly responsible for activities such as slowing the heart rate, digesting food, and eliminating body wastes.

Electron microscopic study reveals an incalculably small space between nerve endings and the effector organ (eg, the muscle, cell, or gland) that is innervated (or controlled) by a nerve fiber. For a nerve impulse to be transmitted from the nerve ending (motor end plate) across the space to the effector organ, a neurohormone is needed.

There are two neurohormones (neurotransmitters) of the parasympathetic nervous system: **acetylcholine** (ACh) and **acetylcholinesterase** (AChE). These two neurohormones are released at nerve endings of parasympathetic nerve fibers, at some nerve endings in the sympathetic nervous system, and at nerve endings of skeletal muscles. These parasympathetic neurohormones are believed to be manufac-

tured by special cells located in the nerve ending. When a parasympathetic nerve fiber is stimulated, the nerve fiber releases acetylcholine, and the nerve impulses pass (travel) from the nerve fiber to the effector organ or structure. After the impulse has crossed over to the effector organ or structure, acetylcholine is inactivated (destroyed) by the neurohormone acetylcholinesterase. When the next nerve impulse is ready to travel along the nerve fiber, acetylcholine is again released and then inactivated by acetylcholinesterase.

▷ Actions of Cholinergic Drugs

Cholinergic drugs may act like the neurohormone acetylcholine, or they may inhibit the release of the neurohormone acetylcholinesterase. Cholinergic drugs that act like acetylcholine are called *direct-acting* cholinergics. If a cholinergic drug inhibits the body's release of acetylcholinesterase, it prolongs the activity of the acetylcholine produced by the body. Cholinergic drugs that prolong the activity of acetylcholine by inhibiting the release of acetylcholinesterase are called *indirect-acting* cholinergics. Although a specific cholinergic drug may act in either of these two ways, the results of drug action are basically the same.

▷ Uses of Cholinergic Drugs

Cholinergic drugs have limited usefulness in medicine, in part because of the adverse reactions that may occur during administration. In some diseases or conditions, however, cholinergic drugs either are definitely indicated or may be of value.

Myasthenia gravis is a disease that involves rapid fatigue of skeletal muscles due to the lack of acetylcholine released at the nerve endings of parasympathetic nerve fibers; it responds to the administration of a cholinergic agent. Drugs used in the treatment of this disorder include ambenonium (Mytelase) and pyridostigmine (Mestinon).

Glaucoma, a disorder of the eye, may be treated by topical application (eg, eye drops) of a cholinergic agent such as carbachol or pilocarpine (Isopto-Carpine). Treatment of glaucoma with a cholinergic agent produces miosis or constriction of the iris, which then opens the blocked channels and allows the normal passage of fluid between the anterior and posterior chamber, thus reducing intraocular pressure.

Urinary retention may be treated with bethanechol chloride (Urecholine), provided the retention is not caused by a mechanical obstruction such as a stone in the bladder or an enlarged prostate. The parasympathetic nervous system partly controls the process of micturition (voiding of urine), which is both a voluntary and involuntary act, by constricting the detrusor muscle and relaxing the bladder sphincter (see Table 6-1 in chap 6). Administration of this drug may result in the spontaneous passage of urine.

▷ Adverse Reactions Associated with the Administration of Cholinergic Drugs

Unless applied topically, as in the treatment of glaucoma, cholinergic agents are not selective in action. Therefore, they may affect many organs and structures of the body, causing a variety of adverse effects.

Oral or parenteral administration can result in nausea, diarrhea, abdominal cramping, salivation, flushing of the skin, cardiac dysrhythmias, and muscle weakness. Topical administration usually produces few adverse effects, but a temporary reduction of visual acuity (sharpness) and headache may occur. Summary Drug Table 8-1 lists the adverse reactions that may be seen with specific cholinergic drugs.

▶ NURSING PROCESS
THE PATIENT RECEIVING A CHOLINERGIC DRUG

ASSESSMENT

Assessment depends on the drug and the reason for administration.

THE PATIENT WITH GLAUCOMA. Before therapy for glaucoma is started, the physician thoroughly examines the eye. The nurse is responsible for reviewing the physician's diagnosis and comments, for taking a general patient health history, and for evaluating the patient's ability to carry out the activities of daily living, especially if the patient is elderly or has limited vision.

THE PATIENT WITH MYASTHENIA GRAVIS. When a cholinergic drug is given to a patient with myasthenia gravis, the patient has a complete neurologic assessment before the therapy is begun. This assessment usually is performed by the physician but the nurse must document any problems (any increase in the symptoms of the disease or adverse drug reactions) before giving each dose of the drug.

When performing an initial assessment, the nurse looks for signs of muscle weakness such as drooling (ie, the lack of ability to swallow); inability to chew and swallow; drooping of the eyelids; inability to perform repetitive movements, such as walking, combing hair, using eating utensils; difficulty breathing; and extreme fatigue.

THE PATIENT WITH URINARY RETENTION. If a patient receives a cholinergic drug for the treatment of urinary retention, assessment includes palpating the bladder to determine its size and taking the blood pressure and pulse rate.

NURSING DIAGNOSIS

Depending on the drug, dose, and reason for administration, one or more of the following nursing diagnoses may apply to a person receiving a cholinergic drug:

SUMMARY DRUG TABLE 8–1
Cholinergic Drugs

GENERIC NAME	TRADE NAME*	USES	ADVERSE REACTIONS	DOSE RANGES
ambenonium	Mytelase	Myasthenia gravis	Increased bronchial secretions, cardiac dysrhythmias, muscle weakness	5–75 mg PO tid, qid
bethanecol chloride	Urecholine, *generic*	Acute nonobstructive urinary retention, neurogenic atony of urinary bladder with retention	Usually due to overdosage or pharmacologic drug activity	10–50 mg PO bid to qid; 2.5–5 mg SC
carbachol, topical	Isopto Carbachol	Glaucoma	Temperary reduction of visual acuity, headache	1–2 drops in eye up to 4 times/d
pilocarpine hydrochloride	Isopto Carpine, Pilocar, *generic*	Glaucoma	Same as carbachol	1 drop in eye 1–6 times/d
pilocarpine ocular therapeutic system	Ocusert Pilo-20, Ocusert Pilo-40	Elevated intraocular pressure	Same as carbachol	1 unit placed in the conjunctival sac, replaced as directed by the physician (usually every 7 d)
neostigmine methylsulfate	Prostigmin, *generic*	Prevention of postoperative distention and urinary retention	Cardiac dysrhythmias, vomiting, bowel cramps, increased peristalsis, urinary frequency, flushing, weakness, diaphoresis, nausea, diarrhea	Prevention of postoperative distention, urinary retention: 1 mL of 1 : 4000 solution (0.25 mg) SC, IM; treatment of urinary retention: 1 mL 1 : 2000 solution (0.5 mg) SC, IM
pyridostigmine bromide	Mestinon	Myasthenia gravis	Same as ambenonium	Average dose is 600 mg/d PO at spaced intervals, with doses as low as 60 mg/d and as high as 1500 mg/d

* The term generic *indicates that the drug is available in a generic form.*

▶ Diarrhea related to adverse drug reaction

▶ Pain (abdominal) related to drug action on cholinergic nerve fibers of the intestines

▶ High risk for injury related to the effects of an ophthalmic medication

▶ Noncompliance related to indifference, lack of knowledge, other factors

▶ Potential altered health maintenance related to inability to comprehend drug regimen, inability to handle the prescribed drug regimen

▶ Knowledge deficit of medication regimen, adverse drug effects, treatment modalities

PLANNING AND IMPLEMENTATION

The major goals of the patient may include an absence of adverse drug effects and an understanding of and compliance to the prescribed treatment regimen.

The major goals of nursing management may include identification of adverse drug effects, competent assessment of the results of drug therapy, and the development and implementation of an effective teaching plan.

THE PATIENT WITH GLAUCOMA. When instilling any ophthalmic preparation, the physician's order and the drug label are checked carefully. It is most important that the drug label indicates that the preparation is for *ophthalmic* use. In addition, the name of the drug and the drug dosage or strength as stated on the label are carefully checked against the physician's orders. The drug is instilled in the lower conjunctival sac unless the physician orders a different method of instillation. The hand holding the eyedropper is supported against the patient's forehead. The tip of the dropper must never touch the eye.

In some instances, the patient may have been using an ophthalmic preparation for glaucoma for a long time, and the physician may allow the hospitalized patient to instill his or her own eye drops. When this is so stated on the patient's order sheet, the medication can be left at the patient's bedside. Even though the drug is self-administered, the patient is checked at intervals to be sure that the medication is instilled at the prescribed time using the correct technique for ophthalmic instillation.

If the pilocarpine ocular system is prescribed for the hospitalized patient, the nurse must check the cheek and eye area several times a day because the system can become displaced from the eye. Most patients are usually aware of displacement of the system, but some patients, the elderly in particular, may not realize that the system has come out of the eye. If displacement does occur, a new system is inserted and the physician is informed of the problem. On occasion, patients cannot insert the system by themselves or cannot retain the system in the eye for the required time. When this occurs, the physician must be notified because it is important that the ocular system remain in place until it is time for it to be changed.

The pilocarpine ocular system is changed every 7 days unless the physician orders otherwise. When this system is used to treat glaucoma, the eye and the area around the eye are checked daily for evidence of redness, inflammation, and excessive secretions. If secretions are present around the eye, they may be removed with a cotton ball or gauze soaked in normal saline or other cleansing solution recommended by the physician. The physician is contacted if the symptoms of glaucoma increase, if the patient is unable to retain the ocular system, or if redness, eye irritation, or excessive secretions are noted.

THE PATIENT WITH MYASTHENIA GRAVIS. In the beginning, it is often difficult to determine the dosage that will control symptoms. In many cases, the dosage must be adjusted upward or downward until optimal drug effects are obtained. Because of this, the patient is observed closely for symptoms of drug overdosage or underdosage. Signs of drug overdosage include muscle rigidity and spasm, salivation, and clenching of the jaw. Signs of drug underdosage are signs of the disease itself, namely, rapid fatigability of the muscles, drooping of the eyelids, and difficulty breathing. If symptoms of drug overdosage or underdosage develop, the physician is contacted immediately because a change in dosage is usually necessary. In the case of overdosage, an antidote, such as atropine, and other treatment may also be necessary.

Assessing the patient for the presence or absence of the symptoms of myasthenia gravis is carried out before each drug dose. In patients with severe myasthenia gravis, these assessments may be carried out between drug doses, as well as immediately before drug administration. It is important to document each symptom, as well as the patient's response or lack or response to drug therapy.

Assessment of the patient is important, because the dosage often has to be frequently increased or decreased early in therapy depending on the patient's response. Regulation of dosage is important in keeping the symptoms of myasthenia gravis from incapacitating the patient. Although this is not always possible for all patients, the symptoms of many patients are fairly well-controlled with drug therapy once the optimal drug dose is determined.

THE PATIENT WITH URINARY RETENTION. After subcutaneous drug administration, voiding may occur in 5 to 15 minutes, and after oral administration, it may occur in 30 to 90 minutes. The call light should be placed within easy reach and the urinal or bedpan should be nearby. If the patient is able to get these aids from the bedside stand or chair, it is important that they be obtained easily and safely. Some patients may not be able to reach or handle these aids easily and thus may require prompt answering of their call light. Intake and output are measured and recorded, and the physician is notified if the patient fails to void after drug administration.

If a cholinergic drug is ordered for the prevention of urinary retention, intake and output are measured and recorded. If the amount of each voiding is insufficient or the patient fails to void, the bladder is palpated to determine its size and the physician is notified.

ADVERSE DRUG EFFECTS. When a cholinergic drug is given by the oral or parenteral route, adverse drug effects may be related to many systems of the body such as the heart, respiratory and gastrointestinal tracts, and the central nervous system. The patient must be closely observed for the appearance of adverse drug effects, a change in vital signs, or an increase in symptoms. Any complaints the patient may have are documented and reported to the physician as soon as possible.

HIGH RISK FOR INJURY. Because drug-induced myopia (nearsightedness) may occur after instillation of a cholinergic ophthalmic drug for the treatment of glaucoma, the patient may require assistance in getting out of bed or ambulating. Night vision may also be decreased so the patient's room should be dimly lit at night. Obstacles such as slippers, chairs, and tables may hinder ambulation or result in falls; they should be placed out of the way, especially during the night. The patient's eyes are checked daily for signs of redness, irritation, or excessive secretions. The physician is notified if these occur or if the patient experiences an increase in the severity of the symptoms of glaucoma.

NONCOMPLIANCE AND ALTERED HEALTH MAINTENANCE. Patients required to take a drug over a long period may incur lapses in their medication schedule.

For some, it is a matter of occasionally forgetting to take a medication, but for others it may be due to other factors such as a failure to understand the importance of drug therapy, inability to instill an eye medication (when the drug is prescribed for glaucoma), cost of the drug, or being unfamiliar with the consequences associated with discontinuing the drug therapy.

When developing a teaching plan for the patient and family, it is most essential that the importance of uninterrupted drug therapy be emphasized. The patient and family should be allowed time to ask questions. Any problems that appear to be associated with the prescribed drug regimen should be explored in depth and then reported to the physician.

KNOWLEDGE DEFICIT. The purpose of the drug therapy as well as the adverse effects that may be seen are reviewed with the patient and family.

THE PATIENT WITH GLAUCOMA. When a cholinergic drug is prescribed for glaucoma, the patient and a family member require instruction in instillation of the eye drops. If a family member is to instill the drug, time must be allowed for instruction as well as practice of the procedure under supervision of a nurse. The patient is warned that the eye drops may sting when instilled into the eye and that this is a normal, but temporary, discomfort that often disappears after a short time. The patient is also advised to observe caution while driving or performing any task that requires visual acuity.

The following points may be included in the teaching plan for a patient using a liquid eye medication:

▶ Keep the bottle tightly closed.
▶ Do not wash the tip of the dropper.
▶ Do not lay the dropper on a table or other surface.
▶ Place the dropper back in the bottle immediately after use.
▶ Tilt the head back and instill the prescribed number of drops in the inner lower eyelid (lower conjunctival sac).
▶ Apply light finger pressure to the inner corner of the eye (lacrimal sac) for about 1 minute after instillation (teaching the use of this maneuver should be approved by the physician).
▶ If unable to instill eye drops, contact the physician immediately.

If the patient is prescribed the pilocarpine ocular system, the physician or nurse must evaluate the patient's ability to insert and remove the system. A package insert is provided with the system and is reviewed with the patient. The patient is also instructed to remove and replace the system every 7 days or as instructed by the physician. Replacement is best done at bedtime (unless the physician orders otherwise) because there is some impairment of vision for a short time after insertion. The patient must also check for placement of the unit before retiring at night and in the morning on arising. The physician is to be notified if eye secretions are excessive or irritation occurs.

THE PATIENT WITH MYASTHENIA GRAVIS. Many patients with myasthenia gravis learn to adjust their drug dosage according to their needs, since dosages may vary slightly from day to day. The patient and family members must be taught to recognize symptoms of overdosage and underdosage, as well as what steps the physician wishes them to take if either occurs. The dosage regimen and how to adjust the dosage upward or downward is explained. The patient should be given a written or printed description of the signs and symptoms of drug overdosage or underdosage. The patient is instructed to keep a record of the response to drug therapy (eg, time of day increased or decreased muscle strength or fatigue is noted) and to bring this to each physician or clinic visit until such time as symptoms are well-controlled and the drug dosage is stabilized. These patients should wear or carry identification (such as Medic-Alert) indicating that they have myasthenia gravis.

EVALUATION

▶ Adverse reactions are identified and reported to the physician
▶ No evidence of injury
▶ Verbalizes importance of complying with the prescribed treatment regimen
▶ Patient complies to the prescribed drug regimen
▶ Patient and family demonstrate understanding of drug regimen

9

Cholinergic Blocking Drugs

On completion of this chapter the student will:

▶ *Discuss the uses and general drug actions of the cholinergic blocking drugs*

▶ *List some of the adverse reactions seen with the administration of cholinergic blocking drugs*

▶ *Use the nursing process when administering a cholinergic blocking drug*

▶ *Discuss the nursing implications to be considered when administering a cholinergic blocking drug*

Cholinergic blocking drugs are also called *anticholinergics* or *parasympathomimetic blocking* drugs. Like adrenergic blocking agents, this group of drugs has an effect on the autonomic nervous system. Cholinergic blocking drugs may be derived from natural sources (eg, plants), for example, atropine and scopolamine, but most drugs in this group are produced synthetically.

▷ Actions of Cholinergic Blocking Drugs

Cholinergic blocking drugs *inhibit* the activity of acetylcholine (ACh; see chap 8) in parasympathetic nerve fibers. When the activity of acetylcholine is inhibited, nerve impulses traveling along parasym-

pathetic nerve fibers cannot pass from the nerve fiber to the effector organ or structure. These drugs are also capable of reversing the action of cholinergic drugs.

Because of the wide distribution of parasympathetic nerves, these drugs affect many organs and structures of the body including the eyes, respiratory and gastrointestinal tracts, the heart, and the bladder (see Table 6-1 in chap 6). Cholinergic blocking agents produce the following responses:

Central nervous system (CNS)—dreamless sleep, drowsiness, atropine may produce mild stimulation in some patients

Eye—dilatation of the pupil (mydriasis), cycloplegia (paralysis of accommodation or inability to focus the eye)

Respiratory tract—drying of the secretions of the

mouth, nose, throat, bronchi, relaxation of smooth muscles of the bronchi resulting in slight bronchodilatation

Gastrointestinal tract—decrease in secretions of the stomach, decrease in gastric and intestinal movement (motility)

Cardiovascular system—increase in pulse rate (most pronounced with atropine administration)

Urinary tract—Dilatation of smooth muscles of the ureters and kidney pelvis, contraction of the detrusor muscle of the bladder

These responses to administration of a cholinergic drug may vary and often depend on the drug as well as the dose used. Occasionally, scopolamine may cause excitement, delirium, and restlessness, which is thought to be a drug idiosyncrasy.

The synthetic cholinergic blocking drugs generally produce the same response as the natural agents. However, the intensity of their effect on one or more body systems is often less than those produced by the natural agents.

▷ Uses of Cholinergic Blocking Drugs

Because of their widespread effect on many organs and structures of the body, cholinergic blocking drugs have a variety of uses. For example, some of the uses of atropine include treatment of pylorospasm, peptic ulcer, ureteral and biliary colic, vagal-induced bradycardia, parkinsonism, and preoperatively to reduce secretions of the upper respiratory tract before the administration of a general anesthetic. Other cholinergic blocking agents have a more selective action, that is, they affect principally one structure of the body. An example of this type of drug is clidinium (Quarzan), which is used only in the treatment of peptic ulcer. Summary Drug Table 9-1 lists the uses of specific cholinergic blocking drugs.

▷ Adverse Reactions Associated with the Administration of Cholinergic Blocking Drugs

Dryness of the mouth with difficulty in swallowing, blurred vision, and an aversion to bright light (photophobia) may be seen with the administration of a cholinergic blocking agent. The severity of many adverse reactions is often dose dependent, that is,

the larger the dose, the more intense the adverse reaction. Even in normal doses, some degree of dryness of the mouth almost always occurs.

Constipation, which is due to a decrease in intestinal motility, may occur in those taking one of these drugs on a regular basis, for example, the patient under treatment for a peptic ulcer. Drowsiness may occur with the use of these drugs, but there are times when this adverse reaction is desirable, as when atropine is used as a preoperative medication to reduce the production of secretions in the respiratory tract.

Other adverse reactions that may be seen with the administration of a cholinergic blocking agent include the following:

CNS—headache, flushing, nervousness, drowsiness, weakness, insomnia, nasal congestion, fever

Eye—blurred vision, mydriasis, photophobia, cycloplegia, increased ocular tension

Gastrointestinal tract—nausea, vomiting, difficulty in swallowing, heartburn

Urinary tract—urinary hesitancy and retention, dysuria

Cardiovascular system—palpitations, bradycardia (following low doses of atropine), tachycardia (after higher doses of atropine)

Other—urticaria, anaphylaxis, other skin manifestations

When these drugs are given to elderly patients, confusion or excitement may be seen even with small doses. Those receiving a cholinergic blocking agent during the hot summer months should be observed for signs of heat prostration (fever, tachycardia, flushing, warm dry skin, mental confusion) because these drugs decrease sweating.

Administration of these drugs can result in urinary retention. Patients with an enlarged prostate are given these drugs with great caution because urinary retention may occur. This caution applies to some over-the-counter (OTC) preparations available for the relief of allergy and cold symptoms and as aids to induce sleep in those who have difficulty falling asleep. Some of these products contain atropine, scopolamine, or other cholinergic blocking agents, and although this warning is given on the container or package, many users fail to read the fine print on drug labels.

Cholinergic blocking agents are also contraindicated in those with glaucoma because use of these drugs may lead to an attack of acute glaucoma. Unfortunately, glaucoma in its early stages may have few, if any, symptoms and the individual is unaware of this disorder until he or she has an eye

SUMMARY DRUG TABLE 9–1
Cholinergic Blocking Drugs

GENERIC NAME	TRADE NAME*	USES	ADVERSE REACTIONS	DOSE RANGES
anisotropine methylbromide	Valpin 50, *generic*	Peptic ulcer	Urinary hesitancy or urgency, blurred vision, dry mouth, nausea, vomiting, palpitation, headache, flushing, drowsiness	50 mg PO tid
atropine sulfate	*Generic*	Pylorospasm, reduction of bronchial and oral secretions, excessive vagal-induced bradycardia, ureteral and biliary colic	Same as anisotropine	0.4–0.6 mg PO; 0.4–1 mg IM, SC, IV
belladonna tincture	*Generic*	Adjunctive therapy for peptic ulcer, digestive disorders, diverticulitis, pancreatitis, diarrhea	Same as anisotropine	0.6–1 mL PO tid, qid
clidinium bromide	Quarzan	Peptic ulcer	Same as anisotropine	2.5–5 mg PO tid, qid ac and hs
glycopyrrolate	Robinul, *generic*	Oral: peptic ulcer Parenteral: in conjunction with anesthesia to reduce bronchial and oral secretions; to block cardiac vagal inhibitory reflexes during induction of anesthesia and intubation	Same as anisotropine	Oral: 1 mg tid or 2 mg bid, tid; parenteral: peptic ulcer 0.1–0.2 mg IM, IV tid, qid; preanesthesia: 0.002 mg/lb IM; intraoperative: 0.1 mg IV
L-hyoscyamine sulfate	Levsin, Anaspaz, Cystospaz	Peptic ulcer, acute rhinitis, renal colic, cystitis, parkinsonism, preoperatively to reduce bronchial and oral secretions	Same as anisotropine	Oral: 0.125–0.25 mg tid, qid; parenteral: 0.25–0.5 mg SC, IM, IV
propantheline bromide	Pro-Banthine, *generic*	Adjunctive therapy for peptic ulcer	Same as anisotropine	15 mg PO 30 min ac and 30 mg PO hs
scopolamine hydrobromide (hyoscine hydrobromide)	*Generic*	Preanesthetic sedation	Same as anisotropine	0.32–0.65 mg SC, IM, and IV when diluted with sterile water for injection

* The term generic *indicates that the drug is available in a generic form.*

examination. The lack of symptoms of early glaucoma plus the fact that many individuals fail to read drug labels can have serious consequences.

▶ NURSING PROCESS
THE PATIENT RECEIVING A CHOLINERGIC BLOCKING AGENT

ASSESSMENT

Before administration of a cholinergic blocking agent for the first time, the nurse obtains a thorough health history as well as a history of the signs and symptoms of the present disorder. The focus of the initial physical assessment depends on the reason for administering the drug. In most instances, the blood pressure, pulse, and respiratory rate are obtained. Additional assessments may include checking the stool of the patient who has a peptic ulcer for color and signs of occult blood, determining visual acuity in the patient with glaucoma, or looking for signs of dehydration and weighing the patient if prolonged diarrhea is one of the patient's symptoms.

NURSING DIAGNOSIS

Depending on the drug, dose, and reason for administration, one or more of the following nursing diagnoses may apply to a person receiving a cholinergic blocking drug:

▶ Anxiety related to diagnosis, drug regimen, other factors (specify)

▶ Altered oral mucous membranes related to drug action on mucous membranes

▶ Noncompliance related to indifference, lack of knowledge, other factors

▶ High risk for injury related to effect of drug

▶ Potential altered health maintenance related to inability to comprehend drug regimen

▶ Knowledge deficit of medication regimen, adverse drug effects, treatment modalities

PLANNING AND IMPLEMENTATION

The major goals of the patient may include maintenance of oral mucous membrane integrity and an understanding of and compliance to the prescribed treatment regimen.

The major goals of nursing management may include identification of adverse drug effects, competent assessment of the results of drug therapy, and the development and implementation of an effective teaching plan.

Daily assessment and observation of the patient receiving a cholinergic blocking agent are necessary and should include checking vital signs, observing for adverse drug reactions, and evaluating the symptoms and complaints related to the patient's diagnosis. For example, the patient with a peptic ulcer is questioned regarding current symptoms, which are then compared to the symptoms present before the start of therapy. Any increase in the severity of symptoms is reported to the physician immediately.

THE PATIENT WITH HEART BLOCK. The patient receiving atropine for third degree heart block should be placed on a cardiac monitor, especially during and after administration of the drug. The monitor is watched for a change in pulse rate. Tachycardia or other cardiac dysrhythmias or failure of the drug to increase the heart rate is reported to the physician immediately because other drugs or medical management may be necessary.

THE PATIENT RECEIVING A PREOPERATIVE MEDICATION. If a cholinergic blocking agent is administered as a preoperative medication, the patient is instructed to void before the drug is given. The patient is told that his or her mouth will become extremely dry, that this is normal, and that fluid is not to be taken. The side rails of the bed are then raised and the patient is told to remain in bed following administration of the preoperative

medication. It is *extremely* important that a preoperative medication is given at the prescribed time because the cholinergic blocking agent must be allowed to produce the greatest effect (ie, the drying of upper respiratory and oral secretions) before the administration of a general anesthetic. If the preoperative medication is given late, the nurse must notify the anesthesiologist.

ADVERSE DRUG REACTIONS. Since this group of drugs may have widespread effects, all patients are closely observed for the appearance of adverse drugs reactions.

The elderly patient receiving a cholinergic blocking agent is observed at frequent intervals for excitement, agitation, mental confusion, drowsiness, urinary retention, or other adverse effects. If any of these should occur, the next dose of the drug is withheld and the physician is contacted. It is also important to ensure patient safety until these adverse reactions disappear. Cholinergic blocking agents are usually not included in the preoperative medication of patients over 60 years of age because of the effects of these agents on the eye and the CNS.

In hot weather, sweating may decrease and may be followed by heat prostration. The patient is observed at frequent intervals for signs of heat prostration (see Adverse Reactions), especially if the patient is elderly or debilitated. The next dose of the drug is withheld and the physician is contacted immediately if heat prostration is suspected.

ANXIETY. Some patients may experience anxiety for reasons such as their diagnosis, impending surgery (when a preoperative cholinergic blocking agent is given as part of the preoperative medication), or necessity for prolonged drug therapy. The nurse can help reduce anxiety by formulating an effective teaching plan, explaining the adverse drug effects that may need to be tolerated, and listening to the concerns of the patient.

ALTERED ORAL MUCOUS MEMBRANES. Dryness of the mouth may be severe and extremely uncomfortable in some patients taking these drugs on a daily basis. The patient may have moderate to extreme difficulty swallowing oral drugs and food. Having the patient take a few sips of water before, as well as while, taking an oral medication and sipping water at intervals during meals may help this problem. If allowed, hard candy slowly dissolved in the mouth and frequent sips of water during the day may help relieve persistent oral dryness. The oral cavity should be checked daily for soreness or ulcerations.

HIGH RISK FOR INJURY. These drugs may cause drowsiness, dizziness, and blurred vision. The patient (especially the elderly) may require assistance with ambulation. For elderly patients, as well as those experiencing visual difficulties, furniture (eg, footstools, chairs, stands) that obstructs ambulatory areas should be placed against the wall. Those with photophobia may be more comfortable in a semidarkened room, especially on sunny days. Overhead lights should be used as little as possible. Mydriasis and cycloplegia, if they occur, may interfere with reading, watching television, and similar activities. If these drug effects upset the patient, this problem is discussed with the physician. At times, the patient will have to tolerate these visual impairments because drug therapy cannot be changed or discontinued. The nurse must attempt to find other forms of diversional therapy such as interaction with other patients, listening to the radio, and so on.

NONCOMPLIANCE AND POTENTIAL ALTERED HEALTH MAINTENANCE. In some instances, a cholinergic blocking agent may be prescribed for a prolonged period. Some patients may discontinue their medication especially if their original symptoms have been relieved. It is most important that the patient and family understand that the prescribed medication is to be taken even though symptoms have been relieved.

KNOWLEDGE DEFICIT. When a cholinergic blocking drug is prescribed for out-patient use, the patient must be made aware of the more common adverse reactions associated with these drugs such as dry mouth, drowsiness, dizziness, and visual impairments. The patient is warned that should drowsiness, dizziness, or blurred vision occur, caution must be observed while driving or performing other tasks requiring alertness and good vision.

At times, some of the adverse reactions associated with the cholinergic blocking agents may be uncomfortable or distressing, and the patient should be encouraged to discuss these problems with the physician. The nurse can also offer suggestions that may lessen the intensity of some of these adverse reactions. Below is a list of adverse reactions that can be included in the teaching plan with the measures that may lessen their intensity or allow the patient to perform tasks at times when these adverse reactions are least likely to occur.

Photophobia—Sunglasses are worn when outside, even on cloudy days; rooms are kept dimly lit; curtains or blinds are closed if there is bright sunlight in the room; soft indirect lighting is usually more comfortable; outdoor activities are scheduled (when necessary) before the first dose of the drug is taken, such as early in the morning.

Dry mouth—Frequent sips of cool water are taken during the day; several sips of water are taken before oral medications; water is sipped frequently during meals; gum may be chewed or hard candy slowly dissolved in the mouth.

Constipation—Plenty of fluids are taken during the day; the individual should exercise; if the physician approves, foods high in fiber are added to the diet.

Heat prostration—Going outside on hot sunny days is avoided; fans are used to cool the body if the day is extremely warm; the skin is sponged with cool water if other cooling measures are not available; loose-fitting clothes are worn in warm weather.

Drowsiness—Tasks requiring alertness are scheduled during times when drowsiness does not occur, such as early in the morning before the first dose of the drug is taken.

THE PATIENT RECEIVING A PREOPERATIVE MEDICATION. When one of these drugs is administered preoperatively, the patient is given an explanation of the preoperative medication, that is, why the drug is being given, when the drug will be given, and when he or she is going to surgery. The patient should be instructed to void before the preoperative medication is administered, and should be given sufficient time to do so. The patient and family members present at this time should be told that drowsiness and extreme dryness of the mouth and nose will occur about 20 to 30 minutes after the drug is given. The importance of remaining in bed after the drug is administered and the use of raised side rails for safety are explained.

THE PATIENT WITH A PEPTIC ULCER. The patient with a peptic ulcer must have a full explanation of the treatment regimen, which may include drugs as well as a special diet. The drug must be taken exactly as prescribed by the physician (eg, 30 minutes before meals or between meals) to obtain the desired results. The patient must receive a full explanation of the special diet (when ordered) and the importance of diet in the treatment of peptic ulcer is stressed.

THE ELDERLY PATIENT. The family of an elderly patient should be advised of possible visual and mental impairments (blurred vision, confusion, agitation) that may occur during therapy with these drugs. Objects or situations that may cause falls such as throw rugs, footstools, and wet or newly waxed floors should be removed or avoided whenever possible. The family must also be warned of the dangers of heat prostration and what steps can be taken to avoid this problem. The patient should also be watched closely during the first few days of therapy, and the physician should be notified if mental changes occur.

EVALUATION

▶ Anxiety is reduced

▶ Oral mucous membranes appear normal

▶ Patient complies to the prescribed drug regimen

▶ No evidence of injury

▶ Patient and family demonstrate understanding of drug regimen

▶ Verbalizes importance of complying with the prescribed treatment regimen

10

The Narcotic Analgesics and the Narcotic Antagonists

On completion of this chapter the student will:

▶ Discuss the general drug action of the narcotic analgesics and the narcotic antagonists

▶ Describe the effects of a narcotic on organs and structures of the body

▶ List the major adverse reactions associated with the administration of a narcotic analgesic

▶ List the uses of the narcotic analgesics and narcotic antagonists

▶ Describe the major adverse reactions associated with the administration of a narcotic analgesic

▶ Use the nursing process when administering a narcotic or narcotic antagonist

▶ List and discuss the nursing activities that are performed before and after a narcotic analgesic is administered

▶ THE NARCOTIC ANALGESICS

The narcotic analgesics are divided into two classes: (1) the narcotic analgesics obtained from raw opium and (2) the synthetic narcotic analgesics.

The narcotics obtained from raw opium (also called the opiates, opioids, or opiate narcotics) include morphine, codeine, hydrochlorides of opium alkaloids (Pantopon), and camphorated tincture of opium (paregoric). Morphine, once extracted from raw opium and treated chemically, yields hydromorphone (Dilaudid), oxymorphone (Numorphan), and heroin. Heroin is an illegal narcotic in the United States and is not used in medicine.

Examples of synthetic narcotic analgesics are butorphanol (Stadol), levorphanol (Levo-Dromoran), and meperidine (Demerol). Additional synthetic narcotics are listed in Summary Drug Table 10-1.

Brompton's cocktail (or mixture) is a mixture of

SUMMARY DRUG TABLE 10–1
Narcotic Analgesic Drugs

GENERIC NAME	TRADE NAME*	USES	ADVERSE REACTIONS	DOSE RANGES†
OPIATE NARCOTICS				
camphorated tincture of opium	paregoric	Diarrhea	Same as morphine but may vary depending on dose	5–10 mL PO up to 4 times/d
codeine	*Generic*	Mild to moderate pain; as an antitussive	Respiratory depression, sedation, nausea, vomiting, anorexia, constipation, dry mouth, hypotension, rash, drug dependency with continued use	Analgesic: 15–60 mg PO, IM, IV, SC; antitussive: 10–20 mg PO
hydrochlorides of opium alkaloids	Pantopon	Moderate to severe pain	Same as morphine‡	5–20 mg IM, SC
hydromorphone hydrochloride	Dilaudid, *generic*	Moderate to severe pain	Same as morphine‡	2–4 mg PO; 2 mg SC, IM; may also be given by slow IV injection
morphine sulfate	*Generic*	Severe pain, preoperatively for sedation, dyspnea associated with acute left ventricular failure and pulmonary edema	CNS depression, anorexia, nausea, vomiting, constipation. See also pages 62–63	10–30 mg PO; 5–20 mg IM, SC; 4–10 mg IV; 10–20 mg rectally
oxymorphone hydrochloride	Numorphan	Moderate to severe pain, preoperative sedation, obstetric analgesia	Same as morphine‡	0.5 mg IV; 1–1.5 mg SC, IM; 5 mg rectally
SYNTHETIC AND SEMISYNTHETIC NARCOTICS				
buprenorphine hydrochloride	Buprenex	Mild to moderate pain	Sedation, dizziness, vertigo, hypotension, nausea, vomiting, sweating, headache	0.3–0.6 mg IM or slow IV
butorphanol tartrate	Stadol	Mild to moderate pain	Sedation, nausea, sweating, headache, vertigo	1–4 mg IM, 0.5–2 mg IV
fentanyl	Sublimaze	Analgesia before, during, or after anesthesia	Same as morphine‡	Preanesthesia: 0.05–0.1 mg IM; postoperative: 0.05–0.1 mg IM; anesthesia: administered by anesthesiologist
levorphanol tartrate	Levo-Dromoran	A moderate to severe pain, preoperatively to relieve apprehension, provide prolonged analgesia, and reduce thiopental requirements	Same as morphine‡	2–3 mg PO, SC
meperidine hydrochloride	Demerol, *generic*	Same as levorphanol	Same as morphine‡	50–150 mg IM, SC, PO
methadone hydrochloride	Dolophine HCL, *generic*	Severe pain, maintenance and treatment of narcotic addiction	Same as morphine‡	Pain: 2.5–10 mg IM, SC, PO; narcotic addiction: 15–120 mg PO
methotrimeprazine hydrochloride	Levoprome	Moderate to marked pain	Orthostatic hypotension, dizziness, nausea, vomiting	5–40 mg deep IM
nalbuphine hydrochloride	Nubain, *generic*	Mild to moderate pain	Sedation, nausea, vomiting, dizziness, dry mouth	10–20 mg IM, SC, IV
pentazocine	Talwin	Mild to moderate pain	Nausea, dizziness, vomiting, euphoria, lightheadedness	50–100 mg PO; up to 60 mg IM, SC; up to 30 mg IV

(continued)

SUMMARY DRUG TABLE 10–1
(continued)

GENERIC NAME	TRADE NAME*	USES	ADVERSE REACTIONS	DOSE RANGES†
SYNTHETIC AND SEMISYNTHETIC NARCOTICS				
propoxyphene hydrochloride	Darvon Pulvules, Dolene, *generic*	Mild to moderate pain	Dizziness, sedation, nausea, vomiting	65 mg PO
propoxyphene napsylate	Darvon-N	Mild to moderate pain	Same as propoxyphene hydrochloride	100 mg PO

* The term generic indicates that the drug is available in a generic form.
† Doses may be administered whenever needed (prn) with intervals depending on the dose and reason for use.
‡ The adverse reactions of some narcotics are basically similar to those of morphine but some of these reactions may be less severe or intense than those seen with morphine. See also section on adverse reactions in this chapter.

an oral narcotic and other drugs. It is used for chronic severe pain such as pain seen in terminal cancer patients. The original formulation used in England contained heroin or morphine, alcohol, water, and syrup (to make the liquid more palatable). The term *Brompton's mixture* is commonly used to identify any solution containing morphine and either cocaine (which is rarely used) or a phenothiazine. Methadone may also be used in the mixture in place of morphine. Various other drugs may also be included in the solution, including antidepressants, stimulants such as amphetamines, and tranquilizers such as diazepam (Valium).

▷ Actions of the Narcotic Analgesics

How the narcotic analgesics relieve pain is not completely understood. What is known is that the relief of pain is a complex physiologic and pharmacologic process.

When pain impulses are transmitted across afferent nerve fibers to the brain (which then interprets the sensation as pain), there is a release of two substances, namely *enkephalins* and *endorphins*. When released, enkephalins and endorphins occupy specific receptors (called opiate receptors) in the brain, brain stem, and spinal cord. When they occupy these receptors, they prevent the release of a neurotransmitter (neurohormone) from the afferent nerve fibers that carry pain impulses to the central nervous system (CNS). If a neurotransmitter is not released from nerve fibers, pain impulses cannot travel along these fibers and reach areas of the brain that interpret a sensation as pain.

Narcotic analgesics can be divided into two

types: (1) those that are pure agonists and (2) those that have both agonist-antagonist properties. An *agonist* is a narcotic capable of occupying the same opiate receptors as do enkephalins and endorphins; therefore, it prevents the release of a neurotransmitter from the afferent nerve fibers carrying pain impulses to the brain. A narcotic possessing agonist *and* antagonist properties has two actions: (1) it acts like the pure narcotic agonists (agonist property); and (2) it blocks the activity of morphine, meperidine, and other opiates (antagonist property). Examples of narcotic agonist-antagonist analgesics are butorphanol, nalbuphine (Nubain), and pentazocine (Talwin).

Administration of a narcotic analgesic elevates the pain threshold and alters the patient's perception of pain. The sedative action of the narcotic analgesics reduces the anxiety that accompanies pain, which appears to help the analgesic activity of the drug.

Morphine is considered the prototype or "model" narcotic, and the actions, uses, and ability to relieve pain of other narcotic analgesics are often compared with morphine. Morphine, as well as other narcotic analgesics, affects the following organs and structures of the body:

CNS—Drowsiness, euphoria, sedation, sleep, lethargy, and mental clouding often occur. The degree to which these occur usually depends on the drug and the dose.

Eye—Morphine and the other opiate narcotics cause constriction of the pupil (miosis). Codeine and the synthetic narcotics have a lesser miotic effect on the pupil.

Respiratory—The respiratory rate and depth are decreased by morphine and to a varying degree by the other opiates. Synthetic narcotics also depress the respiratory rate and depth.

Cough reflex—Morphine and other opiates have an antitussive (depression of the cough reflex) action because of their ability to depress the cough center in the medulla. Codeine has the most noticeable effect on the cough reflex and occasionally is used as an antitussive agent as well as an analgesic.

Medulla—When the chemoreceptor trigger zone (CTZ) located in the medulla is stimulated, nausea and vomiting can occur. To a varying degree, narcotic analgesics may stimulate the CTZ, resulting in nausea and vomiting. The narcotic analgesics also depress the CTZ; therefore, nausea and vomiting may or may not occur when these drugs are given.

Gastrointestinal tract—The opiate narcotics slow peristalsis in the stomach, duodenum, and small and large intestines. After ingestion of food, the emptying time of the stomach is delayed and movement of food through the digestive tract is slowed. Gastric, pancreatic, and biliary secretions are decreased. These drug actions can result in anorexia and constipation.

Gallbladder and common bile duct—Spasm of the biliary tract may occur in some patients after administration of morphine. Other narcotic analgesics have a lesser effect on the biliary tract.

Genitourinary tract—Narcotic analgesics may induce spasms of the ureter. Urinary urgency may also occur due to the action of these drugs on the detrusor muscle of the bladder. Some patients may experience difficulty in voiding due to contraction of the bladder sphincter.

▷ Uses of the Narcotic Analgesics

The ability of a narcotic analgesic to relieve pain depends on several factors such as the drug, the dose, the route of administration, the type of pain, the patient, and the length of time the drug has been administered. Morphine is an effective drug for moderately severe to severe pain. Other narcotics are effective for moderate to severe pain. For mild to moderate pain, the physician may order a narcotic such as codeine or pentazocine.

Some narcotic analgesics may be used as part of a preoperative medication to lessen anxiety and sedate the patient. Patients who are relaxed and sedated when anesthesia is given are easier to anesthetize (and therefore require a smaller dose of an induction anesthetic) as well as to maintain under anesthesia.

In addition to the relief of pain, specific narcotic analgesics may be used for the following reasons:

▷ Treatment of severe diarrhea and intestinal cramping—camphorated tincture of opium

▷ Relief of severe, persistent cough—codeine

▷ Dyspnea associated with acute left ventricular failure and pulmonary edema—morphine

▷ Obstetric analgesia—oxymorphone

Although codeine has the ability to depress the cough reflex, use of the drug for this reason has declined.

Methadone, a synthetic narcotic, may be used for the relief of pain, but it is also used in the detoxification and maintenance treatment of those addicted to narcotics. Detoxification involves withdrawing the patient from the narcotic while at the same time preventing the abstinence syndrome. Maintenance therapy is designed to reduce the patient's desire to return to the drug that caused addiction, as well as prevent the abstinence syndrome. The dosages used vary with the patient, the length of time the individual has been addicted, and the average amount of drug used each day.

Patients enrolled in an outpatient methadone program for detoxification or maintenance therapy on methadone must continue to receive methadone when hospitalized.

▷ Adverse Reactions Associated with the Administration of the Narcotic Analgesics

One of the major hazards of narcotic administration is respiratory depression with a decrease in the respiratory rate and depth. The most frequent adverse reactions include lightheadedness, dizziness, sedation, constipation, anorexia, nausea, vomiting, and sweating. When these effects occur, the physician may lower the dose in an effort to either eliminate or decrease the intensity of the adverse reaction. Other adverse reactions that may be seen with the administration of an *agonist* narcotic analgesic include the following:

CNS—euphoria, weakness, headache, pinpoint pupils, insomnia, agitation, tremor, impairment of mental and physical tasks

Gastrointestinal—dry mouth, biliary tract spasms

Cardiovascular—flushing of the face, peripheral circulatory collapse, tachycardia, bradycardia, palpitations

Genitourinary—spasms of the ureters and bladder sphincter, urinary retention or hesitancy

Allergic—pruritus, rash, urticaria

Other—physical dependence, pain at injection site, local tissue irritation

Administration of a narcotic *agonist-antagonist* may result in symptoms of narcotic withdrawal in those addicted to narcotics. Other adverse reactions associated with the administration of a narcotic agonist-antagonist include sedation, nausea, vomiting, sweating, headache, vertigo, dry mouth, euphoria, and dizziness.

▷ Patient-Controlled Analgesia

Patient-controlled analgesia (PCA) allows patients to administer their own analgesic by means of an intravenous (IV) pump system. The dose and the time interval permitted between doses is programmed into the device to prevent accidental overdosage.

Many postoperative patients require *less* narcotics when they are able to self-administer a narcotic for pain. Because the self-administration system is under control of the nurse, who adds the medication to the infusion pump and sets the time interval (or lockout interval) between doses, the patient cannot receive an overdose of the drug.

▶ NURSING PROCESS
THE PATIENT RECEIVING A NARCOTIC

ASSESSMENT

Before the administration of a narcotic analgesic, the nurse must review the patient's health history, allergy history, and past and present drug therapy. This is especially important when a narcotic is given for the first time because data may be obtained during the initial history and physical assessment that require contacting the physician. For example, the patient may have stated that nausea and vomiting occurred when he or she was given a pain medication several years ago. This information first requires further questioning of the patient, and when reported to the physician may influence a decision regarding administration of a specific narcotic drug. A thorough drug history, as well as physical assessment, may raise a question of drug dependency. Any suspicion of a drug dependency is immediately brought to the physician's attention. Administration of a narcotic with agonist-antagonist properties can result in withdrawal symptoms in those addicted to a narcotic.

Each time the patient requests a narcotic analgesic, the nurse must first determine the exact location of the pain, a description of the pain (eg, sharp, dull, stabbing), and when the pain began. If the pain is of a different type than the patient had been experiencing previously, or if it is in a different area, further questioning and more detailed information about the pain is necessary. Nursing judgment must now be exercised because not all instances of a change in pain type, location, or intensity require notifying the physician. For example, pain in the calf of the leg of the patient with recent abdominal surgery is a change in the location of pain and requires notifying the physician immediately. On the other hand, pain that is slightly worse because the patient has been moving in bed would not require contacting the physician. In addition, it should be determined if there are any controllable factors (eg, uncomfortable position, cold room, drafts, bright lights, noise, thirst) that may decrease the patient's tolerance to pain. If these factors are present, they are corrected as soon as possible, but the patient is not denied or made to wait for the drug.

NURSING DIAGNOSIS

Depending on factors such as the reason for administration (pain, obstetrical analgesia, diarrhea) and the patient's diagnosis, one or more of the following nursing diagnoses may apply to a person receiving a narcotic analgesic:

- ▶ Pain related to medical or surgical disorder
- ▶ Anxiety related to pain
- ▶ High risk for injury related to effect of narcotic on the CNS
- ▶ Altered nutrition: less than body requirements related to anorexia secondary to effects of the narcotic
- ▶ Knowledge deficit of medication regimen, adverse drugs effects, PCA infusion pump

PLANNING AND IMPLEMENTATION

The major goals of the patient may include a relief of pain, reduction in anxiety, absence of injury, an adequate nutrition intake, an understanding of the use of the PCA device (when applicable), and an understanding of and compliance to the prescribed treatment regimen.

The major goals of nursing management may in-

clude relief of pain, reduction in patient anxiety, absence of injury, promotion of an adequate food intake, recognition of adverse drug effects, and the development and implementation of an effective teaching plan.

ADMINISTRATION. Immediately before preparing a narcotic analgesic for administration, the nurse must obtain the patient's blood pressure, pulse, and respiratory rate and evaluate the patient's pain. The drug is withheld (ie, not prepared for administration and then given) and the physician contacted immediately if any of the following is present:

▶ A significant decrease in the respiratory rate or a respiratory rate of 10/min or below

▶ A significant increase or decrease in the pulse rate or a change in the pulse quality

▶ A significant decrease in blood pressure (systolic or diastolic) or a systolic pressure below 100 mmHg

Depending on clinical circumstances and nursing judgment, additional factors may require withholding the drug and contacting the physician. The physician is also notified immediately if the patient's pain is in a different area, if the pain is more intense, or if the character or type of the pain has changed.

PAIN AND ANXIETY. Pain causes anxiety. Anxiety, in some instances, can intensify pain. The analgesic effect of narcotic analgesics is best obtained when a narcotic is given *before* the patient experiences intense pain. This not only keeps the patient more comfortable but also reduces anxiety.

The patient is assessed for relief of pain approximately 1 hour after a narcotic analgesic is given. If the analgesic is ineffective, the physician must be notified because a higher dose or a different narcotic analgesic may be required.

Nursing tasks such as getting the patient out of bed, coughing and deep breathing, and leg exercises (when ordered) are best performed when the drug is producing its greatest analgesic effect, which is usually 1 to 2 hours after the narcotic is administered.

When a narcotic was used for obstetric analgesia, the neonate is observed closely for CNS and respiratory depression at the time of birth and for 4 to 6 hours afterward.

RELIEF OF DIARRHEA. When an opiate is used as an antidiarrheal agent, the nurse must record each bowel movement, as well as appearance, color, and consistency of each stool. If diarrhea is not relieved, if diarrhea becomes worse, or if severe abdominal pain or blood in the stool is noted, the physician is notified immediately.

ADVERSE DRUG EFFECTS. The blood pressure, pulse, and respiratory rate are obtained 15 to 30 minutes after the drug is administered intramuscularly (IM) or subcutaneously (SC), 30 or more minutes if the drug is given orally, and in 5 to 10 minutes if the drug is given IV. Any significant change in these vital signs is reported to the physician immediately. If the respiratory rate is 10 or below, the patient is monitored at frequent intervals and the physician is notified immediately. If the respiratory rate continues to fall, the physician may order the administration of a narcotic antagonist.

Narcotics may depress the cough reflex. Patients receiving a narcotic on a regular basis, even for a few days, must be encouraged to cough and breathe deeply every 2 hours. This task prevents the pooling of secretions in the lungs, which can lead to hypostatic pneumonia and other lung problems.

Constipation may occur with continued use of a narcotic. A daily record of bowel movements is kept and the physician is informed if constipation appears to be a problem. A stool softener, enema, or other means of relieving constipation may be ordered by the physician.

Nausea and vomiting may be seen is some patients receiving a narcotic. If this should occur, the physician is notified immediately because a different analgesic or an antiemetic may be necessary.

HIGH RISK FOR INJURY. Narcotics may produce orthostatic hypotension which, in turn, results in dizziness. The patient should be assisted with ambulatory activities and with rising slowly from a sitting or lying position.

Miosis (pinpoint pupils) may occur with the administration of some narcotics, and is most pronounced with administration of morphine, hydromorphone, and hydrochlorides of opium alkaloids. Miosis decreases the patient's ability to see in dim light. Therefore, the room should be kept well-lighted during daytime hours and the patient should be advised to seek assistance when getting out of bed at night. The bowel elimination pattern is checked daily because constipation can occur with repeated doses of a narcotic.

NUTRITION. When a narcotic is prescribed for a prolonged period of time, anorexia may occur. Those receiving a narcotic for the relief of pain due to terminal cancer often have severe anorexia, which is usually due to the administration of a narcotic as well the disease.

The patient's food intake is assessed after each meal. When anorexia is prolonged, the patient should be weighed weekly or as ordered by the physician. Continued weight loss and anorexia is brought to the attention of the physician.

DRUG DEPENDENCE. Drug dependence can occur when a narcotic is administered over time. If dependence appears to occur, the problem is discussed with the physician. For some patients such as those who are terminally ill and in severe pain, drug addiction may be allowed to occur because the most important task is to keep the patient as comfortable as possible for the time he or she has remaining. When a patient does not have a painful terminal illness, drug dependence must be avoided. Signs of drug dependence may include occurrence of an abstinence syndrome (see chap 13) when the narcotic is discontinued, requests for the narcotic at frequent intervals around the clock, personality changes if the narcotic is not given immediately, and constant complaints of pain and failure of the narcotic to relieve pain. Although these behaviors can have other causes, drug dependence should be considered.

Drug dependence can also occur in a newborn whose mother was dependent on opiates during pregnancy. Withdrawal symptoms usually appear during the first few days of life. Symptoms include irritability, excessive crying, yawning, sneezing, increased respiratory rate, tremors, fever, vomiting, and diarrhea.

BROMPTON'S MIXTURE. If the patient is receiving Brompton's mixture, check with the pharmacist about the ingredients. The patient is then observed for the adverse reactions of *each* drug contained in the solution. The time interval for administration of Brompton's mixture varies. Some physicians may order it on an as-needed basis; others may order it given at regular intervals.

KNOWLEDGE DEFICIT. A patient should be told that the medication he or she is receiving is for pain. The patient may also need to be told additional information such as how often the medication can be given and the name of the drug being given.

Those receiving PCA must be given instruction in its use. The following may be included in the explanation and demonstration given to the patient:

- ▶ Description of how the unit works, for example, the control button that activates the administration of the drug
- ▶ Differentiation between the control button for PCA and the button to call the nurse (when both are similar in appearance and feel)
- ▶ Reassurance that the machine regulates the dose of the drug as well as the time interval between doses
- ▶ Explanation that if the patient uses the control button too soon after the last dose, the machine will not deliver the medication until the correct time
- ▶ Reassurance that pain relief should occur shortly after pushing the button
- ▶ Instruction that if pain relief does not occur after two successive doses call the nurse

Narcotics prescribed for out-patient use are almost always in the oral form. In certain instances, such as terminally ill patients being cared for at home, the family may receive instruction in the parenteral administration of the drug. When a narcotic has been prescribed, the following points are included in a teaching plan:

- ▶ This drug may cause drowsiness, dizziness, and blurring of vision. Caution should be used when driving or performing tasks requiring alertness.
- ▶ The use of alcoholic beverages should be avoided unless use has been approved by the physician. Alcohol may intensify the action of the drug and cause extreme drowsiness or dizziness. In some instances, the use of alcohol and a narcotic can have extremely serious and even life-threatening consequences that may require emergency medical treatment.
- ▶ The drug should be taken as directed on the container label. The prescribed dose should *not* be exceeded. If the drug is not effective, the physician should be contacted.
- ▶ If gastrointestinal upset occurs, the drug may be taken with food.
- ▶ This drug may cause nausea, vomiting, and constipation. The physician should be notified if these problems become severe.

EVALUATION

- ▶ Pain is relieved
- ▶ Anxiety is reduced
- ▶ No evidence of injury
- ▶ Maintains body weight
- ▶ Eats an adequate diet
- ▶ Patient and family demonstrate understanding of drug regimen
- ▶ Demonstrates ability to effectively use PCA

▶ THE NARCOTIC ANTAGONISTS

The two narcotic antagonists in use today are *naloxone* (Narcan) and *naltrexone* (Trexan; Summary Drug Table 10-2). They are called narcotic antagonists because they are capable of reversing the effects of narcotics, particularly their respiratory depressant effects.

SUMMARY DRUG TABLE 10–2
Narcotic Antagonists

GENERIC NAME	TRADE NAME	USES	ADVERSE REACTIONS	DOSE RANGES
naloxone hydrochloride	Narcan	Narcotic overdose, postoperative narcotic depression	Abrupt reversal of narcotic depression may result in nausea, vomiting, sweating, increased blood pressure, tachycardia	0.4–2 mg IV initially with additional doses repeated at 2–3-min intervals; smaller doses used for postoperative narcotic depression
naltrexone hydrochloride	Trexan	Adjunct to maintenance of an opioid-free state in detoxified formerly opioid-dependent patients	Anxiety, difficulty sleeping, abdominal cramps, nasal congestion, joint and muscle pain, nausea, vomiting, dizziness, irritability	Maintenance treatment: 50 mg PO daily and 100 mg PO on Saturdays, or 100 mg PO every other day, or 150 mg PO every third day

▷ Actions of the Narcotic Antagonists

Naloxone

Administration of naloxone prevents or reverses the effects of the opioids (opiates). How this is accomplished is not fully understood, but it is believed that it reverses opioid effects by competing for opiate receptor sites (see Actions of the Narcotic Analgesics). If the individual has taken or received an opiate, the effects of the opiate are reversed. If the individual has *not* taken or received an opiate, naloxone has no drug activity.

Naltrexone

Naltrexone completely blocks the effect of IV opiates as well as drugs with agonist-antagonist actions (butorphanol, nalbuphine, and pentazocine). Its mechanism of action appears to be the same as naloxone.

▷ Uses of Narcotic Antagonists

Naloxone

This drug is used for complete or partial reversal of narcotic depression, including respiratory depression. Drugs causing narcotic depression and responding to naloxone administration include the natural and synthetic opiates, propoxyphene, methadone, nalbuphine, butorphanol, and pentazocine. The causes of narcotic depression may be due to intentional or accidental overdose (self-administration by an individual), accidental overdose by medical personnel, and drug idiosyncrasy. Naloxone may also be used for diagnosis of a suspected acute opioid overdosage.

Naltrexone

Naltrexone is used in the treatment of persons formerly dependent on opioids. Patients receiving naltrexone have been detoxified and are enrolled in a program for treatment of narcotic addiction. Naltrexone, along with other methods of treatment (counseling, psychotherapy, and so on), is used to maintain an opioid-free state. Patients taking naltrexone on a scheduled basis will not experience any *narcotic* drug effects should they use an opioid.

▷ Adverse Reactions Associated with the Administration of Narcotic Antagonists

Naloxone

Although not a true adverse reaction, abrupt reversal of narcotic depression may result in nausea, vomiting, sweating, tachycardia, increased blood pressure, and tremors. In the postoperative patient who has received a narcotic overdose or who experiences narcotic depression due to a drug idiosyncrasy, there may be a reversal of the analgesic effect of the narcotic. This results in a sudden return of pain (for which the narcotic was given) and, in some cases, excitement, hypotension or hypertension, ventricular tachycardia and fibrillation, and pulmonary edema.

Naltrexone

Administration of naltrexone may result in anxiety, difficulty in sleeping, abdominal cramps, nasal congestion, joint and muscle pain, nausea, vomiting, dizziness, irritability, depression, fatigue, and drowsiness.

▶ *NURSING PROCESS*
THE PATIENT RECEIVING A NARCOTIC ANTAGONIST FOR RESPIRATORY DEPRESSION

ASSESSMENT

Before the administration of naloxone, the patient's record is reviewed for the drug suspected of causing the overdosage and the blood pressure, pulse, and respiratory rate are obtained. If there is sufficient time, the patient's initial health history, allergy history, and current treatment modalities are reviewed.

NURSING DIAGNOSIS

▶ Ineffective airway clearance related to administration of a narcotic (specify overdose, drug idiosyncrasy, or other cause)

PLANNING AND IMPLEMENTATION

The major goal of the patient with respiratory depression is a normal respiratory rate, rhythm, and depth.

The major goal of nursing management of the patient with respiratory depression is the return of a normal respiratory rate, rhythm, and depth.

Depending on the patient's condition, cardiac monitoring, artificial ventilation (respirator), and other drugs may be used during and after the administration of naloxone. A patent airway must be maintained. Suction equipment must be readily available because abrupt reversal of narcotic depression may cause vomiting. If naloxone is given by IV infusion, the physician orders the IV fluid and amount, the drug dosage, and the infusion rate. Giving the drug by IV infusion requires use of a secondary line or IV piggyback.

Before and after administration of naloxone, the blood pressure, pulse, and respiratory rate are monitored at frequent intervals, usually every 5 minutes, until the patient responds. These vital signs are then monitored every 5 to 15 minutes after the patient has shown response to the drug.

The physician may order a repeat dose of naloxone if results obtained from the initial dose are unsatisfactory. The duration of close patient observation depends on the patient's response to the administration of the narcotic antagonist. The physician is notified if any adverse drug reactions occur, because additional medical treatment may be needed.

It is most important that a patent airway be maintained and the patient suctioned as needed. The intake and output are monitored and the physician is notified of any change in the intake-output ratio. The physician must always be contacted if there is any sudden change in the patient's condition.

EVALUATION

▶ Respiratory rate, rhythm, and depth are normal
▶ Maintains a clear airway

▶ *NURSING PROCESS*
THE PATIENT RECEIVING A NARCOTIC ANTAGONIST FOR TREATMENT OF OPIOID DEPENDENCY

ASSESSMENT

A complete drug history is obtained. A complete physical examination and psychologic evaluation are usually performed before initiation of therapy. The extent of the pretreatment assessment is usually based on the guidelines set up by the clinic or agency dispensing the drug.

NURSING DIAGNOSIS

▶ Anxiety related to dependency history, effectiveness of treatment program, other factors (specify)
▶ Noncompliance related to anxiety, difficulty in staying drug-free, other factors (specify)
▶ Knowledge deficit of treatment regimen, requirements of treatment program

PLANNING AND IMPLEMENTATION

The major goals of the person formerly dependent on opioids may include reducing anxiety, complying with the treatment program, and remaining drug-free.

The major goals of nursing management of the person formerly dependent on opioids may include reducing patient anxiety, developing and implementing an effective teaching plan, and providing emotional support.

When the patient is receiving naltrexone for opioid

dependency, the administration techniques of the drug treatment program are followed.

ANXIETY. The person entering a program for drug dependency may have anxiety due to many factors. Examples of possible causes of anxiety include the socioeconomic impact of drug dependency, the effectiveness of the treatment program, and concern over remaining drug-free. Individuals vary in their ability to communicate their fears and concerns. At times, the nurse may be able to identify those situations causing anxiety and explore the possible solutions to the many problems faced by these patients.

NONCOMPLIANCE. One of the greatest problems associated with former drug dependency is remaining drug-free. Some people find it difficult to break away from situations, individuals, or pressures that promote drug use. Because of this, some of those entering a drug rehabilitation program that use opiods may, in time, not report to the program or agency to receive their drug and thus are able to return to the use of an opiate.

All staff members of the rehabilitation program should work with the patient, encourage adherence to the medication regimen, and attempt to identify those situations that may encourage a return to drug use.

KNOWLEDGE DEFICIT. Patients under treatment for narcotic addiction, who are receiving naltrexone, are instructed to wear or carry identification indicating that they are receiving this drug. If the patient is taking naltrexone and requires hospitalization, it is important that all medical personnel be aware of therapy with this drug. Narcotics administered to these patients have no effect and therefore do not relieve pain. Patients receiving naltrexone obviously may pose a problem if they develop acute pain. The physician must decide what methods must be used to control pain in these patients.

Patients taking naltrexone must also understand the impact of therapy. They must be informed that while taking the drug, any use of heroin or other opiate results in no effect. Large doses of heroin or other opiates can overcome the drug's effect and result in coma or death.

EVALUATION

▶ Factors causing anxiety are identified

▶ Anxiety is reduced

▶ Complies to the prescribed treatment regimen

▶ Remains drug-free

▶ Demonstrates understanding of the treatment regimen and requirements of the rehabilitation program

11

The Nonnarcotic Analgesics

On completion of this chapter the student will:

▶ *Discuss the types, uses, and general drug actions of the nonnarcotic analgesics*

▶ *List the general adverse reactions associated with the administration of a nonnarcotic analgesic*

▶ *Use the nursing process when administering a nonnarcotic analgesic*

▶ *Discuss the nursing implications to be considered when administering a nonnarcotic analgesic*

The nonnarcotic analgesics are a group of drugs that are used to relieve pain. Use of these drugs does not result in physical dependency, which can occur with the use of a narcotic analgesic.

The nonnarcotic analgesics can be divided into two types—the *salicylates* and the *nonsalicylates*. The salicylates include aspirin (acetylsalicylic acid) and those drugs related to aspirin such as magnesium salicylate and sodium salicylate. The nonsalicylates include drugs that are not related to the salicylates.

▷ Actions of the Nonnarcotic Analgesics

The Salicylates

The salicylates have analgesic, antipyretic, and antiinflammatory effects. All the salicylates are simi-

lar in pharmacologic activity; however, aspirin has a greater antiinflammatory effect than the other salicylates.

The manner in which salicylates relieve pain and reduce inflammation is not fully understood. It is thought that the antiinflammatory action of the salicylates is due to the inhibition of prostaglandins. Prostaglandins are fatty acid derivatives found in almost every tissue of the body and body fluid. Release of prostaglandin is thought to increase the sensitivity of peripheral pain receptors. Salicylates lower an elevated body temperature by dilating peripheral blood vessels, which, in turn, cools the body. Aspirin prolongs the bleeding time by inhibiting the aggregation (clumping) of platelets. When the bleeding time is prolonged, it takes a longer time for the blood to clot after a cut, surgery, or other injury to the skin or mucous membranes. The other salicylates do not have an effect on platelets and therefore do not affect the bleeding time.

The Nonsalicylates

Acetaminophen (Tylenol) is a nonsalicylate nonnarcotic analgesic whose mechanism of action is unknown. Like the salicylates, acetaminophen has analgesic and antipyretic activity. Acetaminophen does not possess antiinflammatory action and therefore is of no value in the treatment of inflammation or inflammatory disorders.

Another type of nonnarcotic analgesic are the nonsteroidal antiinflammatory agents (NSAIDs). Examples of this group of drugs are fenoprofen (Nalfon), ibuprofen (Advil), naproxen (Naprosyn), and ketoprofen (Orudis). Like the salicylates, these drugs have antiinflammatory, antipyretic, and analgesic activity. The exact mode of action of these drugs is not known.

▷ Uses of the Nonnarcotic Analgesics

The Salicylates

The salicylate nonnarcotic analgesics are used for the following reasons:

▷ Relief of mild to moderate pain

▷ Reduction of elevated body temperature (fever)

▷ Treatment of inflammatory conditions such as rheumatoid arthritis, osteoarthritis, and rheumatic fever

▷ Reduction of the risk of myocardial infarction in those with unstable angina—aspirin only

▷ Reduction of the risk transient ischemic attacks (TIAs) or strokes in *males* who have had transient ischemia of the brain due to fibrin platelet emboli—aspirin only

The Nonsalicylates

Acetaminophen is used to relieve mild to moderate pain and to reduce elevated body temperature (fever). This drug is particularly useful for those with aspirin allergy and with bleeding disorders such as bleeding ulcer or hemophilia, those on anticoagulant therapy, and those who have recently had minor surgical procedures. Although acetaminophen has no antiinflammatory action, it may be used to relieve the *pain and discomfort* associated with arthritic disorders, but it is of no value in treating the inflammatory process of the disease.

Nonsteroidal antiinflammatory agents have a variety of uses that vary depending on the drug used.

The uses of individual nonsteroidal antiinflammatory agents are given in Summary Drug Table 11-1 and Summary Drug Table 42-1 in chapter 42.

▷ Adverse Reactions Associated with the Administration of Nonnarcotic Analgesics

The Salicylates

Gastric upset, heartburn, nausea, vomiting, anorexia, and gastrointestinal (GI) bleeding may occur with salicylate use. Although these drugs are relatively safe when taken as recommended on the label or by the physician, use can occasionally result in more serious reactions. Some individuals are allergic to aspirin and the other salicylates. Allergy to the salicylates may be manifested by hives, rash, angioedema, bronchospasm with asthmalike symptoms, and anaphylactoid reactions.

Mild *salicylism* usually occurs with repeated administration of large doses of a salicylate. The symptoms of salicylism include dizziness, tinnitus, difficulty in hearing, nausea, vomiting, diarrhea, mental confusion, and lassitude.

Loss of blood through the GI tract occurs with salicylate use. The amount of blood lost is insignificant when one normal dose is taken. Use of these drugs over a long period, even in normal doses, can result in a significant blood loss. Because the salicylates prolong the bleeding time, they are contraindicated in those with bleeding disorders or bleeding tendencies. This includes patients with GI bleeding (due to any cause), blood dyscrasias, and those receiving anticoagulant or antineoplastic drugs. The use of salicylates must be avoided for at least 1 week before any type of major or minor surgery, including dental surgery, because of the possibility of postoperative bleeding. The salicylates are also not used following any type of surgery until complete healing has occurred. When relief from mild pain is necessary after surgery or a dental procedure, acetaminophen or a nonsteroidal antiinflammatory agent may be used.

Studies suggest that the use of salicylates (especially aspirin) may be involved in the development of Reye's syndrome in children with chickenpox or influenza. This rare but life-threatening disorder is characterized by vomiting and lethargy progressing to coma. Use of salicylates in children with chickenpox, fever, or flulike symptoms is not recommended. Acetaminophen is recommended for the management of symptoms associated with these disorders.

SUMMARY DRUG TABLE 11–1
Non-Narcotic Analgesics

GENERIC NAME	TRADE NAME*	USES	ADVERSE REACTIONS	DOSE RANGES
acetaminophen	Anacin-3, Tylenol, *generic*	Analgesic, antipyretic	Rare; with chronic use skin eruptions, CNS stimulation, hypoglycemia, cyanosis, methemoglobinemia, hemolytic anemia	325–650 mg PO q4–6h; 650-mg rectal suppository
aspirin (acetylsalicylic acid)	Bayer, Ecotrin, Anacin, Empirin, Bufferin, *generic*	Analgesic, antipyretic; as an antiinflammatory	Nausea, vomiting, epigastric distress, GI bleeding, allergic and anaphylactic reactions, salicylism with overuse	325–650 mg PO with up to 8 g/d PO in divided doses for some disorders; 325–650 mg rectally
fenoprofen calcium	Nalfon	Mild to moderate pain, rheumatic disorders	Nausea, vomiting, diarrhea, GI bleeding, jaundice, dizziness, visual disturbances	Pain: 200 mg PO q4–6h; arthritic disorders: see Summary Drug Table 42-1
ibuprofen	Advil, Nuprin, Motrin, Rufen, *generic*	Mild to moderate pain, rheumatic disorders, primary dysmenorrhea	Same as fenoprofen	Pain: 200–400 mg PO q4–6h; dysmenorrhea: 400 mg PO q4h; arthritic disorders: see Summary Drug Table 42-1
ketoprofen	Orudis	Same as ibuprofen	Same as fenoprofen	150–300 mg/d PO in divided doses; arthritic disorders: see Summary Drug Table 42-1
ketorolac	Toradol	Short-term management of pain	Edema, nausea, GI pain, drowsiness, pain at injection site	30–60 mg IM initially, followed by 1/2 the initial dose q6h prn
magnesium salicylate	Original Doan's, Magan	Same as aspirin	Same as aspirin	650 mg PO q4h and up to 4.8 g/d PO in divided doses for some disorders
naproxen	Naprosyn	Same as ibuprofen	Same as fenoprofen	Pain, primary dysmenorrhea: up to 1.25 g/d PO in divided doses; arthritic disorders: see Summary Drug Table 42-1
sodium salicylate	*Generic*	Same as aspirin	Same as aspirin	325–650 mg PO q4h

*The term generic indicates that the drug is available in a generic form.
NOTE: There are many combination analgesic products containing more than one drug, examples of which are aspirin plus an antacid, propoxyphene plus aspirin or acetaminophen, and aspirin plus caffeine. Use of combination-type drugs requires observation for adverse effects that may occur with **each** ingredient.

The Nonsalicylates

Acetaminophen causes few adverse reactions when used as directed on the label or recommended by the physician. Adverse reactions associated with the use of acetaminophen usually occur with chronic use or when exceeding the recommended dosage. Adverse reactions that may be seen with use of this drug include skin eruptions, urticaria, hemolytic anemia, hypoglycemia, cyanosis, methemoglobinemia, pancytopenia, jaundice, drowsiness, and glossitis. Hep-atotoxicity and hepatic failure have been seen in chronic alcoholics taking this drug.

There are many adverse reactions associated with the use of the nonsteroidal antiinflammatory agents. However, many patients take these drugs and experience few, if any, side effects. Some of the adverse reactions associated with the use of these agents include the following:

GI—nausea, vomiting, diarrhea, constipation, epigastric pain, indigestion, abdominal distress or discomfort, intestinal ulceration, stomatitis, jaundice, bloating, anorexia, dry mouth

Central nervous system—dizziness, anxiety, light-headedness, vertigo, headache, drowsiness, insomnia, confusion, depression, psychic disturbances

Cardiovascular—congestive heart failure, decrease or increase in blood pressure, cardiac dysrhythmias

Renal—hematuria, cystitis, elevated blood urea nitrogen, polyuria, dysuria, oliguria, acute renal failure in those with impaired renal function

Special senses—visual disturbances, blurred or diminished vision, diplopia, swollen or irritated eyes, photophobia, reversible loss of color vision, tinnitus, taste change, rhinitis

Hematologic—neutropenia, eosinophilia, leukopenia, pancytopenia, thrombocytopenia, agranulocytosis, aplastic anemia

Skin—rash, erythema, irritation, skin eruptions, exfoliative dermatitis, Stevens-Johnson syndrome, ecchymosis, purpura

Metabolic/endocrinologic—decreased appetite, weight increase or decrease, hyperglycemia, hypoglycemia, increased need for insulin in the diabetic patient, flushing, sweating, menstrual disorders, vaginal bleeding

Other—thirst, fever, chills, vaginitis

▶ NURSING PROCESS
THE PATIENT RECEIVING A NONNARCOTIC ANALGESIC

ASSESSMENT

When a patient is receiving one of the nonnarcotic analgesics for mild to moderate pain, it will be necessary to determine the type, onset, and location of the pain. It is also important to determine if this problem is different in any way from previous episodes of pain or discomfort.

If the patient is receiving a nonnarcotic analgesic for an arthritic or musculoskeletal disorder or soft tissue inflammation, the joints or areas involved are examined. The appearance of the skin over the joint or affected area or any limitation of motion is noted and recorded. The patient's ability to carry out activities of daily living (ADL) is evaluated. This important information is used in the development of a patient care plan as well as in the evaluation of the patient's response to drug therapy.

NURSING DIAGNOSIS

Depending on the drug, dose, and reason for administration, one or more of the following nursing diagnoses may apply to a person receiving a nonnarcotic analgesic:

▶ Anxiety related to pain, discomfort, other factors (specify)

▶ Pain related to physical disorder (name disorder)

▶ High risk for altered body temperature: hyperthermia related to disease process (for example, infection or surgery)

▶ Noncompliance related to indifference, lack of knowledge, other factors

▶ Knowledge deficit of treatment regimen, adverse drug effects

PLANNING AND IMPLEMENTATION

The major goals of the patient may include a reduction in anxiety, relief of pain, and an understanding of and compliance to the prescribed treatment regimen.

The major goals of nursing management may include a reduction in patient anxiety, relief of pain, recognition of adverse drug effects, and the development and implementation of an effective teaching plan.

Patients receiving a nonnarcotic analgesic for a musculoskeletal disorder (eg, osteoarthritis, rheumatoid arthritis, ankylosing spondylitis, gouty arthritis) are observed daily for signs of clinical improvement (see chap 42).

If surgery or a dental procedure such as tooth extraction or gum surgery is anticipated, salicylates are usually discontinued 1 week before the procedure because of the possibility of postoperative bleeding. If emergency surgery is necessary and there is a history of salicylate use, the patient is observed closely during the postoperative period for bleeding tendencies.

ADVERSE DRUG REACTIONS. Patients receiving a salicylate are observed for adverse drug reactions. When high doses of salicylates are administered, for example, to those with severe arthritic disorders, patients are observed for signs of salicylism (see Adverse Reactions). Should signs of salicylism occur, the physician is notified because a reduction in dose or determination of the plasma salicylate level may be necessary. The salicylates may be given with food or milk to prevent gastric upset. If gastric distress occurs despite giving the drug with food or milk, the physician is notified because other drug therapy may be necessary.

The patient receiving a nonsteroidal antiinflammatory agent is observed for adverse drug reactions during initial therapy. Because these drugs have many adverse reactions, inform the physician of *any* complaints the patient may have. GI reactions can occur with these drugs and can be severe and sometimes fatal, especially in those prone to upper GI disease. Withhold the next dose and notify the physician immediately if any GI symptoms, especially nausea, vomiting, diarrhea, evidence of GI bleeding (blood in stool, tarry stools), or abdominal pain occurs. Insulin dosage may require adjustment while the diabetic patient is receiving one of the nonsteroidal antiinflammatory drugs. The physician is notified if there is any change in urine glucose test results or if the patient develops signs of hypoglycemia or hyperglycemia (see chap 20).

ANXIETY. Anxiety related to pain or discomfort may be experienced by some patients, especially those with chronic mild to moderate pain. Anxiety may also occur because the patient is concerned about the ability of the drug to relieve pain. This is especially true in those having minor surgery or dental procedures.

If the patient appears concerned about the ability of the drug to relieve pain or discomfort or if the drug fails to provide relief, the problem is discussed with the physician.

PAIN. The patient's response to the drug is evaluated. If a nonnarcotic analgesic fails to relieve pain or discomfort, the physician is notified because a different drug may be needed.

FEVER. If one of these drugs is used as an antipyretic, the temperature is checked immediately before and 45 to 60 minutes after administration of the drug. If a suppository form of the drug was used, the patient is checked in 30 minutes for retention of the suppository. If the drug fails to lower an elevated temperature, the physician is notified because other means of temperature control, such as a cooling blanket, may be necessary.

NONCOMPLIANCE. In some instances, a nonnarcotic analgesic may be prescribed for a prolonged period, for example, when the patient has arthritis. Some patients may discontinue their medication, fail to take the medication at the prescribed or recommended intervals, increase the dose, or decrease the time interval between doses especially if there is an increase or decrease in their symptoms. The patient and family must understand that the medication is to be taken even though symptoms have been relieved.

KNOWLEDGE DEFICIT. The following points can be included in a patient and family teaching plan. Some of these points apply to a specific nonnarcotic analgesic and are so identified.

► The dose stated on the label of over-the-counter (OTC) nonnarcotic analgesics is not to be exceeded unless a larger dose has been recommended by a physician.

► The use of aspirin or other salicylates is avoided when taking a nonsteroidal antiinflammatory drug.

► If GI upset occurs, the drug is taken with food or milk. If the problem persists, the physician is contacted.

► Nonsteroidal antiinflammatory agents may cause drowsiness, dizziness, or blurred vision. Caution should be exercised while driving or performing tasks that require alertness.

► If the nonsteroidal antiinflammatory agent fails to relieve some or all of the symptoms after 2 weeks of therapy, the medication should be continued but the physician should be contacted as soon as possible.

► If the drug is taken to relieve mild to moderate pain, the physician or dentist should be notified if the pain is not relieved.

► Physicians or dentists are always informed when these drugs are taken on a regular or occasional basis.

► If taking a salicylate, the physician is notified if any of the following occurs: ringing in the ears, GI pain, nausea, vomiting, flushing, sweating, thirst, headache, diarrhea, episodes of unusual bleeding or bruising, or dark-colored stools.

► If taking a nonsteroidal antiinflammatory agent, the physician is notified if any of the following occurs: skin rash, itching, visual disturbances, weight gain, edema, diarrhea, black stools, nausea, vomiting, or persistent headache.

► If the drug is used to reduce a fever, the physician is contacted if the temperature continues to remain elevated for more than 24 hours.

► All drugs deteriorate with age. Salicylates often deteriorate at a more rapid rate than many other drugs. If there is a vinegar odor to the salicylate, the entire contents of the container must be discarded. Salicylates should be purchased in small amounts when used on an occasional basis. The container is kept tightly closed at all times because salicylates deteriorate rapidly when exposed to air, moisture, and heat.

► The ingredients of some OTC drugs contain aspirin. The salicylate name may not appear in the name of the drug, but it is listed on the label. These products should not be used while taking a salicylate, especially during high-dose or long-term salicylate therapy or while taking a nonsteroidal anti-inflammatory drug. If in doubt about a particular product, the pharmacist should be consulted about the product's ingredients before purchasing the drug.

▶ An OTC nonnarcotic analgesic should not be used consistently to treat chronic pain without first consulting a physician.

EVALUATION

▶ Anxiety is reduced

▶ Pain is relieved; discomfort is reduced or eliminated

▶ Body temperature is normal

▶ Verbalizes importance of complying with the prescribed treatment regimen

▶ Demonstrates understanding of treatment regimen, adverse drug effects

12

Sedatives and Hypnotics

On completion of this chapter the student will:

▶ *Differentiate between a sedative and a hypnotic*

▶ *Discuss the types, uses, and general drug actions of the barbiturate and nonbarbiturate sedatives and hypnotics*

▶ *List the general adverse reactions that may be seen with the administration of a sedative or hypnotic*

▶ *Describe how the nurse may assess the patient's need for a sedative or hypnotic*

▶ *Use the nursing process when administering a sedative or hypnotic*

▶ *Discuss the nursing implications to be considered when a patient is given a sedative or hypnotic*

A **sedative** is a drug that produces a relaxing, calming effect. Sedatives are usually given during daytime hours and although they may make the patient drowsy, they usually do not produce sleep.

A **hypnotic** is a drug that induces sleep, that is, it allows the patient to fall asleep and stay asleep. Hypnotics may also be called **soporifics.** Hypnotics are given at night or hour of sleep (HS).

Sedatives and hypnotics may be divided into two classes:

1. Barbiturates
   a. Ultrashort-acting (eg, thiamylal [Surital], thiopental [Pentothal])
   b. Short-acting to intermediate-acting (eg, amobarbital, butabarbital [Butisol], pento-

barbital [Nembutal], secobarbital [Seconal])
   c. Long-acting (eg, phenobarbital)
2. Nonbarbiturates

▷ Actions of the Sedatives and Hypnotics

Barbiturates

All the barbiturates have essentially the same mode of action. Depending on the dose given, these drugs are capable of producing central nervous system (CNS) depression and mood alteration ranging from mild excitation to mild sedation, hypnosis (sleep), and deep coma. These drugs are also respiratory depressants with the degree of depression usually depending on the dose given. When used as hypnotics, the respiratory depressant effect is usually similar to that occurring during sleep.

Sleep induced by a barbiturate reduces the amount of time spent in the rapid eye movement (REM) stage of sleep. This is the dreaming stage of sleep. Dreams appear to be a necessary part of sleep. When an individual is deprived of dreaming for a prolonged period, a psychosis can develop. Use of the barbiturates over time deprives an individual of the dreaming phase of sleep. Examples of barbiturates are given in Summary Drug Table 12-1.

Nonbarbiturates

Most of the nonbarbiturates have essentially the same mode of action as the barbiturates, that is, they depress the CNS. The nonbarbiturates have a varying effect on the respiratory rate and the time spent in REM sleep. Examples of nonbarbiturates are given in Summary Drug Table 12-1.

▷ Uses of the Sedatives and Hypnotics

The primary use of the sedatives and hypnotics is for those conditions that require sedation or that enable the patient to sleep. Sedative doses, usually given during daytime hours, have a variety of uses in the treatment of anxiety and apprehension. Patients with chronic disease may require sedation, not only to reduce anxiety, but also as adjuncts in the treatment of their disease. For example, the patient with a cardiovascular or gastrointestinal disorder may benefit from the use of one of these agents in daytime sedative doses.

When a barbiturate or nonbarbiturate is used as a hypnotic, a dose larger than that required to produce sedation is given. Elderly patients may require a smaller hypnotic dose, and in some instances, a sedative dose produces sleep. Helping the patient sleep is an important part of the management of illness. The patient is in an unfamiliar surrounding that is unlike his or her home situation. There are noises and lights at night which often interfere with or interrupt sleep. Sleep deprivation may interfere with the healing process; therefore, a hypnotic is often given to many patients during hospitalization. These drugs may also be prescribed for short-term use as hypnotics after discharge from the hospital.

Barbiturates and nonbarbiturates are detoxified by the liver. All drugs entering the body ultimately leave the body. Some leave virtually unchanged, whereas others are transformed into other chemicals or compounds before they are eliminated. The liver is the organ that changes these and many other drugs into compounds that are ultimately excreted by the kidney. Patients with liver disease are given these drugs with great caution.

The ultrashort-acting barbiturates are used only as anesthetic agents (see chap 41). In preparation for surgery, a hypnotic is usually given the night before the operation. On the day of surgery, a barbiturate or nonbarbiturate may be used either alone or with other drugs as part of the preoperative medication. The anesthesiologist or surgeon selects a drug that is tailored to the patient's needs.

Paraldehyde, a nonbarbiturate, may be used in the treatment of delirium tremens (DTs) and other psychiatric conditions.

The barbiturates that are used as anticonvulsants are discussed in chapter 31.

▷ Adverse Reactions Associated with the Administration of Sedatives and Hypnotics

Barbiturates

Adverse reactions associated with barbiturate administration include the following:

CNS—somnolence, agitation, confusion, CNS depression, ataxia, nightmares, lethargy, residual sedation (drug hangover), hallucinations, paradoxical excitement

Respiratory—hypoventilation, apnea, respiratory depression, bronchospasm, laryngospasm

Gastrointestinal—nausea, vomiting, constipation, diarrhea, epigastric pain

Cardiovascular—bradycardia, hypotension, syncope

Hypersensitivity—rash, angioneurotic edema, fever, urticaria

Other—headache, liver damage

Nonbarbiturates

Adverse reactions associated with administration of the nonbarbiturates vary depending on the drug used. Some of the adverse reactions that may be seen with nonbarbiturate administration are listed in Summary Drug Table 12-1.

SUMMARY DRUG TABLE 12–1
Sedatives and Hypnotics

GENERIC NAME	TRADE NAME*	USES	ADVERSE REACTIONS	DOSE RANGES
BARBITURATES				
amobarbital, amobarbital sodium	Amytal, Amytal Sodium	Sedation, anxiety, hypnotic, preanesthetic sedation	Somnolence, agitation, confusion, CNS depression, skin rashes, respiratory depression, residual sedation (hangover effect), fever, headache, lethargy	Sedative: 15–120 mg PO; hypnotic: 100–200 mg PO; IV administration: up to 1 mL/min; IM: up to 500 mg
butabarbital sodium	Butisol Sodium, *generic*	As sedative, hypnotic	Same as amobarbital	Sedative: 15–30 mg PO; hypnotic: 50–100 mg PO
pentobarbital, pentobarbital sodium	Nembutal Sodium, Nembutal, *generic*	Same as amobarbital	Same as amobarbital	Sedative: 20 mg PO tid, qid; hypnotic: 100 mg PO; 120–200 mg rectal suppository; IM: 150–200 mg; IV: up to 200 mg
phenobarbital, phenobarbital sodium	Luminal, Solfoton, *generic*	As sedative	Same as amobarbital	30–120 mg/d PO in divided doses; 100–300 mg IM, IV
secobarbital, secobarbital sodium	Seconal, *generic*	As hypnotic, preanesthetic sedative	Same as amobarbital	Hypnotic: 100 mg PO, 100–200 mg IM; preanesthetic sedative: 200–300 mg IM
NONBARBITURATES				
chloral hydrate	Noctec, *generic*	As hypnotic, sedative	Skin rash, GI upset, somnolence, disorientation	Hypnotic: 500 mg–1 g PO; sedative: 250 mg PO tid pc
ethchlorvynol	Placidyl	As hypnotic, sedative	Nausea, vomiting, rash, dizziness, hypotension	Hypnotic: 500 mg PO; sedative: 100–200 mg bid, tid
ethinamate	Valmid	As hypnotic	Rash, mild GI symptoms	500–1000 mg PO
flurazepam hydrochloride	Dalmane, *generic*	As hypnotic	Dizziness, heartburn, nausea, vomiting, weakness	15–30 mg PO
glutethimide	*Generic*	As hypnotic	Skin rash, nausea, blurred vision	250–500 mg PO
methyprylon	Noludar	As hypnotic	Morning drowsiness, gastric upset, dizziness	200–400 mg PO
paraldehyde	Paral	As hypnotic, sedative	GI upset, drowsiness	Up to 10 mL PO; rectal: 10–20 mL mixed with oil
propiomazine	Largon	As sedative (preoperatively, during minor surgery)	Dry mouth, moderate elevation of blood pressure	Preoperative: 20 mg IM; sedation during surgery: 10–20 mg IM, IV; obstetrics: 20–40 mg IM, IV
temazepam	Restoril, *generic*	As hypnotic	Drowsiness, dizziness, lethargy	15–30 mg PO
triazolam	Halcion	As hypnotic	Drowsiness, headache, dizziness, nervousness	0.125–0.5 mg PO

* The term generic indicates that the drug is available in a generic form.

▶ NURSING PROCESS
THE PATIENT RECEIVING A SEDATIVE OR HYPNOTIC

ASSESSMENT

Assessment of the patient receiving a sedative or hypnotic drug depends on the reason for administration and whether the drug is given routinely or whenever necessary (prn). Before administering a barbiturate or nonbarbiturate, the patient's blood pressure, pulse, and respiratory rate are taken and recorded.

If the patient is receiving one of these drugs for daytime sedation, the patient's general mental state and level of consciousness is assessed. If the patient appears sedated and difficult to awaken, the dose of the drug should be withheld and the physician contacted.

Before administering a prn hypnotic, the nurse must assess the following patient needs:

1. Is the patient uncomfortable? If the reason for discomfort is pain, an analgesic rather than a hypnotic may be required.

2. Is it too early for the patient to receive the drug? Is a later hour preferred?

3. On previous nights, has the drug helped the patient sleep? If not, a different drug or dose may be needed, and the physician should be consulted regarding the drug's ineffectiveness.

4. Does the patient receive a narcotic analgesic every 4 to 6 hours? A hypnotic may not be necessary because a narcotic analgesic is also capable of causing drowsiness and sleep.

5. Are there disturbances in the environment that may keep the patient awake and decrease the effectiveness of the drug?

Barbiturates have little analgesic action, and therefore are not given if the patient has pain that can be controlled with an analgesic. Because narcotic analgesics depress the CNS (see chap 10), a barbiturate or nonbarbiturate is not administered shortly before or after administration of a *narcotic analgesic or other CNS depressant*. If the patient has an order for a prn narcotic analgesic or other CNS depressant *and* a hypnotic, the physician is consulted regarding the time interval between administration of these drugs. Usually at least 2 hours should elapse between administration of a hypnotic and any other CNS depressant, but this interval may vary depending on factors such as the patient's age and diagnosis. If the time interval between administration of a narcotic analgesic and a sedative or hypnotic is less than 2 hours, the patient may experience severe respiratory depression, bradycardia, and unresponsiveness.

NURSING DIAGNOSIS

Depending on the drug, dose, and reason for administration, one or more of the following nursing diagnoses may apply to a person receiving a sedative or hypnotic drug:

▶ Anxiety related to inability to sleep, other factors (specify)

▶ Noncompliance related to indifference, lack of knowledge, failure of the drug to produce sedation or sleep, other factors

▶ High risk for injury related to sedative or hypnotic effects of drug

▶ Knowledge deficit of medication regimen, adverse drug effects, warnings regarding use of the drug

PLANNING AND IMPLEMENTATION

The major goals of the patient may include sedation or sleep, reduction in anxiety, and an understanding of and compliance with the postdischarge medication regimen (when applicable).

The major goals of nursing management may include competent assessment of the need for a sedative or hypnotic, recognition of adverse drug effects, reduction in patient anxiety, and the development and implementation of an effective teaching plan when one of these drugs is prescribed for use after discharge from the hospital.

ADMINISTRATION. Hypnotics and sedatives are never left at the bedside to be taken at a later hour. This applies to all drugs except for drugs specifically ordered to be left at the patient's bedside. Hypnotics and sedatives are controlled substances (see chap 3). These drugs should not be left unattended in the nurses' station, hallway, or other areas to which patients, visitors, or hospital personnel have direct access. If these drugs are prepared in advance, they should be placed in a locked cupboard until the time of administration.

Following assessment of the patient, the nurse must make a decision regarding administration of the drug. This is especially true when one of these drugs is ordered to be given as needed. The drug should be withheld and the physician notified if any one or more vital signs significantly varies from the data base, if the respiratory rate is 10 or below, or if the patient appears lethargic. The nurse must also determine if there are any factors (eg, noise, lights, pain, discomfort) that would interfere with sleep and whether these may be controlled or eliminated.

When these drugs are given orally, the patient is encouraged to drink a full glass of water with the medication. When barbiturates are administered intramuscularly (IM), they are given in the gluteus maximus or vastus lateralis or other areas where there is little risk of encountering a nerve trunk or major artery. Injection near or into peripheral nerves may result in permanent nerve damage.

On rare occasions, paraldehyde may be ordered for the patient with signs of alcohol withdrawal (DTs). Intramuscular injection of paraldehyde is painful, and assistance may be needed when the drug is administered by this route. If more than 5 mL is ordered, the dose is divided and given deep IM in both buttocks. When given as an oral liquid, paraldehyde can be mixed with cold orange or tomato juice to eliminate some of the pungent taste.

HIGH RISK FOR INJURY. After administration of a hypnotic, the side rails are raised and the patient is advised to remain in bed and call for assistance if it is necessary to get out of bed. Patients receiving sedative doses may or may not require this safety measure, depending on the patient's response to the drug. The nurse must assess the patient receiving a sedative dose and determine what safety measures must be taken.

The patient receiving a hypnotic is assessed in 1 to 2 hours after the drug is given to evaluate the effect of the drug.

ADVERSE DRUG REACTIONS. As with any drug, the patient is observed for adverse drug reactions. Elderly and debilitated patients are observed for marked excitement, depression, and confusion. If excitement or confusion occurs, the patient is observed at frequent intervals (as often as every 5 to 10 minutes may be necessary) for the duration of this occurrence and safety measures are instituted to prevent injury. The physician should be informed if the patient fails to sleep, awakens one or more times during the night, or develops an adverse drug reaction. In some instances, supplemental doses of a hypnotic may be ordered if the patient awakes during the night.

Excessive drowsiness and headache the morning after a hypnotic has been given (''drug hangover'') may occur in some patients. It should be reported to the physician. A smaller dose or a different drug may be necessary.

DRUG DEPENDENCY. If a barbiturate or nonbarbiturate has been taken for a long time, drug dependency may develop. These drugs must *never* be suddenly discontinued when there is a question of possible dependency. Symptoms of withdrawal can result in serious consequences, especially in those with existing diseases or disorders.

ANXIETY. Many hospitalized patients find it difficult to sleep. The inability to fall asleep or stay asleep often results in varying degrees of anxiety. The nurse should reassure the patient that in most instances the drug being given will help them sleep.

NONCOMPLIANCE AND KNOWLEDGE DEFICIT. The patient and family should have an explanation of the prescribed drug and dosage regimen as well as situations that should be avoided.

The following points should be stressed when a hypnotic or sedative is prescribed:

▶ Do *not* increase or decrease the dose unless a change in dosage is recommended by the physician.

▶ If the drug appears to be ineffective, do *not* increase the dose but contact the physician. Do not repeat the dose during the night unless the physician approves a repeat dose.

▶ Notify the physician if any adverse drug reactions occur.

▶ The physician usually prescribes these drugs for short-term use only.

▶ These drugs may impair the mental and physical abilities required for performing potentially dangerous tasks such as driving a car or operating machinery.

▶ Do not consume alcohol when taking this drug. Use of alcohol and any one of these drugs can result in additive depressant effects. Deaths have been reported with the consumption of alcohol either with the drug or several hours before or after the drug is taken.

▶ Over-the-counter cold, cough, or allergy medication cannot be used unless approved by the physician. Some of these products contain antihistamines or other drugs that also may cause drowsiness. Others may contain an adrenergic drug, which is a mild stimulant, and therefore defeat the purpose of the drug.

To ensure compliance to the prescribed dosage, the nurse must stress the importance of not increasing the dosage of the drug if or when the drug fails to produce the desired effect.

EVALUATION

▶ Anxiety is reduced
▶ Patient obtains optimal benefit from the drug
▶ No evidence of injury
▶ Patient and family demonstrate understanding of drug regimen
▶ Verbalizes importance of complying with the prescribed treatment regimen
▶ Verbalizes understanding of things to avoid while taking the drug

13

Substance Abuse

On completion of this chapter the student will:

▶ *Differentiate between physical and psychological drug dependency*

▶ *Define drug addiction and drug habituation*

▶ *Discuss the dangers associated with substance abuse*

▶ *Describe the methods of treating drug addiction*

Substance (drug) abuse has become one of the leading problems worldwide. The social and economic impact of drug addiction and abuse directly or indirectly affects every member of society. The terms *drug* and *substance* often are used inter. Substance or drug abuse is the use of a natural or synthetic substance to alter mood or behavior in a manner that differs from its generally accepted use.

Substance abuse may be defined as the use of a drug or chemical to produce a change in mood or behavior in a way that departs from approved medical or social patterns.

Compulsive substance abuse is the need to use any drug or chemical substance repeatedly to produce the desired effect. The need to use a drug compulsively may be physical, psychological, or both.

Physical dependency is a compulsive need to use a substance repeatedly to avoid mild to severe withdrawal symptoms; it is the body's dependence on repeated administration of a drug. **Psychological dependency** is a compulsion to use a substance to obtain a pleasurable experience; it is the mind's dependence on the repeated administration of a drug.

Drug tolerance is a need to increase the dose or the frequency of use to obtain the original or desired effect.

When an individual is physically or psychologically dependent on a drug, there is a craving to use the drug repeatedly. If the drug is suddenly withdrawn, symptoms of **drug withdrawal** occur. Symptoms of drug withdrawal are also called the **abstinence syndrome.** Symptoms of the abstinence syndrome can range from very mild to severe, depending on the drug involved, the dose used, the frequency of use, the length of time the drug has been used, and the individual.

Drug addiction may be defined to include the following:

▷ A compulsive desire or craving to use a drug or chemical

▷ An involvement with the drug to the exclusion of all other activities such as work, recreation, family, or school

▷ A strong tendency to return to the drug after withdrawal

▷ A tendency to increase the dose or frequency of use

▷ Physical dependence

▷ The abstinence syndrome produces moderate to severe physical reactions

▷ Detriments to society can exist in the drug and its use, as well as in the user

Drug habituation may be defined to include the following:

▷ A desire to use a drug continually for the effects produced

▷ Little or no tendency to increase the dose

▷ No physical dependence; rather, psychological dependence

▷ When the drug is withdrawn, there is no true abstinence syndrome

▷ The detrimental effect, if any exists, is on the individual rather than society

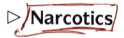

▷ **Narcotics**

Heroin

Heroin (diacetylmorphine) is obtained from morphine (see chap 10), the principal alkaloid of raw opium, and is an illegal drug in the United States. It is the strongest and most addicting of all the opium derivatives, and is not used in the United States as an analgesic. Physical addiction to heroin occurs rapidly, often within several weeks of frequent use, but this varies. Heroin addiction poses serious socioeconomic problems, both to individuals, families, and the community. The cost of a heroin drug habit is high and can deplete finances or require the user to engage in criminal activity (eg, stealing, prostitution) to obtain money to support a drug habit. Continued use of heroin may result in other physical problems such as malnutrition and physical neglect. Those who use the drug intravenously (IV) may develop serious medical disorders. Septicemia may develop if the needle, syringe, or equipment used to prepare the heroin for injection become contaminated. Hepatitis or the acquired immunodeficiency syndrome (AIDS) can be transmitted from one individual to another when contaminated needles and syringes are shared among users.

EFFECTS OF HEROIN

Heroin may be inhaled ("sniffed") or injected subcutaneously (SC; "skin popping") or IV ("mainlining"). The desired effects on the user are euphoria and drowsiness. Mentally, there is an escape from reality. Other effects are those associated with the opiates, namely, anorexia, fixed pinpoint pupils, constipation, and a decreased pulse and respiratory rate. Continued IV use results in scarred veins with skin markings, referred to as tracks.

HEROIN WITHDRAWAL

Signs of heroin withdrawal (abstinence syndrome) are yawning, perspiration, tearing of the eyes, increased nasal discharge, gooseflesh, abdominal cramps, bone and muscle pain, nausea, vomiting, diarrhea, dilatation of the pupils, restlessness, increase in body temperature, increase in pulse and respiratory rate, marked mental depression or despair, and an intense desire (craving) for the drug. The symptoms of withdrawal usually begin when the next dose of heroin is due, reach a peak in 36 to 72 hours, and gradually diminish in 4 or 5 days.

Some individuals accidentally or intentionally take or are given overdoses of heroin. Symptoms of overdose are stupor, pinpoint pupils, nausea, vomiting, decreased pulse and respiratory rate, and signs of shock. Coma may be present. If the overdose is recognized and the individual taken to a hospital, a narcotic antagonist, which will reverse the effects of the heroin, is administered. Other medical treatment is also instituted. Unfortunately, many cases of overdose are never treated and the individual dies.

Heroin crosses the placental barrier. A child born of a mother addicted to heroin is also addicted to the drug and needs immediate treatment. Even after receiving treatment, some infants die.

Other Narcotic Analgesics

Opiates, such as morphine, and other narcotics, such as meperidine (Demerol), are used less frequently than heroin as street drugs (ie, drugs obtained from illegal sources), except as substitutes when heroin is unavailable. Addiction to legal narcotics may occur in those receiving the drug while under the care of a physician, as in the case of a terminally ill cancer patient. Some people become addicted to a narcotic because of a physician's carelessness in prescribing the drug in the treatment of a nonterminal illness.

The Terminally Ill

Terminally ill cancer patients who require a narcotic eventually become addicted to the drug after it has been given for several weeks. Addiction in these patients is morally and legally acceptable. Terminally ill patients in need of pain relief should never be denied a prescribed analgesic because of the potential for addiction. If addiction has occurred, these patients should be given the drug as ordered and on time. Making the patient wait for the drug may result in withdrawal symptoms, which will only add to the pain of her or his illness.

Members of the medical profession administer, prescribe, and dispense narcotics. A few may be tempted to experience the effects of a narcotic and subsequently may continue to use the drug. In some instances, addiction is kept well-hidden and may never be detected. At other times, a change in work performance or personality may give rise to suspicion among fellow workers. Nurses have taken narcotics meant for a patient, and the only clue to misappropriated narcotics is a patient's complaint about failure of the drug to relieve pain. Any suspicion of addiction is brought to the attention of the head nurse or supervisor.

Individuals addicted to opiates and other narcotics experience an abstinence syndrome similar to that experienced by the heroin user. They are also prone to the same dangers, such as hepatitis, septicemia, and AIDS if materials for preparation and administration are shared with others.

▷ Cocaine

Cocaine is an alkaloid obtained from coca leaves. Cocaine is highly addicting and, presently, is the number one substance abuse problem. Use of cocaine has created serious and sometimes deadly consequences that affect the individuals, families, and the community. It still is used in medicine occasionally as a local anesthetic but this use has been largely discontinued.

EFFECTS OF COCAINE

Cocaine stimulates the central nervous system (CNS), producing marked euphoria and excitement. The powder form of cocaine is snorted (inhaled through the nose) or dissolved and injected IV. Crack, a purified form of cocaine with a crystalline or rocklike appearance, is smoked either by placing it in a pipe or by sprinkling it on or mixing it with tobacco. Cocaine may be freebased, which reduces it to its purest form. It is then smoked by sprinkling it on a cigarette or inhaling it through a pipe. Freebasing produces a more immediate rush than when the substance is used by nasal inhalation. The heroin addict usually does not use cocaine as a substitute for heroin but may mix it with heroin and inject it IV to obtain a greater drug effect. This combination is called a "speed-ball."

DANGERS ASSOCIATED WITH THE USE OF COCAINE

Cocaine's danger lies in its ability to cause physical and psychological dependency, as well as permanent damage to the nasal mucosa. The cost of a cocaine habit can reach astounding figures. The individual using cocaine frequently can spend thousands of dollars each month to support his or her drug habit.

Signs and symptoms of acute toxicity include agitation, psychotic behavior, violent behavior, hyperthermia, seizures, dysrhythmias, hypertension, respiratory failure, and dilated pupils. In some individuals, acute toxicity can occur at any time and with any dose. There are times when acute toxicity can result in death.

Signs and symptoms of chronic toxicity include dysrhythmias, hypertension, memory impairment, personality and behavioral changes, ulceration of the nasal mucosa and perforation of the nasal septum (in those who inhale cocaine), needle marks along the pathways of veins (in those who use cocaine IV), anorexia, weight loss, psychosis, and hallucinations.

Cocaine use results in physical dependence. In some people, dependence occurs rapidly—sometimes after one or two uses. How soon physical dependence occurs appears to vary with the individual and pattern of use. Use of this drug also results in psychological dependency. Withdrawal usually is characterized by depression, psychosis, lethargy, restlessness, an intense craving for the drug, inability to concentrate, and irritability.

▷ Marijuana

Marijuana is classified as a hallucinogen, that is, a drug capable of producing a state of delirium characterized by visual and sensory disturbances that are bizarre and distorted. Marijuana belongs to a family of plants called *Cannabis*. The substance or chemical that gives the hallucinogenic effect is a resin from the dried plant tetrahydrocannabinol (THC). The resin extracted from the plant's flowers is called *hashish*, which is 5 to 10 times more potent than the more common variety.

EFFECTS OF MARIJUANA

Users of marijuana may experience a variety of effects that appear to depend on the individual, as well as the amount of THC in the marijuana. The user may experience euphoria, drowsiness, dizziness, light-headedness, visual disturbances, sensory distortions, hunger (especially for sweets), giddiness, and hallucinations. On occasion, other effects such as panic, depression, nausea, vomiting, diarrhea, dryness of the mouth, inflammation and burning of the eyes, decrease in blood pressure, increase in pulse rate, and dilatation of the pupils may occur. Some individuals experience no drug effects, but this may be because the product they used contained fillers and very little marijuana. The effects of the drug usually last 2 to 4 hours, but this is highly variable.

Signs of chronic marijuana use include a lack of interest in school, work, and other people, carelessness in personal hygiene and clothes, a preoccupied appearance, lack of motivation, memory difficulty, and passiveness or apathy.

Marijuana is used medically on a limited basis to lower intraocular pressure in those with glaucoma and in selected terminally ill cancer patients. Specific guidelines in dispensing the drug are required and legal use of the drug is limited to research institutions or physicians who have applied for government approval of marijuana use in certain patients.

▷ Psychotomimetic Drugs

A psychotomimetic (hallucinogenic) drug produces an acute change in the perception of reality. Examples of drugs in this group are mescaline, lysergic acid diethylamide (LSD), 2,5-dimethoxy-4-methylamphetamine (DOM; also called STP), psilocybin, phencyclidine (PCP, angel dust) and dimethyltryptamine (DMT).

Use of these agents causes visual hallucinations and mood changes. The results are inconsistent and differ from person to person—and even within the same person—when the drug is taken under varying circumstances. Psychotic episodes may occur during and after use, and may progress to periodic occurrences even when the drug is not being used. These events take place more frequently in those who have underlying emotional problems. Another problem that may occur for many years after use has

been discontinued is flashbacks, which are more common with LSD use. Flashbacks are brief episodes of the original sensations experienced during use of the substance. The frequency of flashbacks is variable.

Although physical dependence on these drugs does not occur, the user can develop a psychological dependence. No physical withdrawal symptoms occur if use of the substance is discontinued.

▷ **Amphetamines**

Amphetamine, dextroamphetamine, and methamphetamine are adrenergic drugs intended for use as CNS stimulants and anorexiants (drugs that suppress the appetite). Because of the abuse potential of these drugs, their use in medicine in the treatment of obesity has declined. These drugs still have value in the treatment of some obese individuals and in those conditions or diseases requiring CNS stimulation. When medical use of these drugs is necessary, therapy is under the close supervision of a physician.

EFFECTS OF THE AMPHETAMINES

Amphetamines produce euphoria, alertness, and a sense of excitation. The user is talkative, restless, excitable, and perspires freely, and his or her pupils may be dilated. Some use the drug to stay awake for long periods of time or to experience the euphoria produced by the drug. Others may use amphetamines when other illegal substances are not available, or when the drugs are of such a poor quality or strength that the expected effects are decreased.

The drug is usually taken orally, but it is also used IV to produce an instant euphoric effect that is greater in intensity than that produced by the oral route. Some individuals may use an amphetamine for several days, taking the drug every few hours. During this time, the user is in a constant state of euphoria, excitement, and sleeplessness. The drug is usually discontinued because of exhaustion, confusion, or disorientation.

Some substance abusers are involved with more than one drug. Individuals using amphetamines may take a tranquilizer or barbiturate after several days of amphetamine use to reduce the effects produced by the amphetamine. Those using amphetamines may be belligerent and may develop severe psychosis. Depression and suicidal tendencies may occur when the drug is withdrawn. These drugs have addiction potential.

▷ Barbiturates and Nonbarbiturates

Barbiturate and nonbarbiturate drugs have their proper use in medicine but are also subject to abuse. Drug tolerance can develop in the chronic barbiturate user, and these drugs have physical and psychological addiction potential when used for a period of time. Some of the nonbarbiturates have a low addiction potential, but use of large doses for a long time can result in physical and psychological addiction.

When these drugs are subject to abuse or are used under a physician's supervision for a long time, they must *never* be suddenly discontinued. Instead, the dose must be slowly tapered over time. When sudden discontinuation of a barbiturate occurs, there is an abstinence syndrome characterized by abdominal cramps, nausea, vomiting, weakness, and tremors. In some persons, withdrawal from barbiturates can be more harmful physically than withdrawal from heroin.

An overdose of these drugs can result in convulsions, delirium, coma, and in some instances, death.

▷ Tranquilizers

As a group, tranquilizers have been subject to widespread abuse by those involved in substance abuse, as well as by persons who do not consider themselves "drug users." When tranquilizers were first placed on the market, they were not believed to be physically addicting and were frequently prescribed by physicians for mild cases of anxiety and stress. Although they do have a definite use in medicine, they were and perhaps still are overprescribed by some physicians. Unfortunately, the overuse of tranquilizers has resulted in many individuals being physically addicted to these drugs.

Addiction to these drugs appears to occur fairly rapidly, although the time required to produce addiction often depends on the type of tranquilizer, the individual, and the tendency to increase the dose to produce the desired effect. Withdrawal, when it does occur, resembles barbiturate withdrawal, with the intensity of symptoms depending on the length of time the drug was used and the dose most frequently used. Those experiencing withdrawal also experience extreme anxiety and nervousness and a strong desire to return to the drug.

▷ Alcohol

Much has been written about alcohol abuse and alcoholism because it is a major problem. For a wide variety of reasons, alcohol is subject to widespread abuse among all ages and socioeconomic levels. Malnutrition, physical disease, broken marriages, crime, loss of employment, and accidents resulting in injury or death are examples of the many problems associated with alcohol use. The chronic and even occasional alcohol user may additionally use other drugs such as sedatives, tranquilizers, amphetamines, and cocaine. The use of alcohol and one or more of these drugs may have serious consequences because alcohol can potentiate the action of these as well as other drugs. Deaths have been reported with the use of alcohol along with a CNS depressant such as a barbiturate, nonbarbiturate, narcotic, or tranquilizer. Every year many people are killed by drivers who are under the influence of alcohol. Airing television commercials, printing newspaper and magazine articles, and raising the drinking age in some states are methods being used to discourage alcohol abuse. Groups have formed to encourage stricter laws for those convicted of driving while impaired, and businesses have developed programs aimed at helping employees who are compulsive drinkers.

Alcohol is a potentially physically addicting substance. The time or amount of alcohol consumption required to produce physical addiction varies. Signs of withdrawal from alcohol usually appear within 12 to 72 hours, but may appear sooner in some individuals. These signs usually include tremors, weakness, anxiety, restlessness, excessive perspiration, nausea, and vomiting. Seizures may occur in some individuals during the first 24 hours of withdrawal. Hallucinations, which are frequently terrifying, are often experienced. Recovery from withdrawal usually occurs within 5 to 7 days. During the period of alcohol withdrawal ("drying out"), the patient should be under medical supervision.

▷ Methods of Treating Substance Abuse

Methods for treating substance abuse vary not only from drug to drug but in the methods that may be used for a specific drug. Some physicians or drug rehabilitation centers advocate one method of treatment and claim good results, whereas others use a different method and claim equally good or better results. In some instances, the individual addicted to one or more drugs or chemicals may need to try more than one treatment method to achieve results. In the treatment of substance abuse, success depends on the individual's desire to become drug-free. If the individual is forced by parents, by a spouse, or by the court to enter a drug treatment program, there is less chance that treatment will be effective and that the individual will remain drug-free for the rest of his or her life.

Narcotic addiction can be treated in clinics that aim at reducing or eliminating withdrawal symptoms. Methadone, a synthetic narcotic, is used to wean the patient away from and satisfy his craving for the narcotic to which he was addicted. Although addiction to methadone will occur, the patient can be gradually withdrawn from methadone. Methadone withdrawal is less severe than withdrawal from heroin and other narcotics. Counseling and other types of support are provided during and after the treatment period.

Naltrexone (Trexan), a narcotic antagonist (see chap 10), is also used in the treatment of opioid addiction. The drug is used to maintain an opioid-free state in those who have been addicted to an opioid narcotic and are in a detoxified state. Treatment is not begun until the individual has been without a narcotic (opioid-free state) for 7 to 10 days. Individuals taking naltrexone on a regular basis will not obtain any effect from an opioid narcotic should there be an attempt to return to these drugs.

Addiction to other drugs such as cocaine, tranquilizers, or barbiturates may be treated by a physician, in individual clinics, or in public or private drug rehabilitation centers. Withdrawal from these drugs is necessary. Counseling and support therapy is an important part of treatment.

Chronic alcoholism, with or without a history of other substance abuse, may be treated by a physician or in public or private treatment centers. Alcoholics Anonymous (AA) is a support group that has done much to help the alcoholic attain and maintain an alcohol-free state.

▷ Conclusion

As members of the health care professions, nurses must be aware of the signs of substance abuse and overdose. Any patient entering a general hospital may have a hidden history of substance abuse, including alcohol. This includes patients on a pediatric, as well as an adult, hospital unit. Any patient showing unusual behavior, asking for narcotics, or showing physical signs that do not appear related to the diagnosis or disease is closely observed. All observations are carefully documented in the patient's record and reported to the physician and supervisory personnel.

Regardless of the drug used, substance abuse is dangerous. In addition to the danger of physical dependency with many of these agents, the social, legal, and economic implications may be devastating. Substance abuse can lead to various physical and mental disorders such as malnutrition, weight loss, mental changes, and psychotic episodes. Intravenous drug users may develop hepatitis, septicemia, or AIDS, all of which can be fatal.

14

The Cardiotonics and Antiarrhythmic Drugs

On completion of this chapter the student will:

▶ *Discuss the uses and general drug actions of the cardiotonics and antiarrhythmic drugs*

▶ *List the general adverse reactions seen with the administration of a cardiotonic or antiarrhythmic drug*

▶ *Define and list the symptoms of digitalis toxicity*

▶ *Use the nursing process when administering a cardiotonic or antiarrhythmic drug*

▶ *Discuss the nursing implications associated with the administration of a cardiotonic or antiarrhythmic*

▶ THE CARDIOTONICS

The cardiotonics include deslanoside (Cedilanid-D), digitoxin, and digoxin (Lanoxin) and are sometimes called cardiac glycosides or digitalis glycosides. A glycoside is a substance obtained from plants, which when treated chemically yields a sugar and one or more other substances.

digitalis prep depend on Flower used Potency
leave - gardens Purple Flowers

▷ Actions of the Cardiotonics

The heart that is weakened by disease, age, or both is often in need of drug therapy. The cardiotonics all have the same basic drug action; the only difference is in the speed and duration of action of each drug. A

or cardiac glycosides

heart weakened by disease or age sometimes cannot pump a sufficient amount of blood. This results in a decrease in the amount of oxygenated blood leaving the left ventricle during each myocardial contraction. The amount of blood leaving the left ventricle at the time of each contraction is called the *cardiac output*. A marked decrease in cardiac output deprives the kidneys, brain, and other vital organs of an adequate blood supply. When the kidneys are deprived of an adequate blood supply, they are unable to effectively remove water, electrolytes, and waste products from the bloodstream. Excess fluid (edema) may occur in the lungs or tissues. The body then attempts to make up for this deficit by increasing the heart rate, which, in turn, circulates more blood through the kidneys, brain, and other vital organs. In many instances, an increase in the heart rate ultimately fails to deliver an adequate amount of blood to the kidneys, as well as to other vital organs. An increased heart rate also places added strain on the heart's muscle, which may further weaken the heart.

Cardiotonic drugs increase the force of contraction of the muscle (myocardium) of the heart. This is called a *positive inotropic action*. When the force of contraction of the myocardium is increased, cardiac output is increased. When cardiac output is increased, the blood supply to the kidneys and other vital organs is then increased. Water, electrolytes, and waste products are removed in adequate amounts and the symptoms of inadequate heart action or congestive heart failure (CHF) are relieved. In most instances, the heart rate also decreases since vital organs are now receiving an adequate blood supply because of the increased force of myocardial contraction.

The cardiotonics also affect the transmission of electrical impulses along the pathway of the conduction system of the heart. The conduction system of the heart is a group of specialized nerve fibers consisting of the sinoatrial (SA) node, the atrioventricular (AV) node, the bundle of His, and the branches of Purkinje (Fig. 14-1). Each heartbeat (or contraction

Vena cava

SA node

AV node

Left atrium

Bundle of His

Bundle branches

Right atrium

Left ventricle

Purkinje fibers

Papillary muscle

Right ventricle

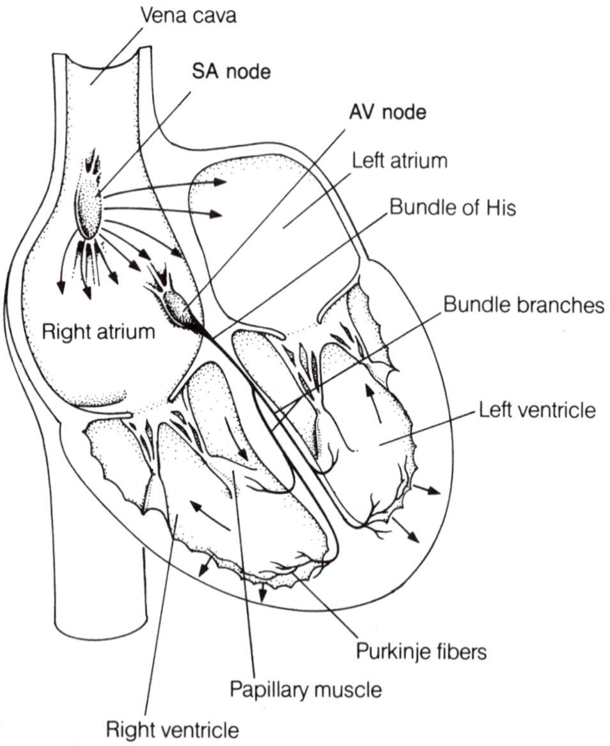

FIGURE 14–1. The conducting system of the heart. Impulses originating in the SA node are transmitted through the atrial bundles to the AV node and down the bundle of His and the bundle branches by way of the Purkinje fibers through the ventricles.

of the ventricles), which is the pulse felt at the wrist and other areas of the body where an artery is close to the surface or lies near a bone, is the result of an electrical impulse that normally starts in the SA node, is then received by the AV node, and then travels down the bundle of His and through the Purkinje fibers (see Fig. 14-1). When the electrical impulse reaches the Purkinje fibers, the ventricles contract. Normally, once the ventricles contract, another electrical impulse is generated by the SA node and the cycle begins again. Cardiotonic drugs depress the SA node and slow conduction of the electrical impulse to the AV node. Slowing this part of the transmission of nerve impulses decreases the number of impulses and the number of ventricular contractions per minute.

▷ Uses of the Cardiotonics

The cardiotonics are used in the treatment of CHF, atrial fibrillation, atrial flutter, and paroxysmal tachycardia.

▷ Adverse Reactions Associated with the Administration of the Cardiotonics

There is a narrow margin of safety between the full therapeutic effects and the toxic effects of cardiotonic drugs. After a time, even normal doses of a cardiotonic can cause toxic drug effects. The term **digitalis toxicity** (digitalis intoxication) is used when toxic drug effects occur when *any* cardiotonic is administered. The signs of digitalis toxicity include the following:

Gastrointestinal (GI)—anorexia, nausea, vomiting, diarrhea

Muscular—weakness (asthenia)

Central nervous system—headache, apathy, drowsiness, visual disturbances (blurred vision, disturbance in yellow/green vision, halo effect around dark objects), mental depression, confusion, disorientation, delirium.

Cardiac—changes in pulse rate or rhythm

Digitalis toxicity often results in electrocardiographic (ECG) changes such as bradycardia, tachycardia, premature ventricular contractions (PVCs), and a bigeminy (two beats followed by a pause) or trigeminy (three beats followed by a pause)

pulse. Other dysrhythmias (abnormal heart rhythm) may also be seen. Any change in the pulse rate or rhythm *may* indicate digitalis toxicity.

The physician may treat digitalis toxicity by temporarily discontinuing the drug until signs of toxicity disappear. The physician may also order a potassium salt to be given orally or intravenously (IV). If severe bradycardia occurs, atropine (see chap 9) may be ordered. If digoxin or digitoxin has been given, the physician may order blood tests to determine drug serum levels. The therapeutic serum level of digoxin is 0.5 to 2 ng/mL (nanogram/milliliter) and the toxic serum level is more than 2.5 ng/mL. The therapeutic serum level of digitoxin is 14 to 26 ng/mL and the toxic serum level is more than 35 ng/mL.

Digoxin has a rapid onset and a short duration of action, whereas digitoxin has a slower onset and longer duration of action. Once the drug is withheld, the toxic effects of digoxin will disappear more rapidly than those of digitoxin. Digitalis has a slow onset and long duration of action. Deslanoside, which is only given parenterally, has an onset and duration of action similar to, but slightly longer than, parenteral digoxin.

▶ NURSING PROCESS
THE PATIENT RECEIVING A CARDIOTONIC

ASSESSMENT

The cardiotonics are potentially toxic drugs, and the patient must be closely observed, especially during initial therapy. Before therapy is started, the physical assessment should include information that will establish a data base for comparison during therapy. The following can be included in the physical assessment:

▶ Blood pressure, apical–radial pulse rate, respiratory rate

▶ Auscultation of the lungs noting any unusual sounds during inspiration and expiration

▶ Examination of the extremities for edema

▶ Checking the jugular veins for distention

▶ Weight

▶ Inspecting sputum raised (if any), and noting the appearance (eg, frothy, pink-tinged, clear, yellow, and so on)

▶ Looking for evidence of other problems such as cyanosis, shortness of breath on exertion (if the patient is allowed out of bed) or when lying flat, mental changes, and so on

The physician may also order laboratory and diagnostic tests such as an ECG, renal and hepatic function tests, complete blood count (CBC), serum enzymes, and serum electrolytes. These tests should be reviewed before the first dose is given. When subsequent laboratory tests are ordered, they also should be reviewed when the results are recorded on the patient's record.

NURSING DIAGNOSIS

Depending on the drug, dose, reason for administration, and possible adverse drug reactions, one or more of the following nursing diagnoses may apply to a person receiving a cardiotonic drug:

▶ Anxiety related to diagnosis, possible lifetime drug therapy, other factors (specify)

▶ Diarrhea related to adverse drug effect

▶ Altered nutrition: less than body requirements related to anorexia secondary to adverse drug effect

▶ Noncompliance related to indifference, lack of knowledge, other factors

▶ Knowledge deficit of treatment regimen, monitoring of response to therapy

PLANNING AND IMPLEMENTATION

The major goals of the patient may include a reduction in anxiety, an absence of adverse drug effects, and an understanding of and compliance with the postdischarge medication regimen.

The major goals of nursing management may include a reduction in patient anxiety, recognition of adverse drug effects and signs of digitalis toxicity, and the development and implementation of an effective teaching plan.

DIGITALIZATION. Patients started on therapy with a cardiotonic are being **digitalized**. Digitalizing doses are also referred to as **loading doses**. Digitalization (the administration of digitalizing doses) is a series of doses given until the drug begins to exert a **full therapeutic effect**. Once a full therapeutic effect is achieved, the patient is usually placed on a **maintenance dose** schedule. The ranges for digitalizing (loading) and maintenance doses are given in Summary Drug Table 14-1. There are variations in digitalizing doses, and the physician may decide to achieve full digitalization rapidly or slowly, depending on the patient's diagnosis, age, present condition, and other factors.

ADMINISTRATION. Before administering *each dose* of a cardiotonic, the pulse rate is taken for 60 seconds; 30

SUMMARY DRUG TABLE 14–1
Cardiotonics and Antiarrhythmic Drugs

GENERIC NAME	TRADE NAME*	USES	ADVERSE REACTIONS	DOSE RANGES
CARDIOTONICS				
deslanoside	Cedilanid-D	Congestive heart failure, atrial fibrillation and flutter, paroxysmal atrial tachycardia	Digitalis toxicity (see text)	Loading dose: 1.6 mg IV, IM given as 1 injection or in portions of 0.8 mg each
digitoxin	Crystodigin, *generic*	Same as deslanoside	Same as deslanoside	Loading dose: rapid digitalization—0.6 mg followed by 0.4 mg PO, then 0.2 mg at 4–6-h intervals; slow digitalization: 0.2 mg PO bid for 4 d; maintenance dose: 0.05–0.3 mg/d PO
digoxin	Lanoxin, Lanoxicaps, *generic*	Same as deslanoside	Same as deslanoside	Loading dose: 0.4–0.6 mg IV or 0.5–0.75 mg PO but dosage for both routes varies; maintenance: based on serum digoxin levels
ANTIARRHYTHMIC DRUGS				
amiodarone	Cordarone	Life-threatening ventricular dysrhythmias	Malaise, fatigue, tremor, nausea, vomiting, constipation, ataxia, anorexia, photosensitivity	Loading dose: 800–1600 mg/d PO in divided doses; maintenance dose: 400–800 mg/d PO
bretylium tosylate	Bretylol	Prophylaxis and ventricular fibrillation, life-threatening ventricular dysrhythmias	Hypotension, nausea, vomiting, vertigo, dizziness	Immediate treatment: 5 mg/kg IV; maintenance: 5–10 mg/kg (diluted) by continuous IV infusion
disopyramide	Norpace, Norpace CR, *generic*	Suppression and treatment of ectopic ventricular contractions, ventricular tachycardia, paired ventricular contractions	Dry mouth, constipation, urinary hesitancy, blurred vision, nausea, dizziness, headache, hypotension, CHF	400–800 mg/d PO in 4 divided doses
encainide hydrochloride	Enkaid	Sustained ventricular tachycardia	Aggravation of ventricular dysrhythmias, dizziness, headache, CHF, blurred or abnormal vision	Initial dose: 25 mg PO q8h; maintenance dose: up to 50 mg PO tid
flecainide acetate	Tambocor	Same as encainide	Dizziness, faintness, unsteadiness, blurred vision, headache, nausea, dyspnea, CHF, fatigue, palpitations, chest pain	Initial dose: 100 mg PO q12h; maintenance dose: up to 200 mg PO q12h
indecainide hydrochloride	Decabid	Same as encainide	Worsening of ventricular dysrhythmias, dyspnea, chest pain, asthenia, dizziness	Initial dose: 50–100 mg PO q12h; maintenance dose: up to 400 mg/d PO
lidocaine hydrochloride	Xylocaine, *generic*	Life-threatening dysrhythmias (particularly those ventricular in origin)	Lightheadedness, soreness at IM injection site, bradycardia, hypotension, drowsiness	300 mg IM; 50–100 mg IV bolus; 1–4 mg/min IV infusion
mexiletine hydrochloride	Mexitil	Symptomatic ventricular dysrhythmias	Palpitations, nausea, vomiting, chest pain, heartburn, dizziness, lightheadedness, rash	Initial dose: 200–300 mg PO q8h; maintenance dose: up to 450 mg PO q12h

(continued)

SUMMARY DRUG TABLE 14–1

(continued)

GENERIC NAME	TRADE NAME*	USES	ADVERSE REACTIONS	DOSE RANGES
ANTIARRHYTHMIC DRUGS				
procainamide hydrochloride	Promine, Pronestyl, Procan SR, generic	Premature ventricular contractions, ventricular tachycardia, atrial fibrillation, paroxysmal atrial tachycardia, cardiac dysrythmias associated with anesthesia and surgery	Hypotension, disturbances of cardiac rhythm, urticaria, fever, chills, nausea, vomiting	Oral: initial dose 1 g or 6 mg/kg q3h; maintenance dose: 50 mg/kg/d q6h; IM: 50 mg/kg/d in divided doses; IV infusion: 500–600 mg
propafenone	Rythmol	Same as encainide	Dizziness, nausea, vomiting, constipation, unusual taste, 1st-degree AV block	Initial dose of 150 mg PO q8h; may be increased to 300 mg PO q8h
propranolol hydrochloride	Inderal, generic	Cardiac dysrhythmias	Bradycardia, dizziness, vertigo, rash, hyperglycemia, bronchospasm, hypotension, agranulocytosis	Dysrhythmias: 10–30 mg PO tid, qid; life-threatening dysrhythmias: up to 1 mg/min IV
quinidine gluconate, quinidine sulfate, quinidine polygalacturonate	Quinaglute Dura-Tabs, generic	Premature atrial and ventricular contractions, atrial tachycardia and flutter, paroxysmal atrial fibrillation	Ringing in the ears, nausea, dizziness, vomiting, headache, disturbed vision	0.2–0.6 mg PO; 400–600 mg IM (quinidine sulfate or gluconate); up to 330 mg IV of quinidine gluconate or its equivalent in other salts
tocainide hydrochloride	Tonocard	Same as mexiletine	Lightheadedness, nausea, tremor, paresthesia/numbness, dizziness	Initial dose: 400 mg PO q8h; may be increased up to 1800 mg/d PO in divided doses

* The term generic indicates that the drug is available in a generic form.

seconds *may* suffice if the patient has been taking the drug for a long time and there is no evidence of digitalis toxicity. The drug should be withheld and the physician notified if the pulse rate is 60 or below unless there is a written order giving different guidelines for withholding the drug. The drug should also be withheld and the physician contacted if there are any signs of digitalis toxicity, if there is any change in the pulse rhythm, if there is a marked increase or decrease in the pulse rate since the last time it was taken, or if the patient's general condition appears to have worsened.

When a cardiotonic is given IV, it is given slowly. When given intramuscularly (IM), the injection sites are rotated. To rotate injection sites correctly, a chart showing the order of rotation is inserted in the Kardex. Each time the drug is given, the injection site is recorded in the patient's chart.

When the patient is being digitalized, the blood pressure, pulse, and respiratory rate are taken every 2 to 4 hours or as ordered by the physician. This time interval may be increased or decreased, depending on the patient's condition and the route used for administration.

DIGITALIS TOXICITY AND ADVERSE DRUG EFFECTS. The patient is observed for signs of digitalis toxicity every 2 to 4 hours during digitalization and one to two times a day when a maintenance dose is being given. *It should be remembered that digitalis toxicity can occur even when normal doses are being administered or when the patient has been receiving a maintenance dose.* Serum levels (digoxin or digitoxin) may be ordered daily during the period of digitalization and periodically during maintenance therapy. Periodic ECGs, serum electrolytes, hepatic, and renal function tests, as well as other laboratory studies, may also be ordered.

Patients receiving a cardiotonic drug are weighed daily or as ordered. Intake and output should be measured especially if the patient has edema, CHF, or is also receiving a diuretic. Diuretics (see chap 18) may be ordered for some patients receiving a cardiotonic drug. Diuretics, as well as other conditions or factors such as GI suction, diarrhea, and old age, may produce low serum potassium levels (hypokalemia). Hypokalemia may alter the effects produced by the cardiotonics. Patients with hypokalemia are observed closely and at frequent intervals for signs of digitalis toxicity.

The patient must also be closely observed for any adverse drug effects (see Adverse Reactions Associated with the Administration of the Cardiotonics), such as anorexia, nausea, vomiting, and diarrhea. Some adverse drug effects are also signs of digitalis toxicity, which can be serious. Any patient complaint or comment should be carefully considered, recorded on the patient's chart, and brought to the attention of the physician.

Great care must be taken in the administration of a cardiotonic drug. References should be consulted for average digitalizing and maintenance doses. The physician's order and the drug container must be checked carefully. If there is any doubt about the dosage or calculation of the dosage, check with the physician or pharmacist before giving the drug.

ANXIETY. Some patients may have varying degrees of anxiety related to their diagnosis or the fact that drug therapy may need to be continued for a long time. The nurse must allow time for the patient to express her or his concerns, as well as to identify any problems that may require a referral to individuals such as the physician, dietitian, or social worker.

NONCOMPLIANCE AND KNOWLEDGE DEFICIT. In some instances, a cardiotonic may be prescribed for a prolonged period. Some patients may discontinue their medication, especially if they feel better and their original symptoms have been relieved. It is most important that the patient and family understand that the prescribed medication must be taken *exactly* as directed by the physician.

The physician may want the patient to monitor his or her pulse rate daily while taking a cardiotonic. The patient or a family member will need to be shown the correct technique for taking the pulse. The physician may also want the patient to omit the next dose of the drug and call him or her if the pulse rate falls below a certain level. These instructions should be reemphasized at the time of patient instruction. Other points that may be included in a teaching plan are the following:

- Do not discontinue this drug without first checking with the physician (unless instructed to do otherwise).
- Take this drug at the *same time* each day.
- Avoid antacids and nonprescription cough, cold, allergy, antidiarrheal, and diet (weight-reducing) drugs unless their use has been approved by the physician. Some of these drugs interfere with the action of the (cardiotonic) drug or cause other, potentially serious, problems.
- Contact the physician if nausea, vomiting, diarrhea, unusual fatigue, weakness, vision changes (such as blurred vision, changes in colors of ob-

jects, or halos around dark objects), or mental depression occurs.
- Follow the dietary recommendations made by the physician (if any).
- The physician will closely monitor therapy. Keep all appointments for physician visits or laboratory or diagnostic tests.

EVALUATION

- Anxiety is reduced
- Adverse reactions are identified and reported to the physician
- Patient and family demonstrate understanding of drug regimen
- Verbalizes importance of continued follow-up care
- Verbalizes importance of complying with the prescribed treatment regimen
- Patient complies to the prescribed drug regimen

▶ ANTIARRHYTHMIC DRUGS

The antiarrhythmic drugs are primarily used to treat cardiac dysrhythmias (arrhythmias). Patients with heart disease may have disturbances in their heart rate, rhythm, or both and require administration of one of these drugs.

▷ Actions of the Antiarrhythmic Drugs

Cardiac muscle (the myocardium) has attributes of both nerve and muscle and therefore has the properties of both. Some cardiac dysrhythmias are caused by the generation of an abnormal number of electrical impulses (stimuli). These abnormal impulses may come from the SA node, whereas others may be generated in other areas of the myocardium.

Quinidine and procainamide (Pronestyl) are unrelated chemically but have similar drug actions. Quinidine and procainamide depress myocardial excitability or the ability of the myocardium to respond to an electrical stimulus. By depressing the myocardium and its ability to respond to some, but not all, electrical stimuli, the pulse rate decreases and the dysrhythmia is corrected. These drugs also prolong or lengthen the **refractory** (resting) **period** of the impulses traveling through the myocardium. Only one impulse can pass along a nerve fiber at any given time. Following the passage of an impulse, there is a brief pause or interval before the next impulse can pass along the nerve fiber. This pause is called the *refractory period*, which is the period between the transmission of nerve impulses along a nerve fiber. By lengthening the refractory period, the number of impulses traveling along a nerve fiber within a given time is decreased. To illustrate this phenomenon, a patient has a pulse rate of 120 beats/ min. By lengthening the refractory period between each impulse, fewer impulses would be generated each minute and the pulse rate would decrease.

Propranolol (Inderal) is a beta-adrenergic blocking agent that has quinidine-like action (see earlier discussion of quinidine). It also decreases myocardial response to epinephrine and norepinephrine (adrenergic neurohormones) because of its ability to block stimulation of beta receptors of the heart (see chap 6). Adrenergic neurohormones stimulate the beta receptors of the myocardium and therefore increase the heart rate. Blocking the effect of these neurohormones decreases the heart rate. This is called a **blockade effect.**

Bretylium (Bretylol) is an adrenergic blocking agent that inhibits the release of norepinephrine. The manner in which this drug corrects certain ventricular dysrhythmias is not well-understood.

Disopyramide (Norpace) decreases the rate of depolarization of myocardial fibers during the diastolic phase of the cardiac cycle. Nerve cells have positive ions on the outside and negative ions on the inside of the cell membrane when they are at rest. This is called **polarization.** When a stimulus passes along the nerve, the positive ions move from outside the cell into the cell and negative ions move from inside the cell to outside the cell. This movement of ions is called **depolarization.** Unless positive ions move into and negative ions move out of a nerve cell, a stimulus (or impulse) cannot pass along the nerve fiber. Once the stimulus has passed along the nerve fiber, the positive and negative ions move back to their original place, that is, the positive ions on the outside and the negative ions on the inside of the nerve cell. This movement back to the original place is called **repolarization.** Disopyramide decreases the rate (or speed) of depolarization and the stimulus must literally wait for this process before it can pass along the nerve fiber. Decreasing the rate of depolarization then decreases the number of impulses that can pass along a nerve fiber during a specific time period.

Lidocaine raises the threshold of the ventricular myocardium. *Threshold* is a term applied to any stimulus of the lowest intensity that will give rise to a response in a nerve fiber. A stimulus must be of a specific intensity (strength, amplitude) in order to

pass along a given nerve fiber; stimuli that are of less intensity will not pass along the nerve fiber. To illustrate this phenomenon using plain figures instead of precise electrical values, a certain nerve fiber has a threshold of 10. If a stimulus rated as nine reaches the fiber, it will not pass along the fiber because its intensity is lower than the fiber's threshold of 10. If another stimulus reaches the fiber and is rated at 14, it will pass along the fiber because its intensity is greater than the fiber's threshold of 10. By raising the threshold of a fiber that was originally 10 to 15, only those stimuli greater than 15 can pass along the nerve fiber.

Some cardiac dysrhythmias result from many stimuli present in the myocardium. Some of these are weak or of low intensity but are still able to excite myocardial tissue. Lidocaine, by raising the threshold of myocardial fibers, reduces the number of stimuli that will pass along these fibers and therefore decreases the pulse rate and corrects the dysrhythmia. Tocainide (Tonocard) and mexiletine (Mexitil) are also antiarrhythmic agents with actions similar to lidocaine.

The actions of encainide (Enkaid) and indecainide (Decabid) are unknown but are believed to be due to their ability to slow the rate of conduction of an electrical impulse along cardiac nerve fibers, as well as to reduce the response of the myocardium to electrical stimulation.

Propafenone (Rythmol) and flecainide (Tambocor) have a direct stabilizing action on the myocardium thus reducing the response of these fibers to electrical stimulation. Amiodarone (Cordarone) appears to prolong the refractory period, as well as to exhibit alpha-adrenergic and beta-adrenergic blocking activity.

Dosage ranges for the antiarrhythmic drugs are given in Summary Drug Table 14-1.

▷ Uses of the Antiarrhythmic Drugs

The uses of the antiarrhythmic drugs are given in Summary Drug Table 14-1.

Propranolol may also be used for those with myocardial infarction. This drug has been shown to reduce the risk of death and repeated myocardial infarctions in those surviving the acute phase of a myocardial infarction. Additional uses include control of tachycardia in those with pheochromocytoma (a tumor of the adrenal gland that secretes excessive amounts of norepinephrine), migraine headaches, angina pectoris caused by atherosclerosis, and hypertrophic subaortic stenosis.

▷ Adverse Reactions Associated with the Administration of Antiarrhythmic Drugs

The more common adverse reactions associated with the administration of antiarrhythmic agents are given in Summary Drug Table 14-1.

 The administration of quinidine may result in **cinchonism**, the signs of which include ringing in the ears, headache, nausea, dizziness, fever, vertigo, and light-headedness.

Procainamide administration may result in transient, but sometimes severe, hypotension and disturbances of cardiac rhythm such as ventricular asystole or fibrillation (when given IV), anorexia, urticaria or pruritus, nausea, and agranulocytosis following repeated use.

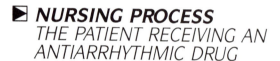

▶ NURSING PROCESS
THE PATIENT RECEIVING AN ANTIARRHYTHMIC DRUG

ASSESSMENT

Antiarrhythmic drugs are used in the treatment of various types of cardiac dysrhythmias. There are initial assessments performed before starting therapy that are the same for all antiarrhythmic drugs and include the following:

1. Blood pressure, an apical and radial pulse, and respiratory rate are taken and recorded. This provides a data base for comparison during therapy.
2. The patient's general condition is assessed and may include observations such as skin color (pale, cyanotic, flushed, and so forth), orientation, level of consciousness, and the patient's general status (appears acutely ill, appears somewhat ill, and so forth). All observations are recorded to provide a means of evaluating the response to drug therapy.
3. Any symptoms (subjective data) described by the patient are recorded.

The physician may also order laboratory and diagnostic tests such as an ECG, renal and hepatic function tests, CBC, serum enzymes, and serum electrolytes. These tests should be reviewed before the first dose is given. When subsequent laboratory tests are ordered, they also should be reviewed when the results are recorded on the patient's record.

NURSING DIAGNOSIS

Depending on the drug, the dose, the patient's diagnosis, and other factors, one or more of the following may apply to the patient receiving an antiarrhythmic drug:

- ▶ Anxiety related to diagnosis, possible lifetime drug therapy, other factors (specify)
- ▶ Altered nutrition: less than body requirements related to anorexia secondary to adverse drug effect
- ▶ Noncompliance related to indifference, lack of knowledge, other factors
- ▶ High risk for injury related to adverse drug reactions (dizziness, light-headedness)
- ▶ Knowledge deficit of medication regimen, adverse drug effects, treatment modalities

PLANNING AND IMPLEMENTATION

The major goals of the patient may include a reduction in anxiety, an absence of injury, an absence of adverse drug effects, and an understanding of and compliance with the postdischarge medication regimen.

The major goals of nursing management may include a reduction in patient anxiety, protection from injury, recognition of adverse drug effects, and the development and implementation of an effective teaching plan.

ADMINISTRATION. During therapy with these drugs, the patient's blood pressure, apical and radial pulse, and respiratory rate are taken at periodic intervals, usually every 1 to 4 hours, depending on the physician's order or on nursing judgment, which is based on the patient's general condition. Significant changes in the blood pressure, the pulse rate or rhythm, respiratory difficulty or change in respiratory rate or rhythm, or a change in the patient's general condition is reported to the physician immediately. Administration of these drugs is withheld and the physician is notified immediately when the pulse rate is above 120 or below 60. In some instances, the physician may establish additional or different guidelines for withholding the drug.

If the patient is acutely ill or is receiving one of these drugs parenterally, the intake and output is measured and recorded.

Additional points of nursing management for these drugs are given below.

QUINIDINE. If the patient is on a cardiac monitor, an ECG strip is taken before treatment with quinidine. If the patient is not on a cardiac monitor, the physician may order an ECG to establish a baseline for comparison during therapy. When the patient is on a cardiac monitor, any changes in the ECG pattern are reported to the physician immediately. If the patient is not being monitored, any changes in the pulse rate or rhythm are reported to the physician. A rise in the pulse rate must be immediately reported to the physician.

PROCAINAMIDE. The physician may order an ECG to provide baseline data for comparison during therapy. If the drug is given IV, continuous and close cardiac monitoring is recommended. When administered IV, the drug is discontinued immediately if changes in the ECG pattern occur. When the drug is given orally, the patient is instructed not to chew the capsule or tablet but to swallow it whole. When given IM, the gluteus muscle is used and the injection sites are rotated. Intravenous administration is by IV piggyback. Hypotension may be seen with IV administration; therefore, the blood pressure is monitored every 15 minutes while the drug is being infused. If hypotension should occur, the drug is discontinued and the primary IV line is run at a rate to keep the vein open (KVO) until the physician sees the patient.

PROPRANOLOL. Cardiac monitoring is recommended when the drug is given IV because severe bradycardia and hypotension may be seen.

BRETYLIUM. Bretylium is a drug used in the emergency treatment of life-threatening ventricular dysrhythmias. Baseline data will come from routine assessments made before the emergency. This drug is administered IM or IV, and the patient must be on continuous cardiac monitoring. The patient is placed in a supine position and suction equipment is made readily available in case vomiting should occur. After administration of the drug, close patient observation is necessary. The blood pressure and respiratory rate are taken every 5 minutes and the pulse rate is obtained from the cardiac monitor. These activities are continued until the dysrhythmia is corrected.

DISOPYRAMIDE. Because of the cholinergic blocking effects of disopyramide (see chap 9), urinary retention may occur. The urinary output should be closely monitored, especially during the initial period of therapy. If the patient's intake is sufficient but the output is low, the lower abdomen is palpated for bladder distention. If urinary retention does occur, catheterization may be necessary.

Dryness of the mouth and throat due to the cholinergic blocking action of this drug also may be seen. Dryness can often be relieved by frequent sips of water. The patient is provided with an adequate amount of fluid and is instructed to take sips of water to relieve this problem.

Postural hypotension may occur during the first few weeks of therapy, and the patient is advised to make position changes slowly. In some instances, the patient may require assistance in getting out of the bed or chair.

LIDOCAINE. Lidocaine is an emergency drug used in the treatment of life-threatening dysrhythmias. Constant cardiac monitoring is essential when this drug is administered by the IV or IM routes. The patient is closely observed for signs of respiratory depression, respiratory arrest, convulsions, and hypotension. An oropharyngeal airway and suction equipment is kept at the bedside in case convulsions should occur. The blood pressure and respiratory rate are monitored every 2 to 5 minutes when the drug is given IV and every 5 to 10 minutes when the drug is given IM. The pulse rate is continually checked by means of the cardiac monitor. The physician is contacted immediately if there are any changes in the vital signs or the ECG pattern or if respiratory problems or convulsions occur. If pronounced bradycardia does occur, the physician may order emergency measures such as the administration of IV atropine (see chap 9) or isoproterenol (see chap 6).

TOCAINIDE AND MEXILETINE. The dosage of this drug must be individualized; therefore, the vital signs are monitored at frequent intervals during initial therapy. Changes in the pulse rate or rhythm are reported to the physician. Adverse effects related to the CNS or GI tract may occur during initial therapy and must be reported to the physician.

ENCAINIDE, INDECAINIDE, FLECAINIDE, AND PROPAFENONE. The patient is observed closely for a response to drug therapy, signs of CHF, the development of a new cardiac dysrhythmia, or worsening of the dysrhythmia being treated.

AMIODARONE. This drug is only used when the patient dose not respond to other antiarrhythmic drugs. The patient is *closely* monitored for adverse effects especially CHF. The patient should be placed on intake and output to detect early signs of fluid retention. This drug is best given with food to reduce GI irritation. Changes in the pulse rate or rhythm are noted and reported to the physician.

ADVERSE DRUG REACTIONS. The patient is observed for adverse drug reactions. Nursing judgment is necessary in reporting these to the physician. For example, the patient with a dry mouth is in no danger, even though the condition is uncomfortable. Although the occurrence of this is reported to the physician, it is not of an emergency nature. In some instances, minor adverse reactions must be tolerated by the patient. On the other hand, the patient with severe bradycardia or prolonged nausea and vomiting is in a potentially dangerous situation, and the physician must be contacted immediately because additional treatment may be necessary.

ANXIETY. Varying degrees of anxiety may be seen in those with a cardiac disorder. The nurse must allow time for the patients to express their concerns, as well as to identify any problems that may require a referral to individuals such as the physician, dietitian, or social worker.

HIGH RISK FOR INJURY. Some of these drugs may cause dizziness and light-headedness, especially during early therapy. Patients not on complete bed rest should be assisted with ambulatory activities until these symptoms are no longer present.

NONCOMPLIANCE AND KNOWLEDGE DEFICIT. The adverse drug effects that may occur are explained to the patient and family. To ensure compliance to the prescribed drug regimen, the importance of taking these drugs as prescribed is emphasized.

▶ Take the drug at the prescribed intervals. Do not omit a dose or increase or decrease the dose unless advised to do so by the physician. Do not stop the drug unless advised to do so by the physician.

▶ Do not take any nonprescription drug unless the use of a specific drug is approved by the physician.

▶ Avoid drinking alcoholic beverages or smoking unless these have been approved by the physician.

▶ When applicable, follow the directions on the label, such as taking the drug with food.

▶ Do not chew tablets or capsules; swallow them whole.

▶ Do not attempt to drive or perform hazardous tasks if light-headedness or dizziness should occur.

▶ Notify the physician as soon as possible should any adverse effects occur.

▶ If a dry mouth should occur, take frequent sips of water, allow ice chips to dissolve in the mouth, or chew (sugar-free) gum.

▶ The wax matrix of sustained release tablets of procainamide (Procan SR only) is not absorbed by the body and may be found in the stool. This is normal.

▶ Keep all physician, clinic, or laboratory appointments because therapy will be closely monitored.

▶ Diabetic patients taking propranolol: adhere to the prescribed diet and check the urine one to two times a day (or as recommended by the physician). Report positive glucose or ketones to the physician as soon as possible because an adjustment in the dosage of insulin or oral hypoglycemic agent may be necessary.

EVALUATION

▶ Anxiety is reduced

▶ Adverse reactions are identified and reported to the physician

▶ No evidence of injury

▶ Patient and family demonstrate understanding of drug regimen

▶ Verbalizes importance of continued follow-up care

▶ Verbalizes importance of complying with the prescribed treatment regimen

▶ Patient complies to the prescribed drug regimen

15

Anticoagulant and Thrombolytic Drugs

On completion of this chapter the student will:

▶ *Discuss the uses and general drug actions of the oral anticoagulants and heparin preparations*

▶ *List the adverse effects associated with the administration of anticoagulants*

▶ *Discuss the areas to be checked for evidence of bleeding when the patient is receiving an anticoagulant*

▶ *Use the nursing process when administering an anticoagulant or thrombolytic drug*

▶ *Discuss the nursing implications to be considered when administering an anticoagulant or thrombolytic drug*

Anticoagulants are used to prevent the formation of a thrombus (blood clot). Although they do not thin the blood, they are sometimes called *blood thinners* by patients. The anticoagulants are a group of drugs that include the oral anticoagulants and heparin preparations.

Thrombolytic drugs are those used to dissolve blood clots that have already formed within the walls of a blood vessel.

▶ THE ORAL ANTICOAGULANTS

The oral anticoagulants consist of dicumarol, anisindione (Miradon) and warfarin (Coumadin; Summary Drug Table 15-1).

▷ Actions of the Oral Anticoagulants

All anticoagulants interfere with the clotting mechanism of the blood, which is a complex chemical process. Oral anticoagulants interfere with the manufacture of vitamin K–dependent clotting factors by the liver. This results in the depletion of clotting factors II (prothrombin), VII, IX, and X. It is the depletion of prothrombin (Fig. 15-1), a substance that is essential for the clotting of blood, that accounts for most of the action of the oral anticoagulants. The oral anticoagulants have no effect on clots that have already formed.

SUMMARY DRUG TABLE 15—1
Anticoagulant and Thrombolytic Drugs

(handwritten margin notes: "Greatest risk is hemorrhage ē anti-coagulants")

GENERIC NAME	TRADE NAME*	USES	ADVERSE REACTIONS	DOSE RANGES
ANTICOAGULANTS				
anisindione	Miradon	Prophylaxis of venous thrombosis, pulmonary embolism, atrial fibrillation with embolization	Hemorrhage	300 mg PO first day, 200 mg PO second day, 100 mg PO third day; maintenance dose: 25–250 mg/d PO
dicumarol (bishydroxy- coumarin)	Generic	Same as anisindione	Same as anisindione	200–300 mg PO first day; 25–200 mg on subsequent days depending on prothrombin time
heparin sodium	Liquaemin, generic	Prophylaxis of venous thrombosis, pulmonary embolus, peripheral arterial embolism, atrial fibrillation with embolization; disseminated intravascular coagulation	Hemorrhage, pain at injection site, thrombocytopenia	Dosage adjusted to individual patient according to coagulation test results
heparin sodium lock flush solution	Hep-Lock, generic	As IV flush to maintain patency of indwelling IV catheters used in intermittent IV therapy	Rare	1–2.5 mL as directed by the physician
warfarin sodium	Coumadin, Panwarfin, generic	Same as anisindione	Same as anisindione	Initial dose: 10–15 mg/d PO, 20–60 mg IM; maintenance: 2–15 mg/d depending on prothrombin time
ANTICOAGULANT ANTAGONISTS *Coagulant*				
phytonadione (vitamin K₁)	Aquamephyton, Konakion, Mephyton	Anticoagulant-induced prothrombin deficiency (oral anticoagulants)	Hypersensitivity, anaphylaxis, nausea, vomiting (with oral use), rash	2.5–50 mg IM, SC, IV, PO; dose may be repeated
protamine sulfate	Generic	Heparin overdosage	Sudden fall in blood pressure, bradycardia, dyspnea, feeling of warmth, anaphylaxis	1 mg neutralizes 90–115 U heparin; dosage is individualized
THROMBOLYTIC DRUGS				
alteplase, recombinant	Activase	Acute myocardial infarction	Bleeding, urticaria	60 mg IV the first hour, 20 mg IV the second and third hours
anistreplase	Eminase	Same as alteplase	Bleeding, hypotension, cardiac dysrhythmias	30 U IV
streptokinase	Streptase	Acute transmural myocardial infarction, deep vein thrombosis, arterial thrombosis or embolism, occluded fever, arteriovenous cannula	Major or minor bleeding episodes, allergic reactions, bronchospasm	20,000–1,500,000 IU by IV infusion
urokinase	Abbokinase	Pulmonary emboli, coronary artery thrombosis; as IV catheter clearance	Bleeding, fever	IV infusion: 2000 IU/lb initially, followed by 2000 IU/ lb/h at 15 mL/h for 12 h; coronary artery thrombi: 6000 IU/min for up to 2 h

* The term generic indicates that the drug is available in a generic form.

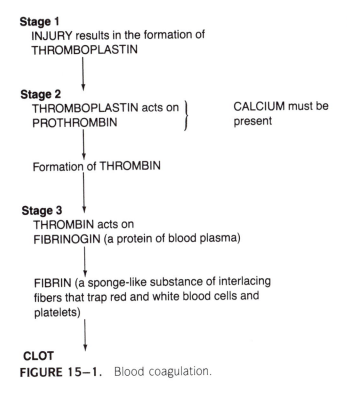

Stage 1
INJURY results in the formation of
THROMBOPLASTIN

Stage 2
THROMBOPLASTIN acts on }
PROTHROMBIN

CALCIUM must be
present

Formation of THROMBIN

Stage 3
THROMBIN acts on
FIBRINOGIN (a protein of blood plasma)

FIBRIN (a sponge-like substance of interlacing
fibers that trap red and white blood cells and
platelets)

CLOT

FIGURE 15–1. Blood coagulation.

▷ Uses of the Oral Anticoagulants

The oral anticoagulants are used for the following:

▷ Prevention (prophylaxis) and treatment of venous thrombosis

▷ Treatment of atrial fibrillation with thrombus formation

▷ Prevention and treatment of pulmonary embolus

▷ As part of the treatment of coronary occlusion

▷ Adverse Reactions Associated with the Administration of the Oral Anticoagulants

The principal adverse reaction associated with the oral anticoagulants is bleeding, which may range from very mild to severe. Bleeding may be seen in many areas of the body such as the bladder, bowel, stomach, uterus, and mucous membranes. Other adverse reactions are rare but may include nausea, vomiting, alopecia, urticaria, abdominal cramping, diarrhea, rash, hepatitis, jaundice, and blood dyscrasias.

▶ NURSING PROCESS
THE PATIENT RECEIVING AN ORAL ANTICOAGULANT

ASSESSMENT

Before administering the first dose of an oral anticoagulant, the nurse must question the patient about *all* drugs taken during the previous 2 to 3 weeks (if the patient was recently admitted to the hospital). The activity of the oral anticoagulants is influenced by many prescription and nonprescription drugs. If any drugs have been taken before admission, the physician is contacted before the first dose is administered.

If the patient has a thrombus in an extremity, the area is examined for color and skin temperature. Any areas of redness or tenderness are noted and the patient is asked to describe any symptoms he or she presently has. Vital signs are also taken and recorded.

NURSING DIAGNOSIS

Depending on the patient's diagnosis, one or more of the following may apply to the patient receiving an oral anticoagulant:

▶ Anxiety related to diagnosis, treatment regimen, other factors (specify)

▶ Knowledge deficit of dose regimen, adverse drug effects

PLANNING AND IMPLEMENTATION

The major goals of the patient may include a reduction in anxiety and an understanding of the postdischarge medication regimen.

The major goals of nursing management may include a reduction of patient anxiety, recognition of adverse drug effects (especially bleeding), and the development and implementation of an effective teaching plan.

LABORATORY TESTS. A prothrombin time is ordered before and during oral anticoagulant therapy. The first dose of the oral anticoagulant is *not* given until blood for a baseline prothrombin time is drawn.

Patients receiving an oral anticoagulant for the first time often require daily adjustment of the dose, which is based on the daily prothrombin time results. The results of the prothrombin time are recorded on a flow sheet and reported as two figures. One figure is the patient's prothrombin time in seconds and the other is the control value in seconds. The control value is a method of laboratory standardization of the materials used to determine the prothrombin time. The daily dose of the oral anticoagulant is based on the patient's daily prothrombin time. Optimal therapeutic results are obtained when the patient's prothrombin time is 1.5 to 2.5 times the control value.

ADMINISTRATION. Before giving *each dose* of an oral anticoagulant, the nurse must check the prothrombin flow sheet, as well as patient for any evidence of bleeding. The drug is withheld and the physician is contacted immediately if either of the following occurs:

1. The prothrombin time exceeds 2.5 times (30% of normal) the control value.

2. There is evidence of bleeding.

ADVERSE DRUG REACTIONS. Bleeding can occur any time during therapy with an oral anticoagulant, even when the prothrombin time appears to be within a safe limit (eg, <2.5 times the control value). All nursing personnel and medical team members must be made aware of all patients receiving oral anticoagulants and the observations made when a patient is receiving one of these drugs. The following are checked for signs of bleeding:

Urinal, bedpan, catheter drainage unit—The urine is inspected for a pink to red color; the stool is inspected for signs of gastrointestinal (GI) bleeding (bright red to black stools); the catheter drainage units are visually checked every 2 to 4 hours and when emptied. Oral anticoagulants may impart a red-orange color to alkaline urine, making it difficult to visually detect hematuria. A urinalysis may be necessary to determine if blood is in the urine.

Emesis basin, nasogastric suction units—A nasogastric suction unit is visually checked every 2 to 4 hours and whenever it is emptied. The emesis basin is checked each time it is emptied.

Skin, mucous membranes—The patient's skin is inspected daily for evidence of easy bruising or bleeding. The nurse should be alert to bleeding from minor cuts and scratches, nosebleeds, or excessive bleeding following intramuscular (IM), subcutaneous (SC), or intravenous (IV) injections or following a venipuncture. After oral care, the toothbrush and gums are checked for signs of bleeding.

Prolonged pressure is applied to the needle or catheter site after venipuncture, removal of central or peripheral IV lines, and IM and SC injections. Laboratory personnel or those responsible for drawing blood for laboratory tests are made aware of oral anticoagulant therapy because prolonged pressure on the venipuncture site will be necessary. All laboratory request slips require a notation stating the patient is receiving anticoagulant therapy.

If bleeding occurs or if the prothrombin time ex-

ceeds 2.5 times the control value, the physician may either discontinue the anticoagulant for a few days or order vitamin K₁ (phytonadione), an oral anticoagulant antagonist, which must always be readily available when a patient is receiving an oral anticoagulant. The patient is also closely observed for further evidence of bleeding until the prothrombin time is below 2.5 times the control value or until the bleeding episodes cease.

ANXIETY. Patients may be concerned over their need for an anticoagulant or the possibility that bleeding may occur. The patient should be reassured that therapy will be closely monitored by members of the health team. Because use of an anticoagulant signifies a potentially serious problem, patients should be allowed time to discuss their concerns.

KNOWLEDGE DEFICIT. Patients taking an oral anticoagulant require a full explanation of their drug regimen, as well as an explanation of the problems that can occur during therapy. A thorough review of the dose regimen, possible adverse drug reactions, and early signs of bleeding tendencies help the patient cooperate with the prescribed therapy.

The following points may be included in a patient and family teaching plan:

► Follow the dosage schedule prescribed by the physician.

► It is necessary to periodically monitor the prothrombin time. Keep all physician and laboratory appointments because dosage changes may be necessary during therapy.

► Do not take or discontinue other medications except on the advice of the physician. This includes nonprescription drugs, as well as those prescribed by a physician or dentist.

► Inform the dentist or other physicians of therapy with this drug *before* any treatment or procedure is started or medications are prescribed.

► Take the drug at the same time each day.

► Avoid alcohol unless use has been approved by the physician. Avoid eating excessive amounts of leafy green vegetables because they may contain large amounts of vitamin K that can interfere with the anticoagulant's effect.

► If evidence of bleeding should occur, for example, unusual bleeding or bruising, bleeding gums, blood in the urine or stool, black stool, or diarrhea, omit the next dose of the drug and contact the physician immediately.

► Use a soft toothbrush and consult a dentist regarding routine oral hygiene including the use of dental floss. Use an electric razor whenever possible to avoid small skin cuts.

▶ Wear or carry identification, such as Medic-Alert, to inform medical personnel and others of therapy with this drug.

EVALUATION

▶ Anxiety is reduced
▶ Patient and family demonstrate understanding of the drug regimen
▶ Verbalizes importance of complying with the prescribed treatment regimen
▶ Lists or describes early signs of bleeding

▶ HEPARIN PREPARATIONS

Heparin preparations are available as heparin calcium and heparin sodium (see Summary Drug Table 15-1).

▷ Actions of Heparin

Heparin inhibits the formation of fibrin clots, inhibits the conversion of fibrinogen to fibrin, and inactivates several of the factors necessary for the clotting of blood. Heparin cannot be taken orally because it is inactivated by gastric acid in the stomach; therefore, it must be given by injection. Heparin has no effect on clots that have already formed and aids only in preventing the formation of new blood clots (thrombi).

▷ Uses of Heparin

Heparin is used for the following:

▷ Prevention and treatment of venous thrombosis
▷ Atrial fibrillation with embolus formation
▷ Prevention of postoperative venous thrombosis and pulmonary embolism in certain patients undergoing surgical procedures such as major abdominal surgery
▷ Prevention of clotting in arterial and heart surgery, in blood transfusions and dialysis procedures, and in blood samples for laboratory purposes
▷ Prevention of a repeat cerebral thrombosis in some stroke patients
▷ Treatment of coronary occlusion, acute myocardial infarction, and peripheral arterial embolism

▷ Adverse Reactions Associated with the Administration of Heparin

Hemorrhage is the chief complication of heparin administration. Other adverse reactions include local irritation when heparin is given by the SC route. Hypersensitivity reactions may also occur with any route of administration and include fever, chills, and urticaria. More serious hypersensitivity reactions include an asthmalike reaction and an anaphylactoid reaction.

▶ NURSING PROCESS
THE PATIENT RECEIVING HEPARIN

ASSESSMENT

Before administering the first dose of heparin, vital signs are obtained. Laboratory studies related to heparin therapy include a partial thromboplastin time (PTT) and whole blood clotting time (WBCT). Blood for laboratory studies must be drawn *before* the first dose of heparin is given.

NURSING DIAGNOSIS

Depending on the reason for administration, one or more of the following nursing diagnoses may apply to a person receiving heparin:

▶ Anxiety related to diagnosis, drug therapy, other factors (specify)
▶ Knowledge deficit of treatment regimen

PLANNING AND IMPLEMENTATION

The major goals of the patient may include a reduction in anxiety and an understanding of the treatment regimen.

The major goals of nursing management may include a reduction in patient anxiety, recognition of adverse drug effects (especially bleeding), and a clear explanation of the treatment regimen.

Heparin is given to prevent the formation of a thrombus, and the patient is observed for signs of thrombus formation every 2 to 4 hours. Because the signs and symptoms of thrombus formation vary and depend on the area or organ involved, any complaint the patient may have or any change in the patient's condition is carefully evaluated and then reported to the physician.

LABORATORY TESTS. Blood coagulation tests are usually ordered before and during heparin therapy, and the dose of heparin is adjusted to the test results. Optimal results of therapy are obtained when the PTT is 1.5 to 2.5 times the control value or the WBCT is two and one-half to three times the control value. Blood for a blood coagulation test is usually drawn about 30 minutes before the next intermittent IV or SC dose is due. Laboratory personnel must be given sufficient notice for the timing of the blood coagulation test. Blood coagulation tests for those receiving heparin by continuous IV infusion are taken at periodic intervals that are determined by the physician. If the patient is on prolonged heparin therapy, blood coagulation tests may be performed at less frequent intervals.

ADMINISTRATION. The dosage of heparin is measured in **units** and is available in various dosage strengths as units per milliliter (U/mL), for example, 10,000 U/mL. When selecting the strength used for administration, the strength closest to the prescribed dose is chosen. As an example, if 5000 U are ordered and the available strengths are 1000, 5000, 20,000, and 40,000 U/mL, 1 mL of the 5000 U/mL is used for administration.

Heparin may be given by intermittent IV administration, continuous IV infusion, and the SC route. Intramuscular administration is avoided.

INTERMITTENT IV INFUSION. Intermittent IV administration (heparin lock, heparin trap) requires the use of an intermittent IV infusion set. After insertion of the intermittent IV infusion set, the date and time of insertion is printed on a small piece of tape that is used to anchor the loop of tubing. Intermittent infusion sets are changed at the time intervals ordered by the physician or according to hospital policy.

A solution called a lock flush may be ordered to be injected before and after the administration of the intermittent dose of heparin. The lock flush solution, which may be sterile normal saline or a heparin solution of 10 or 100 U/mL, aids in preventing small clots from obstructing the needle of the intermittent administration set. The physician or hospital policy dictates the use and type of lock flush solution.

Each time heparin is given, the needle site is inspected for signs of inflammation, pain, and tenderness along the pathway of the vein. If these should occur, it is usually necessary to discontinue use of this site and insert a new intermittent set at a different site.

If the patient is receiving heparin by intermittent or continuous IV infusion, other drugs administered by the IV route are *not* given through the IV tubing or injection port or piggybacked into the continuous IV line unless the physician orders the drug given in this manner. In addition, other drugs are *not* mixed with heparin when heparin is given by any route.

CONTINUOUS IV INFUSION. An infusion pump is recommended for the administration of heparin by continuous IV infusion. If an infusion pump is not used, the IV flow rate must be monitored every 15 to 30 minutes because the flow rate, which must be maintained at a steady rate, can be affected by movement of the extremity or changes in position. The needle site is inspected every 4 hours for signs of inflammation, pain, and tenderness along the pathway of the vein. If these should occur, it is usually necessary to discontinue the infusion and restart it in another vein.

DEEP SC ADMINISTRATION. Subcutaneous administration sites are rotated and the site used is recorded on the patient's chart. The recommended sites of administration include the abdominal fat layer and the area above the iliac crest.

Ice may be applied to the injection site for 10 to 15 minutes before administration to reduce the possibility of bleeding or oozing (hematoma formation) at the injection site. The application of ice requires a physician's order or a written hospital policy. Each time heparin is given by this route, all recent injection sites are inspected for signs of inflammation (redness, swelling, tenderness) and hematoma formation.

ADVERSE DRUG REACTIONS. Bleeding can occur during therapy with heparin. Vital signs are monitored every 2 to 4 hours or as ordered by the physician. If a decided drop in blood pressure or rise in the pulse rate occurs, the physician is notified because this may indicate internal bleeding. Because hemorrhage may begin as a slight bleeding or bruising tendency, the patient is observed frequently for these occurrences (see earlier discussion of the oral anticoagulants). At times, hemorrhage can occur without warning. If bleeding should occur, the physician may either decrease the dose, discontinue the heparin for a time, or order the administration of protamine sulfate. Protamine sulfate, a heparin antagonist, counteracts the effects of heparin and thus brings blood coagulation tests within normal limits. If administration of this drug is necessary, the blood pressure and pulse rate are monitored every 15 to 30 minutes for 2 or more hours after administration of the heparin antagonist. Any sudden decrease in blood pressure or increase in the pulse rate is reported to the physician immediately. The patient is also observed for new evidence of bleeding until blood coagulation tests are within normal limits.

When other drugs are given IM, SC, or IV, prolonged pressure must be applied to the injection site to prevent hematoma formation. Prolonged pressure is also applied when IV needles or catheters are removed.

In some instances, application of a small pressure dressing may be necessary after venipuncture or removal of an IV needle or catheter. Laboratory personnel or those responsible for drawing blood for laboratory tests must be made aware of heparin therapy by a notation on all laboratory request slips.

ANXIETY AND KNOWLEDGE DEFICIT. The diagnosis, as well as the insertion of an IV line or SC injection at scheduled intervals, may result in varying degrees of anxiety. The treatment regimen should be thoroughly explained to the patient. Although the physician may explain the reason for heparin administration, the nurse should explain the procedure and when the injections will be given. Patient should be allowed time to ask questions or discuss their concerns.

EVALUATION

▶ Anxiety is reduced

▶ Verbalizes an understanding of treatment modalities

▶ THROMBOLYTIC DRUGS

Alteplase, recombinant (Activase),* anistreplase (Eminase), urokinase (Abbokinase), and streptokinase (Streptase) are a group of drugs used to dissolve certain types of blood clots.

▷ Actions of Thrombolytic Drugs

Although their exact action is slightly different, these drugs break down fibrin clots by converting plasminogen to plasmin (fibrolysin). Plasmin is an enzyme that breaks down the fibrin (see Fig. 15-1) of a blood clot.

▷ Uses of Thrombolytic Drugs

These drugs are used in the treatment of acute myocardial infarction (AMI) to lyse (dissolve) a blood clot in a coronary artery. Urokinase is also used in

---

Alteplase is a tissue plasminogen activator (tPA) that is produced by recombinant DNA. Recombinant DNA is obtained by using gene splicing. Specific DNA segments of one organism are placed in the DNA of another organism. The genetic material of the recipient organism then reproduces itself and contains genetic material of its own plus the genetic material from the donor organism.

the treatment of pulmonary emboli and for clearance of IV catheters obstructed by a blood clot. Streptokinase is also used in the treatment of deep vein thrombosis and obstructed arteriovenous cannulae.

▷ Adverse Reactions Associated with the Administration of Thrombolytic Drugs

Bleeding is the most frequent adverse reaction seen with the use of these drugs. Bleeding may be internal and involve areas such as the GI tract, genitourinary tract, and the brain. Bleeding may also be external (superficial) and be seen at areas of broken skin such as venipuncture sites and recent surgical wounds. Allergic reactions may also be seen.

▶ NURSING PROCESS
THE PATIENT RECEIVING A THROMBOLYTIC DRUG

ASSESSMENT

These drugs are used as soon as possible, preferably within 6 hours, after the formation of a thrombus. Initial patient assessments would include vital signs and a review of the diagnostic tests performed to establish a diagnosis. Most of these patients are admitted or transferred to an intensive care unit because close monitoring for 48 or more hours after therapy is usually necessary.

NURSING DIAGNOSIS

Depending on the patient's diagnosis, one or more of the following may apply to the patient receiving a thrombolytic drug:

▶ Anxiety related to pain (AMI, pulmonary embolus, deep vein thrombosis), seriousness of disorder, other factors (specify)

▶ Pain related to obstruction of blood vessel

▶ Knowledge deficit of thrombolytic regimen

PLANNING AND IMPLEMENTATION

The major goals of the patient may include a reduction in anxiety, relief of pain, and an understanding of the treatment regimen.

The major goals of nursing management may in-

clude a reduction in patient anxiety, relief of pain (when applicable), recognition of adverse drug effects (especially bleeding), and a clear explanation of the treatment regimen.

ADMINISTRATION. The physician's orders regarding dosage and time of administration must be precisely followed. These drugs are available in powder form and must be reconstituted according to the directions in the package insert.

ADVERSE DRUG REACTIONS. Bleeding is the most common adverse reaction. The patient must be *closely observed* the first few hours after administration for signs of internal and external bleeding (see earlier discussion the oral anticoagulants). If any bleeding is noted, the physician is contacted immediately because whole blood, packed red cells, or fresh, frozen plasma may be required.

The patient is monitored for signs of an allergic (hypersensitivity) reaction, namely difficulty breathing, wheezing, hives, skin rash, and hypotension. Vital signs are monitored as ordered and the physician contacted if there is a marked change in one or more of the vital signs.

PAIN. If pain is present, the physician may order a narcotic analgesic. Once the clot is dissolved and blood flows freely through the obstructed blood vessel, severe pain usually decreases.

ANXIETY AND KNOWLEDGE DEFICIT. If the patient is conscious, the procedure is explained to the patient and family. The patient also should be told that frequent monitoring techniques are necessary during and after therapy with the drug.

EVALUATION

▶ Anxiety is reduced

▶ Pain is relieved

▶ Patient and family demonstrate understanding of treatment and techniques necessary to monitor therapy

16

Antianginal Agents and Peripheral Vasodilating Drugs

On completion of this chapter the student will:

▶ *Discuss the general actions, uses, and adverse reactions of vasodilating drugs*

▶ *List the initial assessments made before a vasodilating drug is given*

▶ *Use the nursing process when administering an antianginal or peripheral vasodilating drug*

▶ *Discuss the nursing implications to be considered when administering an antianginal or peripheral vasodilating drug*

Diseases of the arteries can cause serious problems, namely coronary artery disease, cerebral vascular disease, and peripheral vascular disease. Vasodilating agents sometimes relieve the symptoms of these diseases, but in some cases drug therapy only gives minimal and temporary relief.

The vasodilating agents can be divided into two groups according to their use:

Peripheral vasodilators—used mainly in the treatment of peripheral vascular diseases but may also be used for other vascular disorders

Antianginal agents—used in the treatment of angina

The antianginal agents consist of the nitrates and a newer group of drugs called calcium channel blockers. See also chapter 7 and Summary Drug Table 7-1 for the adrenergic blocking agents that are also used in the treatment of angina.

▷ Actions of Antianginal Agents and Peripheral Vasodilators

A vasodilating agent relaxes the smooth muscle layer of arterial blood vessels, which results in *vasodilation*. Because peripheral, cerebral, or coronary artery disease usually results in decreased blood flow to an area, drugs that *dilate* narrowed arterial blood vessels will carry more blood followed by an increase in blood flow to the affected area. It is hoped that increasing the blood flow to an area then results in complete or partial relief of symptoms.

Peripheral Vasodilators

The peripheral vasodilators, such as cyclandelate (Cyclan) and isoxsuprine (Vasodilan) act on the smooth muscle layers of peripheral blood vessels primarily by blocking alpha-adrenergic nerves and stimulating beta-adrenergic nerves. For a review of the effect of stimulation and blocking (or blockade) effects on adrenergic nerve fibers, see chapters 6 and 7 and Summary Drug Table 6-1.

Nitrates

The nitrates, for example, nitroglycerin and isosorbide (Isordil), have a direct relaxing effect on the smooth muscle layer of blood vessels, thereby producing vasodilation.

Calcium Channel Blockers

Calcium is involved in the transmission of nerve impulses. Calcium channel blockers, for example, nifedipine (Procardia), nicardipine (Cardene), di-

ltiazem (Cardizem), and verapamil (Calan), inhibit the movement of calcium ions across cell membranes; therefore, less calcium is available for the transmission of nerve impulses. This drug action of the calcium channel blockers (also known as slow channel blockers) has several effects on the heart, including an effect on vascular smooth muscle. These drugs dilate coronary arteries and arterioles, which, in turn, deliver more oxygen to cardiac muscle. The end effect of these drugs is the same as the nitrates and peripheral vasodilators.

▷ Uses of Vasodilating Agents

Peripheral Vasodilators

The peripheral vasodilators are chiefly used in the treatment of peripheral vascular diseases such as arteriosclerosis obliterans, Raynaud's phenomenon, and spastic peripheral vascular disorders. These drugs also have other uses, such as the relief of symptoms associated with cerebral vascular insufficiency and circulatory disturbances of the inner ear. More specific uses of individual peripheral vasodilating agents are given in Summary Drug Table 16-1.

SUMMARY DRUG TABLE 16–1
Antianginal Agents and Peripheral Vasodilating Drugs

GENERIC NAME	TRADE NAME*	USES	ADVERSE REACTIONS	DOSE RANGES
ANTIANGINAL AGENTS				
NITRATES				
amyl nitrite	*Generic*	Angina pectoris	Flushing, headache, dizziness, vertigo, palpitation, weakness	0.18 or 0.3 mL by inhalation
erythrityl tetra-nitrate (sublingual, oral)	Cardilate	Prophylaxis and long-term management of angina pectoris	Same as amyl nitrite	5–10 mg PO, sublingually
isosorbide di-nitrate (oral)	Isordil, *generic*	Treatment and prevention of angina pectoris	Same as amyl nitrite	5–40 mg PO
isosorbide di-nitrate (sub-lingual, chewable)	Isordil, Sorbi-trate, *generic*	Same as oral isosorbide	Same as amyl nitrite	2.5–10 mg
nitroglycerin (sublingual)	Nitrostat, *generic*	Prophylaxis, and treatment of angina pectoris	Same as amyl nitrite	1 tablet dissolved under the tongue or buccal area and repeated every 5 min until relief obtained (various dosage strengths are available)

(continued)

SUMMARY DRUG TABLE 16–1
(continued)

GENERIC NAME	TRADE NAME*	USES	ADVERSE REACTIONS	DOSE RANGES
ANTIANGINAL AGENTS				
nitroglycerin (sustained release)	Nitro-Bid, Nitrospan, Nitrostat, *generic*	Prevention of angina pectoris	Same as amyl nitrite	Initial dose: 2.5–2.6 mg PO tid, qid; up to 26 mg PO qid
nitroglycerin (topical)	Nitro-Bid, Nitrostat, *generic*	Prevention and treatment of angina pectoris	Same as amyl nitrite	1–5 inches q4–8h
nitroglycerin (transdermal systems)	Nitrodisc, Nitro-Dur, Transderm-Nitro	Same as topical nitroglycerin	Same as amyl nitrite	Apply pad daily
pentaerythritol tetranitrate	Pentylan, Peri-trate, *generic*	Prophylactic management of angina pectoris	Same as amyl nitrite	10–40 mg PO tid, qid
CALCIUM-CHANNEL BLOCKERS				
diltiazem hydrochloride	Cardizem	Angina due to coronary artery spasm, chronic stable angina	Peripheral edema, dizziness, lightheadedness, nausea, dermatitis, rash, sweating, constipation, hypotension	30 mg PO qid ac and hs and increased up to a total of 180–240 mg/d in divided doses
nicardipine hydrochloride	Cardene	Chronic stable angina	Same as diltiazem	20–40 mg PO tid
nifedipine	Procardia	Prinzmetal's angina, chronic stable angina	Same as diltiazem	10–20 mg PO tid and increased as needed up to 120 mg/d in divided doses
verapamil	Calan, Isoptin	Angina	Same as diltiazem	80–120 mg PO tid and increased prn
PERIPHERAL VASODILATING AGENTS				
cyclandelate	Cyclan, *generic*	Intermittent claudication, arteriosclerosis obliterans, nocturnal leg cramps, Raynaud's phenomenon	GI distress, headache, mild flushing, tachycardia	400–1600 mg/d PO in divided doses
isoxsuprine hydrochloride	Vasodilan, *generic*	Symptoms associated with cerebral vascular insufficiency, peripheral vascular disease	Hypotension, tachycardia, nausea, vomiting, dizziness, rash	10–20 mg PO tid, qid
papaverine hydrochloride	Pavabid, *generic*	Oral: cerebral and peripheral ischemia; parenteral: spasm associated with acute myocardial infarction, angina pectoris, peripheral vascular disease	Nausea, abdominal distress, flushing of the face, vertigo, drowsiness, headache, rash	Oral: 100–300 mg PO 3–5 times/d; parenteral: 30–120 mg IM, IV

* *The term* generic *indicates that the drug is available in a generic form.*

Nitrates

The nitrates are used in the treatment of angina pectoris. Some agents, for example, erythrityl tetranitrate (Cardilate), are used for prophylaxis (prevention) and long-term treatment of angina, whereas others are used to treat acute anginal attacks when they occur.

Calcium Channel Blockers

Calcium channel blockers are primarily used in the treatment of certain forms of angina such as Prinzmetal's angina. When angina is due to coronary artery spasm, these drugs are recommended when the patient cannot tolerate therapy with the beta-adrenergic blocking agents or the nitrates.

Verapamil affects the conduction system of the heart and also may be used as an antiarrhythmic agent. Nifedipine, verapamil, nicardipine, and diltiazem are also used in the treatment of essential hypertension (see chap 18).

The uses of specific antianginal agents are given in Summary Drug Table 16-1.

▷ Adverse Reactions Associated with the Administration of Vasodilators

Peripheral Vasodilators

Adverse reactions associated with the peripheral vasodilators are variable. Some of the more common adverse reactions are listed in Summary Drug Table 16-1. Because these drugs dilate peripheral arteries, some degree of hypotension is often associated with their administration. Along with hypotension, there is a physiologic increase in the pulse rate (tachycardia). Some of these agents also cause flushing of the skin, which can range from mild to moderately severe. Nausea and vomiting may also be seen with these drugs.

Nitrates

The nitrate antianginal agents all have the same adverse reactions, although the intensity of some reactions may vary with the drug as well as the dose. A common adverse reaction seen with these drugs is headache, especially early in therapy. Associated with headache there may be dizziness, vertigo, weakness, and flushing due to dilatation of small capillaries near the surface of the skin. In many instances, the adverse reactions associated with these drugs lessen and often disappear with prolonged use of the drug. For some patients, these adverse reactions become severe, and the physician may lower the dose until symptoms subside. The dose may then be slowly increased if the lower dosage does not provide relief from the symptoms of angina.

Calcium Channel Blockers

Adverse reactions to these drugs are usually not serious and rarely require discontinuation of the drug. The more common adverse reactions seen include peripheral edema, dizziness, light-headedness, nausea, dermatitis, skin rash, and fever, and chills (see Summary Drug Table 16-1).

▶ NURSING PROCESS
THE PATIENT RECEIVING A PERIPHERAL VASODILATOR

ASSESSMENT

Before the first dose of a peripheral vasodilator, assessment should include a thorough history of the patient's symptoms. After patient history is taken, the physical assessment is based on the patient's diagnosis. If cerebral vascular disease is present, the patient's mental status is evaluated. If the diagnosis is a peripheral vascular disorder, the involved areas are examined for general appearance, such as the color of the skin and evidence of drying or scaling. The skin temperature (warm, cool, cold) of the involved area is noted and compared to other areas of the body and to the extremities not affected by peripheral vascular disease. These findings are described in the patient's record. The peripheral pulses in the affected extremities are palpated and the strength and amplitude of each peripheral pulse is recorded in the patient's record. Vital signs are obtained and recorded.

NURSING DIAGNOSIS

Depending on the reason for administration, one or more of the following nursing diagnoses may apply to a person receiving a peripheral vasodilator:

▶ Anxiety related to pain or discomfort, diagnosis, other factors (specify)

▶ Pain related to narrowing of peripheral arteries

▶ Noncompliance related to indifference, lack of knowledge, other factors

▶ High risk for injury related to hypotension, dizziness, light-headedness secondary to drug action

▶ Knowledge deficit of medication regimen, adverse drug effects

PLANNING AND IMPLEMENTATION

The major goals of the patient may include a reduction in anxiety, relief of pain, absence of injury, and an understanding of and compliance to the prescribed treatment regimen.

The major goals of nursing management may include relief of pain, reduction in patient anxiety, recognition of adverse drug effects, protection from injury, and the development and implementation of an effective teaching plan.

ANXIETY. An evaluation of the patient's response to the drug is important. To reduce anxiety associated with a slow response to therapy, the patient may need to be reminded that signs of improvement may be rapid, but improvement usually occurs slowly over many weeks. The anticipated result of therapy for cerebral vascular disease is an improvement in the mental status.

PAIN. Positive results of therapy for a peripheral vascular disorder may include a decrease in pain, discomfort, and cramping, increased warmth in the extremities, and an increase in amplitude of the peripheral pulses. These assessments may be made every 2 or 3 days because the results of drug therapy usually occur slowly. The blood pressure and pulse are monitored one to two times per day because these drugs can cause a decrease in blood pressure in some instances.

ADVERSE DRUG REACTIONS. If adverse reactions occur, the physician is notified. It is important to note the severity of the adverse reactions on the patient's record. In some instances, adverse reactions are mild and may need to be tolerated.

HIGH RISK FOR INJURY. Some patients may experience dizziness and light-headedness, especially during early therapy. If these effects should occur, assistance with ambulatory activities will be required.

NONCOMPLIANCE AND KNOWLEDGE DEFICIT. To ensure compliance to the drug regimen, the patient and family should be told that improvement will most likely be gradual, although some improvement may be noted in a few days. Other points that may be included in the teaching plan are the following:

- ▶ If nausea, vomiting, or diarrhea occurs, contact the physician.
- ▶ Dizziness may occur. Avoid driving and other potentially dangerous tasks, as well as sudden changes in position. Dangle the legs over the side of the bed for a few minutes when getting up in the morning or after lying down. If dizziness persists, contact the physician.
- ▶ Use caution when walking up or down stairs or when walking on ice, snow, a slick pavement, or slippery floors.
- ▶ Stop smoking (if applicable).
- ▶ Peripheral vascular disease: follow the physician's recommendations regarding exercise, avoid exposure to cold, keep the extremities warm, and take care of the extremities.

EVALUATION

- ▶ Anxiety is reduced
- ▶ Pain is relieved
- ▶ No evidence of injury

- ▶ Patient and family demonstrate understanding of drug regimen
- ▶ Verbalizes importance of complying with the prescribed treatment regimen

▶ NURSING PROCESS
THE PATIENT RECEIVING AN ANTIANGINAL AGENT

ASSESSMENT

Before administration of an antianginal drug, a thorough description of the patient's anginal pain is recorded. Information regarding the anginal pain should include a description of the type of pain (eg, sharp, dull, squeezing), whether the pain radiates and to where, events that appear to cause anginal pain (eg, exercise, emotion), and events that appear to relieve the pain (eg, resting). Physical assessments include the blood pressure, an apical/radial pulse rate, and respiratory rate, after the patient has been at rest for about 10 minutes. Depending on the type of heart disease, additional physical assessments such as weight, inspection of the extremities for edema, and auscultation of the lungs may be appropriate.

NURSING DIAGNOSIS

Depending on whether the antianginal drug is used each time anginal pain occurs or for prophylaxis of anginal, one or more of the following nursing diagnoses may apply to a person receiving one of these drugs:

- ▶ Anxiety related to diagnosis, pain, other factors (specify)
- ▶ Fear related to diagnosis, chest pain
- ▶ Pain related to myocardial ischemia secondary to narrowing of the coronary arteries
- ▶ Knowledge deficit of medication regimen, adverse drug effects

PLANNING AND IMPLEMENTATION

The major goals of the patient may include a reduction in anxiety and fear, relief of pain and an understanding of the postdischarge medication regimen.

The major goals of nursing management may include a reduction in patient fear and anxiety, relief of pain, recognition of adverse drug effects, and the development and implementation of an effective teaching plan.

ADMINISTRATION. If the *sublingual* form of nitroglycerin has been prescribed, patients must be shown how and where to place the tablet in the mouth. This form of nitroglycerin also may be ordered to be left at the bedside and taken as needed. Usually 6 to 10 tablets are left in a closed container for the patient's use. If the physician orders the drug left at the bedside, the nurse should inquire as to the number of tablets to be given to the patient if an order for a definite number has not been written. The nurse is also responsible for replacing the patient's supply, as well as recording the number of tablets used over a given time. The nitroglycerin supply should be checked every 2 to 6 hours depending on the average number of tablets given to the patient and the frequency of use. The dose usually may be repeated every 5 minutes until pain is relieved but patients should be told to call the nurse if the pain is not relieved after three doses, 5 minutes apart. The physician is notified if the patient has frequent anginal pain, if the pain worsens, or if the pain is not relieved after three doses within a 15 minute period because a change in the dose or the drug or other treatment may be necessary.

The dose of the *topical* form of nitroglycerin is measured in inches or millimeters (mm); about 25 mm equals 1 inch. Before the drug is measured and applied and after the ambulatory patient has rested for 10 to 15 minutes, the blood pressure and pulse rate are obtained and compared with the baseline and previous vital signs. If the blood pressure is appreciably lower or the pulse rate higher than the resting baseline, the physician is contacted before the drug is applied. Applicator paper is supplied with the drug and one paper is used for each application. While holding the paper with the printed side down, the prescribed amount of ointment is expressed from the tube onto the paper. The plastic wrap and paper from the previous application are removed and the area is cleansed as needed. The applicator paper is then used to apply the ointment to the skin and spread over a 6 × 6-inch area in a thin, uniform layer. Application sites are rotated to prevent inflammation of the skin. Areas that may be used for application include the chest (front and back), abdomen, and upper or lower arms and legs. The ointment is *not rubbed into the patient's skin*. The area is then covered with plastic wrap and held in place with tape. The nurse must exercise care in applying topical nitroglycerin and must not allow the ointment to come in contact with the fingers or hands while measuring or applying the ointment. Disposable plastic gloves may be used if drug contact is a problem.

Nitroglycerin *transdermal systems* are more convenient and easier to use. These systems have the drug impregnated in a pad, which is applied to the skin once a day. The skin site should be free of hair, dry, and not subject to excessive rubbing or movement. If needed, the application site can be shaved. Transdermal systems are applied at the same time each day and the placement sites are rotated. The best time to apply the transdermal system is after morning care (bed bath, shower, tub bath) because it is important that the skin be thoroughly dry before applying the system. When removing the pad from the previous day, the area is cleansed as needed.

Nitroglycerin is also available as *oral tablets* that are swallowed, and are given on an empty stomach unless the physician orders otherwise. If nausea occurs following administration, the physician is notified. Taking the tablet or capsule with food may be ordered to relieve nausea.

RELIEF OF PAIN. When a patient is receiving an antianginal agent, the blood pressure and pulse rate are monitored every 3 to 4 hours or as ordered by the physician. In addition, the patient's response to therapy is evaluated by questioning the patient about his or her anginal pain. In some patients, the pain may be entirely relieved, whereas in others it may be less intense or less frequent or may only occur with prolonged exercise. All information is carefully recorded in the patient's chart because this helps the physician plan future therapy, as well as dose adjustment if required.

ADVERSE DRUG REACTIONS. Patients receiving these drugs are observed for adverse reactions. During initial therapy, headache and postural hypotension are not uncommon. If these reactions occur, the physician is notified because a dose change may be necessary. If the patient has episodes of postural hypotension, he or she must be assisted with all ambulatory activities. Postural hypotension may also be relieved by instructing the patient to take the drug in a sitting or lying down position and to remain in that position until symptoms disappear. In many instances, headache, flushing, and postural hypotension that are seen with the administration of the nitrates become less severe or even disappear after a time.

ANXIETY AND FEAR. The patient is reassured that the medication will relieve pain and if pain is not relieved, his or her physician will be contacted immediately. Patients must also be allowed time to discuss their concerns about their diagnosis and treatment.

KNOWLEDGE DEFICIT. The patient and family must have a thorough understanding of the treatment of chest pain with an antianginal agent. These drugs are used to prevent angina from occurring. The treatment regimen (dose, time of day the drug is taken) is explained to the patient.

The teaching plan must be adapted to the type of prescribed antianginal agent. The following are general areas included in a teaching plan, as well as those points relevant to specific forms of the drug.

Nitrates

▶ Avoid alcohol unless use has been permitted by the physician.

▶ This drug may cause headache, flushing, and dizziness. Notify the physician if these or other reactions become severe.

▶ Notify the physician if the drug does not appear to relieve the pain of if the pain becomes more intense despite use of this drug.

▶ Follow the recommendations of the physician regarding frequency of use.

▶ Take oral capsules or tablets (except sublingual) on an empty stomach unless the physician directs otherwise.

▶ Keep an adequate supply of the drug on hand for events such as vacations, bad weather conditions, holidays, and so on.

▶ When taking nitroglycerin for an acute attack of angina, sit or lie down. To relieve severe light-headedness or dizziness, lie down, elevate the extremities, move the extremities, and breathe deeply.

▶ Keep capsules and tablets in their original containers. Do not mix this drug with any other drug in a container.

▶ Always replace the cover or cap of the container for the oral form as soon as the drug is removed from the container. Replace caps or covers tightly because this drug deteriorates on contact with air.

▶ Keep a record of the frequency of acute anginal attacks (date, time of the attack, drug and dose used to relieve the acute pain) bring this record to each physician or clinic visit.

▶ Do not handle the sublingual tablets any more than necessary.

▶ Check the expiration date on the container of sublingual tablets. If it is past the expiration date, do not use the tablets. Instead, purchase a new supply.

▶ Do not swallow or chew sublingual tablets; allow them to dissolve slowly under the tongue.

▶ Instructions for application of the topical ointment or transdermal system are available with the product.

▶ Apply the topical ointment or transdermal system at approximately the same time each day.

▶ Be sure the area is clean and *thoroughly dry* before applying the system. Application sites should be rotated when the topical ointment or transdermal system is used.

▶ When using the topical ointment form or transdermal system, cleanse old application sites with soap and warm water.

▶ To use the topical ointment, apply a thin layer on the skin using the paper applicator (the patient or family member may need instructions regarding this technique). Avoid finger contact with the ointment.

▶ Wash the hands before and after applying the ointment. Replace the cap on the container and tighten securely after each use.

Calcium Channel Blockers

▶ Notify the physician if any of the following occurs: increased severity of chest pain or discomfort, irregular heartbeat, shortness of breath, swelling of the hands or feet, severe and prolonged episodes of light-headedness and dizziness, and nausea.

▶ Diltiazem: take this drug *before* meals and before going to bed.

▶ If the physician prescribes one of these drugs plus a nitrate, take both exactly as directed to obtain the best results of the combined drug therapy.

EVALUATION

▶ Anxiety is reduced

▶ Fear is reduced

▶ Pain is relieved

▶ Verbalizes an understanding of treatment modalities

▶ Adverse reactions are identified and reported to the physician

▶ Patient and family demonstrate understanding of drug regimen

17

The Management of Body Fluids

On completion of this chapter the student will:

▶ *List the types and uses of solutions used in the management of body fluids*

▶ *Use the nursing process when administering solutions used in the management of body fluids*

▶ *Discuss the nursing implications to be considered when administering a solution used in the management of body fluids*

▶ *List the types and uses of electrolytes and their salts used in the management of electrolyte imbalances*

▶ *Discuss the more common signs and symptoms of electrolyte imbalance*

▶ *Use the nursing process when administering electrolytes and their salts*

▶ *Discuss the nursing implications to be considered when administering electrolytes and their salts*

The composition of body fluids remains relatively constant despite the many demands placed on the body each day. On occasion, these demands cannot be met and electrolytes or electrolyte salts and fluids must be given in an attempt to restore equilibrium.

Two major areas are covered in this chapter: (1) the solutions used in the management of body fluids and (2) the electrolytes and electrolyte salts that may be administered to replace the one or more electrolytes that may be lost by the body.

▶ SOLUTIONS USED IN THE MANAGEMENT OF BODY FLUIDS

Blood plasma, plasma protein fractions, protein substrates, plasma expanders, and **parenteral nutrients** are used to correct nutritional or fluid deficiencies, as well as to treat certain diseases and conditions.

▷ Types and Uses of Solutions Used in the Management of Body Fluids

Blood Plasma

Plasma is the liquid part of blood, containing in solution, water, sugar, electrolytes, fats, gases, proteins, bile pigment, and clotting factors. Human plasma, also called human *pooled* plasma, is obtained from donated blood. Although whole blood must be typed and crossmatched because it contains red blood cells carrying blood type and Rh factors, human plasma does not require this procedure. Because of this, plasma can be given in acute emergencies. Plasma administered intravenously (IV) is used to increase blood volume when severe hemorrhage has occurred and it is necessary to partially restore blood volume while waiting for whole blood to be typed and crossmatched. Another use of plasma is in treating conditions when plasma alone has been lost, as may be seen in severe burns.

Plasma Protein Fractions

Plasma protein fractions include human plasma protein fraction 5% and normal serum albumin 5% and 25%. Human plasma protein fraction 5% is an IV solution containing 5% human plasma proteins in sodium chloride 0.9%. Serum albumin is obtained from donated whole blood and is a protein found in plasma. Plasma protein fractions are used to treat hypoproteinemia (a deficiency of protein in the blood), as might be seen in patients with the nephrotic syndrome and hepatic cirrhosis, as well as other diseases or disorders. Plasma protein fractions are also used to treat hypovolemic (low blood volume) shock. As with human pooled plasma, blood type and crossmatch is not needed when plasma protein fractions are given.

Protein Substrates

Protein substrates are amino acids, which are essential to life. Amino acids promote the production of proteins, enhance tissue repair and wound healing, and reduce the rate of protein breakdown. Amino acids are used in certain disease states such as severe kidney and liver disease, as well as in total parenteral nutrition solutions. Total parenteral nutrition may be used in conditions such as impairment of gastrointestinal (GI) absorption of protein and as increased requirement for protein as seen in those with extensive burns or infections, and when the oral route for nutritional intake cannot be used.

Plasma Expanders

Intravenous solutions of plasma expanders include hetastarch (Hespan), low-molecular-weight dextran (Dextran 40), and high-molecular-weight dextran (Dextran 70, Dextran 75). Plasma expanders are used to expand plasma volume when shock is due to burns, hemorrhage, surgery, and other trauma. When used in the treatment of shock, plasma expanders are not a substitute for whole blood or plasma but are of value as emergency measures until the latter substances can be used.

Parenteral Nutrients

Solutions used to supply nutrients and fluid include dextrose (glucose), fructose (levulose), invert sugar, and IV fat emulsion. Dextrose, fructose, and invert sugar, which is a combination of equal parts of fructose and dextrose, are carbohydrates. Carbohydrates are used to provide a source of calories and fluid. These products are available in various strengths (or percent of the carbohydrate) in a fluid, which may be water or sodium chloride (saline). Calories provided by these solutions are listed in Table 17-1.

Intravenous fat emulsion contains soybean or safflower oil and a mixture of natural triglycerides, predominately unsaturated fatty acids. It is used in the prevention and treatment of essential fatty acid deficiency. It also provides nonprotein calories for those receiving parenteral nutrition when calorie requirements cannot be met by glucose.

▷ Adverse Reactions Associated with the Administration of Solutions Used in the Management of Body Fluids

One adverse reaction common to all solutions administered by the parenteral route is fluid overload, that is, the administration of more fluid than the body is able to handle. The term *fluid overload* (circulatory overload) is not a specific amount of fluid that is given, but it describes a condition when the body's fluid requirements are met and the administration of fluid occurs at a rate that is greater than the rate at which the body can use or eliminate the fluid. Thus, the amount of fluid and the rate of administration of fluid that will cause fluid overload depends on several factors, such as the cardiac status and the adequacy of renal function. The signs and symptoms of fluid overload are listed in Table 17-2.

TABLE 17—1
Calories Provided in Intravenous
Carbohydrate Solutions

CARBOHYDRATE	PERCENTAGE	CALORIES/1000 mL
Dextrose	2.5	85
Dextrose	5	170
Dextrose	10	340
Fructose	10	375
Invert sugar	10	375

Adverse reactions are rare when plasma protein fractions are administered but nausea, chills, fever, urticaria, and hypotensive episodes may occasionally be seen. Administration of protein substrates (amino acids) may result in nausea, fever, flushing of the skin, metabolic acidosis or alkalosis, and decreased phosphorus and calcium blood levels.

Administration of hetastarch, a plasma expander, may be accompanied by vomiting, a mild temperature elevation, itching, and allergic reactions. Allergic reactions are evidenced by wheezing, edema around the eyes (periorbital edema), and urticaria. Low- or high-molecular-weight dextran administration may result in allergic reactions, which are evidenced by urticaria, hypotension, nasal congestion, and wheezing.

Hyperglycemia and phlebitis may be seen with administration of glucose, fructose, and invert sugar.

▶ NURSING PROCESS
THE PATIENT RECEIVING A SOLUTION FOR MANAGEMENT OF BODY FLUIDS

ASSESSMENT

Before administration of IV solutions used for the management of body fluids, assessments will include an evaluation of the patient's general status, a review of recent laboratory test results (when appropriate), the patient's weight (when appropriate), and vital signs. The blood pressure, pulse, and respiratory rate provide a baseline, which is especially important when the patient is receiving blood plasma, plasma expanders, or plasma protein fractions for shock or other serious disorders.

NURSING DIAGNOSIS

Depending on the diagnosis, type of fluid, and reason for administration, one or more of the following nursing diagnoses may apply to a person receiving one of these preparations:

▶ Anxiety related to diagnosis, invasive procedure (venipuncture), other factors (specify)

▶ Fluid volume deficit related to inability to take oral fluids, abnormal fluid loss, other factors (specify cause of fluid volume deficit)

▶ Altered nutrition: less than body requirements related to inability to eat, recent surgery, other factors (specify cause of altered nutrition)

▶ Knowledge deficit of administration procedure

PLANNING AND IMPLEMENTATION

The major goals of the patient may include a reduction in anxiety, correction of the fluid volume deficit (where appropriate), improved oral nutrition (where appropriate), and an understanding of the administration procedure.

The major goals of nursing management may include a reduction in patient anxiety, correction of the fluid volume and nutrition deficit, and an appropriate explanation of the administration procedure.

ANXIETY. Some patients may exhibit anxiety related to their diagnosis or the need to administer a drug by the IV route. The procedure, as well as the need for medical personnel to frequently inspect the solution and needle site, should be explained to the patient.

FLUID VOLUME DEFICIT AND ALTERED NUTRITION. Many times the solutions used in the management of body fluids are given to correct a fluid volume deficit and to supply carbohydrates. The nurse should review the patient's chart for a full understanding of the rationale for administration of the specific solution.

When appropriate, planning and implementation

TABLE 17—2
Signs and Symptoms of Fluid Overload

Headache	Hyponatremia
Weakness	Rapid breathing
Blurred vision	Wheezing
Behavioral changes (confusion, disorientation, delirium, drowsiness)	Coughing
	Rise in blood pressure
Weight gain	Distended neck veins
Isolated muscle twitching	Elevated CVP
	Convulsions

should include nursing measures that may be instituted to correct a fluid volume and carbohydrate deficit. Examples of these measures include offering oral fluids at frequent intervals and encouraging the patient to take small amounts of food.

ADMINISTRATION. An IV infusion pump may be ordered for the administration of these solutions. The alarm of the infusion pump should be set and the functioning of the unit checked every hour. The needle site is checked every 15 to 30 minutes and more frequently if the patient is restless or confused. When one of these agents is given with a regular IV infusion set, the infusion rate is checked every 15 minutes.

The needle site is inspected for signs of extravasation every 30 minutes. More frequent inspection may be necessary if the patient is confused or restless. If signs of extravasation are apparent, the infusion must be restarted in another vein.

Patients receiving an IV fluid should be made as comfortable as possible, although under some circumstances this may be difficult. The extremity used for administration should be made comfortable and supported as needed by a small pillow or other device.

All IV solutions are administered with great care. At no time should *any* IV solution be infused at a rapid rate. The average length of time for infusion of 1000 mL of an IV solution is 4 to 8 hours. The only exception is when there is a written or verbal order by the physician to give the solution at a rapid rate because of an emergency situation. In this instance, the order should specifically state the rate of administration (as drops per minute) or the period of time over which a specific amount of fluid is to be infused.

When these solutions are given, a central venous pressure (CVP) line may be inserted to monitor the patient's response to therapy. CVP readings are taken and recorded as ordered. During administration, the blood pressure, pulse, and respiratory rate are taken as ordered or at intervals determined by the patient's clinical condition. For example, a patient in shock and receiving a plasma expander may require monitoring of the blood pressure and pulse rate every 5 to 15 minutes, whereas the patient receiving dextrose 3 days after surgery may require monitoring every 30 to 60 minutes.

The rate of IV infusion ordered by the physician may be stated as drops per minute, milliliters per minute, or a given volume administered over a specified period, for example, 125 mL/h or 1000 mL in 8 hours. Calculation of IV flow rates is discussed in chapter 2.

Patients receiving IV solutions are observed at frequent intervals for signs of fluid overload (Table 17-2). If signs of fluid overload are observed, the IV infusion rate is slowed and the physician is notified immediately.

KNOWLEDGE DEFICIT. The patient or family should have a brief explanation of the reason for and the method of administration of an IV solution. Patients and families have been known to tamper with or adjust the rate of flow of IV administration sets. The importance of not touching the IV administration set should be emphasized.

EVALUATION

▶ Anxiety is reduced

▶ Fluid volume deficit is corrected

▶ Nutrition deficit is corrected

▶ Patient and family demonstrate understanding of the procedure

▶ ELECTROLYTES AND ELECTROLYTE SALTS

Along with a disturbance in fluid volume (eg, loss of plasma, blood, or water) or a need for providing parenteral nutrition with the previously discussed solutions, an electrolyte imbalance may exist. In some instances, an electrolyte imbalance may be present without an appreciable disturbance in fluid balance. For example, a patient taking a diuretic is able to maintain fluid balance by an adequate oral intake of water, which replaces the water lost through diuresis, but is unable to replace the potassium that is also lost during diuresis. Commonly used electrolytes are listed in Summary Drug Table 17-1.

▷ Types and Uses of Electrolytes and Electrolyte Salts

Bicarbonate (HCO_3^-)

This electrolyte plays a vital role in the acid–base balance of the body. Bicarbonate may be given IV as sodium bicarbonate ($NaHCO_3$) in the treatment of metabolic acidosis, a state of imbalance that may be seen, for example, in diseases or situations such as cardiac arrest, severe shock, diabetic acidosis, and severe renal disease. Oral sodium bicarbonate is used as a gastric and urinary alkalinizer, and may be used as a single drug or may be found as one of the ingredients in some antacid preparations. It is also useful as part of the treatment for gout because it is capable of minimizing the formation of uric acid crystals in the urine.

SUMMARY DRUG TABLE 17–1
Drugs Used in the Management of Body Fluids

GENERIC NAME	TRADE NAME*	USES	ADVERSE REACTIONS	DOSE RANGES
calcium carbonate	Os-Cal 500, *generic*	Hypoparathyroidism, post-menopausal and senile osteoporosis, rickets, osteomalacia; as a dietary supplement when calcium intake may be inadequate	Symptoms of hypercalcemia	Oral: 0.5–2 g/d PO in divided doses
calcium gluconate	Kalcinate, *generic*	Same as calcium carbonate	Same as calcium carbonate; parenteral use: local skin reactions, a calcium taste, tingling sensation, "heat waves"	0.5–2 g/d PO; IV infusion administered at a rate of 0.5–2 mL/min
dibasic calcium phosphate dihydrate	*Generic*	Same as calcium carbonate	Same as calcium carbonate	Same as calcim carbonate
electrolyte mixture	Lytren	Electrolyte and water deficiency	Rare	Dosage calculated on water requirements
magnesium	*Generic*	Hypomagnesemia, prevention; and control of seizures in severe eclampsia and convulsions associated with epilepsy	Symptoms of hypermagnesemia	Oral: up to 400 mg qid; anticonvulsant, see Summary Drug Table 32-1
potassium chloride	Kaon, K-Lyte, *generic*	Hypokalemia	Symptoms of hyperkalemia, nausea, vomiting, diarrhea, local tissue necrosis if extravasation of parenteral form occurs	Oral: 16–100 mEq/d and adjusted to patient's need; parenteral: 40–80 mEq/L of IV fluid (usual dose) and adjusted to patient's need
potassium gluconate	Kaon-Cl, *generic*	Same as potassium chloride	Symptoms of hyperkalemia, nausea, vomiting, diarrhea	Same as oral potassium chloride
sodium bicarbonate, parenteral	Neut, *generic*	Acidosis	Symptoms of alkalosis	Varies with degree of acidosis
sodium chloride, oral	Slo-Salt, *generic*	Deficiency of sodium and chloride	Symptoms of hypernatremia	0.5–1 g PO and up to 4.8 g/d
sodium chloride, parenteral	*Generic*	Same as oral sodium chloride	Same as oral sodium chloride	Adjusted to patient's needs

* The term generic *indicates that the drug is available in a generic form.*

Calcium (Ca^{2+})

Calcium is necessary for the functioning of nerves and muscles, the clotting of blood (see Fig. 15-1), the building of bones and teeth, and other physiologic processes. Examples of calcium salts are calcium gluconate and calcium carbonate. Calcium may be given for the treatment of *hypocalcemia,* which may be seen in those with parathyroid disease or following accidental removal of the parathyroid glands during surgery of the thyroid gland. Calcium may also be recommended for those eating a diet low in calcium or as a dietary supplement when there is an increased need for calcium, such as during pregnancy. Calcium may also be given during cardiopulmonary resuscitation.

Magnesium (Mg^{2+})

Magnesium plays an important role in the transmission of nerve impulses. It is also important in the activity of many enzyme reactions, for example, carbohydrate metabolism. Magnesium sulfate (MgSO$_4$) is used in the prevention and control of seizures in obstetrical patients with preeclampsia or eclampsia. It may also be added to TPN mixtures.

Potassium (K$^+$)

Potassium is necessary for the transmission of impulses, the contraction of smooth, cardiac, and skeletal muscles, and other important physiologic processes. Potassium as a drug is available as potassium chloride (KCl) and potassium gluconate and is measured in milliequivalents (mEq), for example, 40 mEq in 20 mL. Potassium may be given for *hypokalemia* (low blood potassium). Examples of causes of hypokalemia are a marked loss of GI fluids (severe vomiting, diarrhea, nasogastric suction, draining intestinal fistulas), diabetic acidosis, marked diuresis, and severe malnutrition.

Sodium (Na$^+$)

Sodium is essential for the maintenance of normal heart action and in the regulation of osmotic pressure in body cells. Sodium, as sodium chloride (NaCl), may be given alone or as a mixture with dextrose and other IV carbohydrates. A solution containing 0.9% sodium chloride is called *normal saline* and a solution containing 0.45% sodium chloride is called *half-normal saline.* An example of a sodium chloride and carbohydrate solution is 5% dextrose in 0.9% sodium chloride.

Sodium is administered for *hyponatremia* (low blood sodium). Examples of causes of hyponatremia are excessive diaphoresis, severe vomiting or diarrhea, excessive diuresis, and draining intestinal fistulas.

Combined Electrolyte Solutions

Combined electrolyte solutions are available for oral and IV administration. The IV solutions contain various electrolytes, as well as dextrose, fructose, or invert sugar. The amount of electrolytes, given as mEq per liter, also varies. The IV solutions are used to replace fluid and electrolytes that have been lost and to provide calories by means of their carbohydrate content. Examples of IV electrolyte solutions are 5% dextrose in Ringer's, 5% dextrose in lactated Ringer's, and Plasma-Lyte 148. The physician selects the type of combined electrolyte solution that will meet the patient's needs.

Oral electrolyte solutions contain a carbohydrate and various electrolytes. Examples of combined oral electrolyte solutions are Pedialyte and Lytren. Oral electrolyte solutions are most often used to replace lost electrolytes, carbohydrates, and fluid in conditions such as severe vomiting or diarrhea.

▷ Adverse Reactions Associated with the Administration of Electrolytes and Electrolyte Salts

Many adverse reactions associated with the administration of electrolytes and electrolyte salts are related to overdose, which result in, as example, signs of *hyper*kalemia or *hyper*natremia (Table 17-3). Adverse reactions other than those related to overdose are discussed later.

Calcium

Irritation of the vein used for administration, tingling, a calcium taste, and "heat waves" may occur when calcium is given IV. Oral administration may result in GI disturbances.

Magnesium

Adverse reactions seen with magnesium administration are rare. If they do occur, they are most likely related to overdose and may include flushing, sweating, hypotension, depressed reflexes, muscle weakness, and circulatory collapse.

Potassium

Nausea, vomiting, diarrhea, abdominal pain, and phlebitis have been seen with oral and IV administration of potassium. If extravasation of the IV solution should occur, local tissue necrosis may be seen. If this should occur, the physician is immediately contacted and the infusion slowed to a rate that keeps the vein open.

Sodium

Sodium as the salt (eg, sodium chloride) has no adverse reactions except those related to overdose. In some instances, excessive oral use may produce nausea and vomiting.

Sodium Bicarbonate

Some individuals may use sodium bicarbonate (baking soda) for the relief of gastric disturbances such as pain, discomfort, symptoms of indigestion, and gas. Prolonged use of oral sodium bicarbonate or excessive doses of IV sodium bicarbonate may result in systemic alkalosis.

TABLE 17—3
Signs and Symptoms of Electrolyte Imbalances

CALCIUM

Normal laboratory values—4.5–5.3 mEq/L or 9–11 mg/dL*

HYPOCALCEMIA

Hyperactive reflexes, carpopedal spasm, perioral paresthesias, positive Trousseau's signs, positive Chvostek's sign, muscle twitching, muscle cramps, tetany, laryngospasm, cardiac dysrhythmias, nausea, vomiting, anxiety, confusion, emotional lability, convulsions

HYPERCALCEMIA

Anorexia, nausea, vomiting, lethargy, bone tenderness or pain, polyuria, polydipsia, constipation, dehydration, muscle weakness and atrophy, stupor, coma, cardiac arrest

MAGNESIUM

Normal laboratory values—1.5–2.5 mEq/L or 1.8–3 mg/dL*

HYPOMAGNESEMIA

Leg and foot cramps, hypertension, tachycardia, neuromuscular irritability, tremor, hyperactive deep tendon reflexes, confusion, disorientation, visual or auditory hallucinations, painful paresthesias, positive Trousseau's sign, positive Chvostek's sign, convulsions

HYPERMAGNESEMIA

Lethargy, drowsiness, impaired respiration, flushing, sweating, hypotension, weak to absent deep tendon reflexes

POTASSIUM

Normal laboratory values—3.5–5 mEq/L*

HYPOKALEMIA

Anorexia, nausea, vomiting, mental depression, confusion, delayed or impaired thought processes, drowsiness, abdominal distention, decreased bowel sounds, paralytic ileus, muscle weakness or fatigue, flaccid paralysis, absent or diminished deep tendon reflexes, weak irregular pulse, paresthesias, leg cramps, ECG changes

HYPERKALEMIA

Irritability, anxiety, listlessness, mental confusion, nausea, diarrhea, abdominal distress, gastrointestinal hyperactivity, paresthesias, weakness and heaviness of the legs, flaccid paralysis, hypotension, cardiac dysrhythmias, ECG changes

SODIUM

Normal laboratory values—132–145 mEq/L*

HYPONATREMIA

Cold clammy skin, decreased skin turgor, apprehension, confusion, irritability, anxiety, hypotension, postural hypotension, tachycardia, headache, tremors, convulsions, abdominal cramps, nausea, vomiting, diarrhea

HYPERNATREMIA

Fever, hot dry skin, dry sticky mucous membranes, rough dry tongue, edema, weight gain, intense thirst, excitement, restlessness, agitation, oliguria or anuria

* These laboratory values may not concur with the normal range of values in all hospitals and laboratories. The hospital policy manual or laboratory values sheet should be consulted for the normal ranges of all laboratory tests.

► NURSING PROCESS
THE PATIENT RECEIVING AN ELECTROLYTE OR ELECTROLYTE SALT

ASSESSMENT

Before the administration of any electrolyte, electrolyte salt, or a combined electrolyte solution, the patient is assessed for signs of an electrolyte imbalance (see Table 17-3), if an imbalance is present. The nurse also reviews all recent laboratory and diagnostic tests appropriate to the imbalance. Vital signs are obtained to provide a data base.

In some situations, electrolytes are administered when an electrolyte imbalance may *potentially* occur. For example, the patient with nasogastric suction is prescribed one or more electrolytes added to an IV solution such as 5% dextrose or a combined electrolyte solution to be given IV to make up for the electrolytes that are lost through nasogastric suction. In other instances, electrolytes are given to replace those already lost, such as the patient admitted to the hospital with severe diarrhea for several days.

NURSING DIAGNOSIS

Depending on the drug, dose, route of administration, and reason for administration, one or more of the following nursing diagnoses may apply to a person receiving an electrolyte or electrolyte salt:

► Anxiety related to diagnosis, method of administration (IV), other factors (specify)

► Noncompliance related to indifference, lack of knowledge, other factors

► Knowledge deficit of medication regimen, adverse drug effects

PLANNING AND IMPLEMENTATION

The major goals of the patient may include a reduction in anxiety, compliance to the prescribed treatment regimen, and an understanding of the medication regimen and adverse drug effects.

The major goals of nursing management may include a reduction in patient anxiety, correct administration of the electrolyte, recognition of adverse drug effects, and the development and implementation of an effective teaching plan.

ADMINISTRATION OF CALCIUM. When calcium is administered IV, the solution is warmed to body temperature immediately before administration and the drug is administered *slowly*. In some clinical situations, the physician may order the patient to be placed on a cardiac monitor because additional drug administration may be determined by electrocardiographic changes. Before, during, and after the administration of IV calcium, the blood pressure, pulse, and respiratory rate are monitored every 30 minutes until the patient's condition has stabilized. After administration of calcium, the patient is observed for signs of hypercalcemia (see Table 17-3).

ADMINISTRATION OF POTASSIUM. When given orally, potassium may cause GI distress. Therefore, it is given immediately after meals or with food and a full glass of water. Tablets must *not* be crushed or chewed. If the patient has difficulty swallowing the tablets, the physician should be consulted regarding the use of a solution or an effervescent tablet, which effervesces (fizzes) and dissolves on contact with water. Potassium in the form of an effervescent tablet, powder, or liquid must be thoroughly mixed with 4 to 8 oz of cold water, juice, or another beverage. Effervescent tablets must stop fizzing before the solution is swallowed. The patient is instructed to sip the liquid over 5 to 20 minutes. Patients should be advised that liquid potassium solutions have a salty taste. Some of these products have a flavoring added, which makes the solution more palatable.

Patients receiving oral potassium should have their blood pressure and pulse monitored every 4 hours, especially during early therapy. The nurse also observes the patient for signs of hyperkalemia (see Table 17-3), which would indicate that the dose of potassium is too high. Signs of hypokalemia may also occur during therapy and may indicate that the dose of potassium is too low and must be increased. If signs of hypokalemia or hyperkalemia are apparent or suspected, the physician is notified. In some instances, frequent laboratory monitoring of the serum potassium may be ordered.

When potassium is given IV, it is *always diluted* in 500 or 1000 mL of an IV solution. The maximum recommended concentration of potassium is 80 mEq in 1000 mL of IV solution, although certain acute emergency situations may require a larger concentration of potassium. The physician orders the dose of the potassium salt (in mEq) and the amount and type of IV solution, as well as the time interval over which the solution is to be infused. After addition of the drug to the IV container, it is gently rotated to ensure mixture in the solution. A large vein is used for administration; the veins on the back of the hand should be avoided. An IV containing potassium should infuse in *no less than* 3 to 4 hours, thus requiring frequent monitoring of the IV infusion rate even when an IV infusion pump is used. The IV needle site is also inspected every 30 minutes for signs of extravasation. Potassium is irritating to the tissues. If extravasation does occur, the IV must be discontinued immediately and the physician notified. The acutely ill patient and the patient with severe hypokalemia will require monitoring of the blood pressure and pulse rate every 15 to 30 minutes during the time of the IV infusion. Intake and output is measured every 8 hours. The infusion rate is slowed to KVO and the physician is notified if an irregular pulse is noted.

ADMINISTRATION OF MAGNESIUM. Magnesium sulfate may be ordered intramuscularly (IM), IV, or by IV infusion diluted in a specified type and amount of IV solution. When ordered to be given IM, this drug is given undiluted as a 50% solution for adults and a 20% solution for children. The drug is given deep IM in a large muscle mass such as the gluteus muscle.

When magnesium sulfate is ordered to treat convulsions or severe hypomagnesemia, the patient requires constant observation. The blood pressure, pulse, and respiratory rate are obtained immediately before the drug is administered, as well as every 5 to 10 minutes during the time of IV infusion or after the drug is given direct IV. Monitoring of these vital signs is continued at frequent intervals until the patient's condition has stabilized. The patient is closely observed for early signs of hypermagnesemia (see Table 17-3) and the physician is contacted immediately if this imbalance is suspected. Frequent plasma magnesium levels are usually ordered. Laboratory request slips for this procedure are marked "emergency" because results must be obtained as soon as possible. The physician is notified if the magnesium level is higher or lower than the normal range.

ADMINISTRATION OF SODIUM. When sodium chloride is administered by IV infusion, the patient is observed during and after administration for signs of hypernatremia (see Table 17-3). The rate of IV infusion as ordered by the physician is checked every 15 to 30 minutes. More frequent monitoring of the infusion rate may be necessary when the patient is restless or confused. Patients receiving a 3% or 5% sodium chloride solution by IV infusion are observed closely for signs of pulmonary edema (dyspnea, cough, restlessness, bradycardia). If any one or more of these symptoms should occur, the IV infusion is slowed to KVO and the physician is contacted immediately. Patients receiving sodium chloride by the IV route should have their intake and output measured every 8 hours. The patient is observed for signs of hypernatremia every 3 to 4 hours and the physician is contacted if this condition is suspected.

ADMINISTRATION OF BICARBONATE. Oral sodium bicarbonate tablets are given with a full glass of water; the powdered form is dissolved in a full glass of water. If oral sodium bicarbonate is used to alkalinize the urine, the urine pH is checked two or three times a day or as ordered by the physician. If the urine remains acidic, the physician is notified because an increase in the dose of the drug may be necessary.

Intravenous sodium bicarbonate is given in emergency situations such as cardiac arrest or certain types of drug overdose when alkalinization of the urine is necessary to hasten drug elimination. The blood pressure, pulse, and respiratory rate are obtained immediately before administration of the drug (an exception may be cardiac arrest or other emergency situations), and then monitored at frequent intervals thereafter. In cardiac arrest, the initial and subsequent doses are given by IV push. Doses are repeated at intervals of about 5 minutes until the patient's condition has stabilized. Extravasation of the drug requires selection of another needle site because the drug is irritating to the tissues.

When given in the treatment of metabolic acidosis, the drug may be added to the IV fluid or given as a prepared IV sodium bicarbonate solution. Frequent laboratory monitoring of the blood pH and blood gases is usually ordered because dosage and length of therapy depend on test results. The patient is observed for signs of clinical improvement and the blood pressure, pulse, and respiratory rate are monitored every 15 to 30 minutes or as ordered by the physician.

ANXIETY. Some patients may exhibit anxiety related to their diagnosis or the method of administration of the drug (IV). The procedure, as well as the need for medical personnel to frequently inspect the solution and needle site, should be explained to the patient.

NONCOMPLIANCE AND KNOWLEDGE DEFICIT. The dose and time intervals are carefully explained to the patient or a family member. Because overdose (which can be serious) may occur if the patient does not adhere to the prescribed dosage and schedule, it is most important that the patient completely understands how much and when to take the drug. The importance of adhering to the prescribed dosage schedule is stressed during patient teaching.

The physician may order periodic laboratory and diagnostic tests for some patients receiving oral electrolytes. The patient is encouraged to keep all appointments for these tests, as well as physician or clinic visits.

Individuals with a history of using sodium bicarbonate (baking soda) as an antacid should be warned that overuse can result in alkalosis and could disguise a more serious problem. Those with a history of using salt tablets (sodium chloride) during hot weather are advised not to use the drug unless it is recommended by a physician. Excessive use of salt tablets can result in a serious electrolyte imbalance.

Additional teaching points for specific electrolytes are the following:

Calcium Salts

▶ Contact the physician if nausea, vomiting, anorexia, constipation, abdominal pain, dry mouth, thirst, polyuria (symptoms of hypercalcemia) occurs.

▶ Do not exceed the dosage recommendations.

Potassium Salts

▶ Take the drug *exactly* as directed on the prescription container. Do *not* increase, decrease, or omit the drug unless advised to do so by the physician. This drug is best taken immediately after meals or with food and a full glass of water. Avoid the use of nonprescription drugs and salt substitutes (many contain potassium) unless use of a specific drug or product has been approved by the physician.

▶ Contact the physician if tingling of the hands or feet, a feeling of heaviness in the legs, vomiting, nausea, abdominal pain, or black stools should occur.

▶ If the tablet has a coating (enteric-coated tablets), swallow it whole. Do not chew or crush the tablet.

▶ If effervescent tablets are prescribed, place the tablet in 4 to 8 oz of cold water or juice. Wait until the fizzing stops before drinking. Sip the liquid over 5 to 10 minutes.

▶ If oral liquids or a powder is prescribed, add the dose to 4 to 8 oz of cold water or juice and sip slowly over a 5 to 10 minutes. Measure the dose accurately.

EVALUATION

▶ Anxiety is reduced

▶ Patient complies to the prescribed drug regimen

▶ Patient and family demonstrate understanding of drug regimen

▶ Verbalizes importance of complying with the prescribed treatment regimen

18

Diuretics and Antihypertensive Drugs

On completion of this chapter the student will:

▶ *List the general types, actions, and uses of the diuretics*

▶ *Discuss the major adverse reactions associated with the administration of a diuretic*

▶ *Use the nursing process when administering a diuretic*

▶ *Discuss the nursing implications to be considered when a diuretic is give*

▶ *List the general types, actions, and uses of the antihypertensive drugs*

▶ *Discuss the major adverse reactions associated with the administration of an antihypertensive drug*

▶ *Use the nursing process when administering an antihypertensive agent*

▶ *Discuss the nursing implications to be considered when an antihypertensive drug is given*

▶ DIURETICS

Many conditions or diseases, such as heart failure, endocrine disturbances, and kidney and liver diseases can cause retention of excess fluid (edema). When the retention of excess fluid occurs, the physician may order a diuretic, an agent that promotes the excretion of water and electrolytes. There are various types of diuretic agents, and the physician selects the agent that best suits the patient's needs and effectively reduces the amount of excess fluid in body tissues.

The types of diuretic agents are **carbonic anhydrase inhibitors, thiazides and related diuretics, loop diuretics, osmotic diuretics,** and **potassium-sparing diuretics.** Onset and duration of the activity of diuretic agents are listed in Table 18-1. Summary Drug Table 18-1 lists examples of the different types of diuretic agents.

TABLE 18–1
Examples of Onset and Duration of Activity
of Diuretic Agents

DRUG	ONSET	DURATION OF ACTIVITY
acetazolamide		
tablets	1–1.5 h	8–12 h
sustained-release capsules	2 h	18–24 h
IV	2 min	4–5 h
amiloride	2 h	24 h
bumetanide	30–60 min	4–6 h
dichlorphenamide	Within 1 h	6–12 h
ethacrynic acid		
PO	Within 30 min	6–8 h
IV	Within 5 min	2 h
furosemide		
PO	Within 1 h	6–8 h
IV	Within 5 min	2 h
Mannitol (IV)	30–60 min	6–8 h
spironolactone	24–48 h	48–72 h
thiazides and related diuretics	1–2 h	*
triamterene	2–4 h	12–16 h
urea (V)	30–45 min	5–6 h

Duration varies with drug used. Average duration is 12–24 h with poly-thiazide, chlorthalidone, and indapamide having a duration of more than 24 h.

▷ Actions of Diuretic Agents

Most diuretics act on the tubules of the kidney neph-ron. There are approximately one million nephrons in each kidney, filtering the bloodstream to remove waste products. During this process, water and elec-trolytes are also selectively removed.

The filtrate (ie, the fluid removed from the blood) normally contains ions (potassium, sodium, chloride), waste products (ammonia, urea), water, and, at times, other substances that are being ex-creted from the body, such as drugs. The filtrate then passes through the proximal tubule, the loop of Henle, and the distal tubules. At these points, selec-tive reabsorption of amino acids, glucose, some elec-trolytes, and water takes place. Ions and water that are required by the body to maintain fluid and elec-trolyte balance are returned to the bloodstream by means of the minute capillaries that surround the distal and proximal tubules and the loop of Henle. Ions and water that are not needed by the body are then excreted in the urine.

Carbonic Anhydrase Inhibitors

Carbonic anhydrase is an enzyme that produces free hydrogen ions, which are then exchanged for so-dium ions in the kidney tubules. Carbonic an-hydrase inhibitors inhibit the action of the enzyme carbonic anhydrase. This effect results in the excre-tion of sodium, potassium, bicarbonate, and water. Carbonic anhydrase inhibitors also decrease the se-cretion of aqueous humor in the eye. Administration of these drugs results in a decrease in intraocular pressure.

Thiazides and Related Diuretics

Thiazides and related diuretics increase the excre-tion of sodium and chloride by inhibiting reabsorp-tion of these ions in the distal tubule of the kidney. This results in secretion of sodium, chloride, and water.

Loop Diuretics

The loop diuretics increase the excretion of sodium and chloride by inhibiting reabsorption of these ions in the distal and proximal tubules and in the loop of Henle. This mechanism of action at these three sites appears to increase their effectiveness as diuretics.

Osmotic Diuretics

Osmotic diuretics increase the density of the filtrate in the glomerulus. This prevents selective reabsorp-tion of water, and water is excreted. Sodium and chloride excretion is also increased.

Potassium-Sparing Diuretics

Potassium-sparing diuretics may work in two ways. Triamterene (Dyrenium) and amiloride (Midamor) depress the reabsorption of sodium in the kidney tubules, and therefore increase sodium and water excretion. Both drugs additionally depress the ex-cretion of potassium, and therefore are called po-tassium-sparing (or potassium-saving) diuretics. Spironolactone (Aldactone), also a potassium-spar-ing diuretic, antagonizes the action of aldosterone. Aldosterone, a hormone produced by the adrenal cortex, enhances the reabsorption of sodium in the distal convoluted tubules of the kidney. When this activity of aldosterone is blocked, sodium (but not potassium) and water are excreted.

SUMMARY DRUG TABLE 18–1
Diuretic Agents

GENERIC NAME	TRADE NAME*	USES	ADVERSE REACTIONS	DOSE RANGES
CARBONIC ANHYDRASE INHIBITORS				
acetazolamide	Diamox	Adjunctive treatment of simple (open-angle) glaucoma, drug-induced edema, petit mal epilepsy	Fever, rash, paresthesias, anorexia, crystalluria	Glaucoma: 250 mg–1 g/d in divided doses; CHF: 250–375 mg PO; edema: 250–375 mg PO; epilepsy: 8–30 mg/kg/d PO in divided doses
dichlorphenamide	Daranide	Glaucoma	Same as acetazolamide	Initially: 100–200 mg PO; maintenance dose: 25–50 mg PO 1–3 times/d
methazolamide	Neptazane	Glaucoma	Same as acetazolamide	50–100 mg PO bid, tid
THIAZIDES AND RELATED DIURETICS				
bendroflu-methiazide	Naturetin	Edema due to: CHF, cirrhosis, corticosteroid and estrogen therapy, renal dysfunction, hypertension	Anorexia, leukopenia, orthostatic hypotension, muscle cramps or spasm, fluid or electrolyte imbalance, nausea, vomiting, frequent urination	Edema: 5–20 mg/d PO; hypertension: 2.5–20 mg/d PO
benzthiazide	Exna	Same as bendroflumethiazide	Same as bendroflumethiazide	Edema: 50–200 mg/d PO; hypertension: 50–200 mg/d PO
chlorothiazide	Diachlor, Diuril, *generic*	Same as bendroflumethiazide	Same as bendroflumethiazide	Edema: 0.5–2 g PO, IV 1–2 times/d; hypertension: 0.5–2 g/d PO as a single dose or divided doses
chlorthalidone	Hygroton, *generic*	Same as bendroflumethiazide	Same as bendroflumethiazide	Edema: 50–100 mg/d or every other day PO; hypertension: 25–100 mg/d PO
cyclothiazide	Anhydron	Same as bendroflumethiazide	Same as bendroflumethiazide	Edema: 1–2 mg PO daily, every other day, or 2–3 times/wk; hypertension: 2.5–5 mg/d PO
hydrochloro-thiazide	Esidrlx, HydroDIURIL, *generic*	Same as bendroflumethiazide	Same as bendroflumethiazide	Edema: 25–200 mg/d PO (may also be given 2–3 times/wk); hypertension: 50–200 mg/d PO
hydroflu-methiazide	Diucardin, Saluron, *generic*	Same as bendroflumethiazide	Same as bendroflumethiazide	Edema: 25–200 mg/d PO; hypertension: 50–200 mg/d PO
indapamide	Lozol	Edema associated with CHF, hypertension	Same as bendroflumethiazide	Initially 2.5 mg/d PO; may be increased to 5 mg/d
methyclo-thiazide	Enduron, Aquatensen, *generic*	Same as bendroflumethiazide	Same as bendroflumethiazide	Edema: 2.5–10 mg/d PO hypertension: 2.5–5 mg/d PO
metolazone	Diulin, Zaroxolyn	Same as bendroflumethiazide	Same as bendroflumethiazide	Edema: 5–20 mg/d PO; hypertension: 2.5–5 mg/d PO
polythiazide	Renese	Same as bendroflumethiazide	Same as bendroflumethiazide	Edema: 1–4 mg/d PO; hypertension: 2–4 mg/d PO
trichlor-methiazide	Metahydrin, Naqua, *generic*	Same as bendroflumethiazide	Same as bendroflumethiazide	Edema: 1–4 mg/d PO; hypertension: 2–4 mg/d PO

(continued)

SUMMARY DRUG TABLE 18-1
(continued)

GENERIC NAME	TRADE NAME*	USES	ADVERSE REACTIONS	DOSE RANGES
LOOP DIURETICS				
bumetanide	Bumex	Edema associated with CHF, cirrhosis, renal disease	Anorexia, nausea, vomiting, dry mouth, weakness, hypotension, pruritus	Oral: 0.5–10 mg/d; parenteral: 0.5–1 mg IM, IV, not to exceed 10 mg/d
ethacrynic acid	Edecrin, Edecrin Sodium	Same as bumetanide plus ascites due to a malignancy, cirrhosis, idiopathic edema	Profuse diarrhea, anorexia, nausea, vomiting, vertigo, headache, neutropenia	Oral: 50–200 mg/d, bid; parenteral 50–100 mg IV
furosemide	Lasix, *generic*	Same as bumetanide; used orally for hypertension	Oral and gastric irritation, paresthesia, anemia, orthostatic hypotension	Edema: 20–80 mg/d PO; 20–40 mg IM, IV; acute pulmonary edema: 40–80 mg IV; hypertension: 40 mg/d PO and adjusted prn
OSMOTIC DIURETICS				
mannitol	Osmitrol, *generic*	Promotion of diuresis in acute renal failure, reduction of intracranial pressure, urinary excretion of toxic substances, reduction of intraocular pressure, cerebral edema	Fluid and electrolyte imbalance, pulmonary edema, urinary retention, dry mouth, thirst	Renal failure: 50–100 g IV infusion; reduction of intracranial pressure: 1.5–2 g/kg infused over a period of 30–60 min; reduction of intraocular pressure: 1.5–2 g/kg IV; excretion of toxic substances: up to 200 g IV
urea	Ureaphil	Reduction of intracranial and intraocular pressure	Headache, nausea, vomiting, syncope	1–1.5 g/kg IV infusion
POTASSIUM-SPARING DIURETICS				
amiloride	Midamor, *generic*	CHF, hypertension	Headache, dizziness, anorexia, weakness, nausea, elevated serum potassium	5–20 mg/d PO
spironolactone	Aldactone, Spiractone, *generic*	Hypertension, edema due to CHF, cirrhosis, nephrotic syndrome	Hypokalemia, diarrhea, drowsiness, headache, mental confusion, abdominal cramping	25–200 mg/d PO
spironolactone with hydrochlorothiazide	Alazide, Aldactazide, *generic*	Hypertension, edema due to CHF, cirrhosis, nephrotic syndrome	Same as spironolactone and hydrochlorothiazide	1–8 tablets/d
triamterene	Dyrenium	Edema due to CHF, nephrotic syndrome, cirrhosis, steroid therapy	Hyperkalemia, weakness, dry mouth, diarrhea, nausea, vomiting, headache	100 mg PO bid pc and up to 300 mg/d total daily dosage
triamterene with hydrochlorothiazide	Dyazide	Edema and hypertension	Same as triamterene and hydrochlorothiazide	1–2 capsules, tablets bid pc

* *The term* generic *indicates that the drug is available in a generic form.*

▷ Uses of Diuretic Agents

Carbonic Anhydrase Inhibitors

Glaucoma is an increase in intraocular pressure in the eye that, if left untreated, can result in blindness. These drugs are used in the treatment of simple (open-angle) glaucoma, secondary glaucoma, and preoperatively in acute angle-closure glaucoma when delay of surgery is desired to lower intraocular pressure. These drugs are also used in the treatment of edema due to congestive heart failure (CHF), drug-induced edema, and control of epilepsy (petit mal and unlocalized seizures).

Thiazides and Related Diuretics

Thiazides and related diuretics are used in the treatment of hypertension and edema caused by CHF, hepatic cirrhosis, corticosteroid and estrogen therapy, and renal dysfunction.

Loop Diuretics

Loop diuretics are used in the treatment of edema associated with CHF, cirrhosis of the liver, and renal disease, including the nephrotic syndrome. These drugs are particularly useful when a greater diuretic effect is desired. Furosemide (Lasix) is also used to treat hypertension. Ethacrynic acid (Edecrin) is also used for the short-term management of ascites due to a malignancy, idiopathic edema, and lymphedema.

Osmotic Diuretics

Mannitol (Osmitrol) is used for the promotion of diuresis in the prevention and treatment of the oliguric phase of acute renal failure, as well as the reduction of intraocular pressure in the eye and the treatment of cerebral edema. Urea, also an osmotic diuretic, is useful in reducing cerebral edema and in the reduction of intraocular pressure.

Potassium-Sparing Diuretics

Potassium-sparing diuretics may be used in the treatment of some disorders because of their ability to conserve potassium. Amiloride is used in the treatment of CHF and hypertension and is often used with a thiazide diuretic. Spironolactone and triamterene are also used in the treatment of hypertension and edema due to CHF, cirrhosis, and the nephrotic syndrome. Both spironolactone and triamterene are also available with hydrochlorothiazide, a thiazide diuretic which enhances the diuretic effect of the drug combination while still conserving potassium.

▷ Adverse Reactions Associated with the Administration of Diuretics

The administration of any diuretic may result in electrolyte imbalance. The most common imbalance is a loss of potassium and water. When too much potassium is lost, hypokalemia occurs. When too much water is lost, dehydration occurs. Other electrolytes, for example sodium and chlorides, are also lost. Whether a fluid or electrolyte imbalance occurs depends on the amount of fluid and electrolytes lost and the ability of the individual to replace the lost fluid and electrolytes. For example, if a patient receiving a diuretic eats poorly and does not drink extra fluids, an electrolyte and water imbalance is likely to occur. However, even in a patient drinking adequate amounts of fluid and eating a well-balanced diet, an electrolyte imbalance may still occur and require electrolyte replacement (see chap 17).

Carbonic Anhydrase Inhibitors

Adverse reactions associated with short-term therapy with carbonic anhydrase inhibitors are rare. Long-term use of these drugs may result in fever, rash, paresthesias, anorexia, and crystalluria (crystals in the urine). On occasion, acidosis may occur and oral sodium bicarbonate may be used to correct this imbalance.

Thiazides and Related Diuretics

Administration of thiazides and related diuretics may be associated with numerous adverse reactions. However, many patients take these drugs without experiencing side effects other than excessive fluid and electrolyte loss, which can be corrected with an adequate fluid intake, a well-balanced diet, supplemental oral electrolytes, or the eating of foods or fluids high in the electrolytes that are being lost. In addition to the adverse reactions listed in Summary Drug Table 18-1, some of the adverse reactions that may be seen include gastric irritation, abdominal bloating, reduced libido, dizziness, vertigo, headache, photosensitivity, and weakness.

Loop Diuretics, Osmotic Diuretics, Potassium-Sparing Diuretics

Adverse reactions seen with the **loop diuretics, osmotic diuretics,** and the **potassium-sparing diuretics** are listed in Summary Drug Table 18-1. When a potassium-sparing and thiazide diuretic are given together, the adverse reactions associated with both agents may be seen.

▶ NURSING PROCESS
THE PATIENT RECEIVING A DIURETIC

ASSESSMENT

Before the administration of a diuretic for edema, the vital signs are taken and the patient is weighed. Current laboratory tests, especially the levels of serum electrolytes, are reviewed. If the patient has peripheral edema, the involved areas are inspected and the degree and extent of edema is recorded in the patient's chart. If the patient is receiving a carbonic anhydrase inhibitor for increased intraocular pressure, it is necessary to record the patient's description of pain and to obtain vital signs. The physical assessment of the patient receiving a diuretic for epilepsy includes vital signs and weight. The patient's chart is reviewed for a description of the seizures and the frequency of their occurrence.

If the patient is to receive an osmotic diuretic, assessment focuses on the patient's disease or disorder and the symptoms being treated. For example, if the patient has a low urinary output and the osmotic diuretic is given to increase urinary output, a review of the intake and output ratio and symptoms the patient is experiencing plus the patient's weight and vital signs are part of the physical assessment before starting drug therapy.

NURSING DIAGNOSIS

Depending on the drug, dose, and reason for administration, one or more of the following nursing diagnoses may apply to a person receiving a diuretic:

▶ Anxiety related to diagnosis, frequent urination, other factors (specify)

▶ High risk for fluid volume deficit related to excessive diuresis secondary to administration of a diuretic

▶ High risk for injury related to adverse drug effects (light-headedness, dizziness)

▶ Noncompliance related to indifference, lack of knowledge, other factors

▶ Knowledge deficit of medication regimen, adverse drug effects

PLANNING AND IMPLEMENTATION

The major goals of the patient may include a reduction in anxiety, correction of a fluid volume deficit, absence of injury, and an understanding of and compliance with the postdischarge medication regimen.

The major goals of nursing management may include a reduction in patient anxiety, recognition of adverse drug effects, prevention of injury, and the development and implementation of an effective teaching plan.

OBSERVATIONS AND NURSING MANAGEMENT.

During initial therapy, the patient must be observed for the effects of drug therapy. The type of assessments will depend on the reason for the administration of the diuretic, as discussed later. Intake and output are measured and recorded when any patient is receiving a diuretic. Any marked decrease in the patient's intake or output is reported to the physician.

THE PATIENT WITH EDEMA. Patients with edema are weighed daily or as ordered by the physician. The intake and output is measured and recorded every 8 hours. The critically ill patient or the patient with renal disease may require more frequent measurements of urinary output. The blood pressure, pulse, and respiratory rate are obtained every 1 to 4 hours or as ordered by the physician. An acutely ill patient may require more frequent monitoring of the vital signs.

Areas of edema are examined daily to evaluate the effectiveness of drug therapy. The findings are recorded in the patient's chart. The patient's general appearance and condition are evaluated daily or more often if the patient is acutely ill.

THE PATIENT WITH GLAUCOMA. If a diuretic is given for glaucoma, the patient's response to drug therapy (relief of eye pain) is evaluated every 2 hours. The physician is notified immediately if eye pain increases or if it has not begun to decrease 3 to 4 hours after the first dose. If the patient has acute closed-angle glaucoma, the pupil of the affected eye is checked for dilation and response to light every 2 hours. If the patient is ambulatory and has reduced vision because of glaucoma, assistance may be needed with ambulatory and self-care activities.

THE PATIENT WITH EPILEPSY. If a diuretic is being given for epilepsy, the patient is assessed at frequent intervals for the occurrence of seizures, especially early in therapy and in those known to have seizures at frequent intervals. If a seizure does occur, a description of the seizure and the time the seizure began and ended are recorded in the patient's chart. Accurate descriptions of the pattern and the number of seizures occurring each day helps the physician plan future therapy and adjust drug dosage as needed.

THE PATIENT WITH INCREASED INTRACRANIAL PRESSURE. If a patient is receiving a diuretic for increased intracranial pressure due to cerebral edema, the blood pressure, pulse, and respiratory rate are monitored every 30 to 60 minutes or as ordered by the physician. Any increase in blood pressure or decreases in the pulse or respiratory rate or neurological status is immediately reported to the physician. Neurologic assessments (vital signs, response of the pupils to light, level of consciousness, response to a painful stimulus, and so on) are performed at the time intervals ordered by the physician. The patient's response to the drug, that is, the signs and symptoms that may indicate a *decrease* in intracranial pressure, is evaluated and recorded.

ADVERSE DRUG REACTIONS. The most common adverse reaction associated with the administration of a diuretic is the loss of fluid and electrolytes. In some patients, the diuretic effect is moderate, whereas in others a large volume of fluid is lost. Regardless of the amount of fluid lost, there is always the possibility of excessive electrolyte loss, which can be potentially serious. Any patient receiving a diuretic is observed for adverse drug reactions, as well as the signs and symptoms of fluid and electrolyte imbalance (see chap 17).

ANXIETY. Some patients may exhibit anxiety related to their diagnosis or the fact that it will be necessary to urinate at frequent intervals. To reduce anxiety, the purpose and effects of the drug are explained. The patient should also be told that the need to urinate frequently will probably decrease. For some patients, the need to urinate frequently decreases after several days to a week of therapy. The patient on bed rest is provided with a call light and, when necessary, a bedpan or urinal that is placed within easy reach.

The patient is informed that the drug will be given early in the day so that nighttime sleep will not be interrupted. Although the duration of activity of most diuretics is around 8 hours or less, some diuretics have a longer activity which may result in a need to urinate during nighttime hours. This is especially true early in therapy.

FLUID VOLUME DEFICIT. On occasion, a fluid volume deficit may occur if the patient experiences diuresis but fails to take a sufficient amount of fluid orally to correct the deficit. This is especially true in the elderly or confused patient. To prevent a fluid volume deficit in these patients, oral fluids are encouraged during waking hours.

HIGH RISK FOR INJURY. Some patients experience dizziness or light-headedness, especially during the first few days of therapy or when a rapid diuresis has occurred. The patient allowed out of bed should be assisted with ambulatory activities until these adverse drug effects disappear.

NONCOMPLIANCE AND KNOWLEDGE DEFICIT. Before the first dose of a diuretic is given, the purpose of the drug (ie, to rid the body of excess fluid), when diuresis may be expected to occur, and how long diuresis will last (see Table 18-1) is explained to the patient.

The patient and the family require a full explanation of the prescribed drug therapy including when to take the drug (diuretics taken once a day are best taken early in the morning), if the drug is to be taken with food, and the importance of following the dosage schedule printed on the container label. The onset and duration of the drug's diuretic effect are also explained. The patient and family must also be made aware of the signs and symptoms of the fluid and electrolyte imbalances and adverse reactions that may occur when using a diuretic. To ensure compliance to the prescribed drug regimen, the importance of diuretic therapy in treating the patient's disorder is stressed.

Additional teaching points include the following:

▶ Do not stop the drug except on the advice of a physician.

▶ Take the drug early in the morning (once a day dosage, only) unless directed otherwise.

▶ Avoid alcohol and nonprescription drugs unless their use has been approved by the physician.

▶ Notify the physician if any of the following should occur: muscle cramps or weakness, dizziness, nausea, vomiting, diarrhea, dry mouth, thirst, general weakness, rapid pulse, or GI distress.

▶ Weigh self weekly or as recommended by the physician. Keep a record of these weekly weights and contact the physician if weight loss exceeds three to five pounds per week.

▶ If foods or fluids high in potassium are recommended by the physician: eat the amount of food or fluid high in potassium as recommended by the physician. Do not exceed this amount or eliminate from the diet for more than 1 day except when told to do so by the physician.

▶ After a time, the diuretic effect of the drug may be minimal because most of the body's excess fluid has been removed. Continue therapy to prevent further accumulation of fluid.

▶ The patient with glaucoma: contact the physician immediately if eye pain is not relieved or if it increases.

▶ A family member of the patient with epilepsy should keep a record of all seizures witnessed and bring this to the physician at the time of the next visit. Contact the physician immediately if the seizures increase in number.

EVALUATION

▶ Anxiety is reduced

▶ Fluid volume deficit (if present) is corrected

▶ No evidence of injury

▶ Patient complies to the prescribed drug regimen

▶ Patient and family demonstrate understanding of drug regimen

▶ Verbalizes importance of complying with the prescribed treatment regimen

▶ ANTIHYPERTENSIVE AGENTS

Most cases of hypertension have no known cause. As in many other diseases and conditions, there is no one best drug, drug combination, or medical regimen for treatment of hypertension. Following examination and evaluation of the patient, the physician selects the antihypertensive drug that will probably be most effective. In some instances, it may be necessary to change to another antihypertensive drug when the patient does not respond to therapy. In addition to drug therapy, the physician may also recommend additional measures such as weight loss (if the patient is overweight) and dietary changes such as the elimination of some salt from food.

The types of agents used for the treatment of hypertension include the following:

Alpha/beta-adrenergic blocking agent—for example, labetalol (Normodyne)

Angiotensin converting enzyme inhibitors—for example, captopril (Capoten), enalapril (Vasotec I.V.), lisinopril (Prinivil)

Antiadrenergic agents (centrally acting)—for example, methyldopa (Aldomet), clonidine (Catapres-TTS-1, Catapres-TTS-2, or Catapres-TTS-3), guanfacine (Tenex)

Antiadrenergic agents (peripherally acting)—for example, guanethidine (Ismelin), guanadrel (Hylorel)

Beta-adrenergic blocking agents—for example, metoprolol (Lopressor), atenolol (Tenormin), propranolol (Inderal)

Diuretics—for example, furosemide (Lasix), hydrochlorothiazide (HydroDIURIL)

Vasodilators—for example, minoxidil (Loniten), hydralazine (Apresoline)

Calcium channel blocking agents—for example, verapamil (Calan), nicardipine (Cardene)

▷ Actions of Antihypertensive Agents

Many antihypertensive agents lower the blood pressure by dilating arterial blood vessels. Dilation creates an increase in the lumen of the arterial blood vessels, which in turn increases the amount of space available for the blood to circulate. Because blood volume (the amount of blood) remains relatively constant, an increase in the space in which the blood circulates (ie, the blood vessels) lowers the blood pressure. Although the method by which antihypertensive agents dilate blood vessels varies, the result remains basically the same. Antihypertensive agents that have vasodilating activity include the **alpha/beta-adrenergic blocking agents, antiadrenergic agents, beta-adrenergic blocking agents, calcium channel blocking agents,** and the **vasodilators.** See chapter 7 for additional discussion of adrenergic blocking agents and antiandrenergic agents.

The ability of thiazides and related diuretics to reduce an elevated blood pressure is unknown, but is thought to be due, in part, to their ability to increase the excretion of sodium from the body.

The mechanism of action of the angiotensin converting enzyme inhibitors is not fully understood. It is believed these drugs may prevent (or inhibit) the activity of the angiotensin-converting enzyme (ACE) that converts angiotensin I to angiotensin II, which is a powerful vasoconstrictor. Both angiotensin I and ACE are produced by the body; therefore, they are called *endogenous* substances.

▷ Uses of Antihypertensive Agents

These drugs are used in the treatment of hypertension. Although there is a variety of antihypertensive drugs available, not all drugs may work equally well in a given patient. In some instances, the physician may find it necessary to prescribe a different antihypertensive drug when the patient fails to respond to therapy. Some antihypertensive drugs are used only in severe cases of hypertension and when other less potent agents have failed to lower the blood pressure.

▷ **Adverse Reactions Associated with the Administration of Antihypertensive Agents**

The adverse reactions that may be seen when an antihypertensive agent is administered are listed in Summary Drug Table 18-2. For the adverse reactions seen when a diuretic is used as an antihypertensive agent, see Summary Drug Table 18-1.

Postural or orthostatic hypotension may be seen in some patients, especially early in therapy. Postural hypotension is the occurrence of dizziness and light-headedness when the individual rises suddenly from a lying or sitting position. Orthostatic hypotension occurs when the individual has been standing in one place for a long time. These reactions can be avoided or minimized by having the patient rise slowly from a lying or sitting position and avoid standing in one place for a prolonged period.

SUMMARY DRUG TABLE 18—2
Antihypertensive Agents

GENERIC NAME	TRADE NAME*	USES	ADVERSE REACTIONS	DOSE RANGES
ALPHA/BETA-ADRENERGIC BLOCKING AGENTS				
labetalol hydrochloride	Normodyne	Hypertension	Fatigue, headache, nausea, vomiting, muscle weakness, diarrhea, drowsiness	100 mg—1.2 g PO bid; 20—50 mg IV; 50—300 mg IV infusion
ANGIOTENSIN-CONVERTING ENZYME INHIBITORS				
captopril	Capoten	Hypertension	Rash, hypotension, gastric irritation, dizziness, renal insufficiency	25—150 mg PO bid, tid
enalapril maleate	Vasotec, Vasotec IV	Hypertension	Chest pain, nervousness, nausea, diarrhea	Oral: 2.5—40 mg/d; IV: 0.625—1.25 mg slow IV infusion over 5 min
lisinopril	Prinivil, Zestril	Hypertension	Hypotension, chest pain, cough, dyspnea, nausea, vomiting	10—40 mg/d PO
ANTIADRENERGIC AGENTS				
clonidine hydrochloride	Catapres-TTS	Mild to moderate hypertension	Dry mouth, drowsiness, anorexia, rash, malaise, constipation, dizziness, sedation	0.2—2.4 mg/d PO in divided doses
guanabenz acetate	Wytensin	Hypertension	Drowsiness, sedation, dry mouth, weakness, headache	4—32 mg PO bid
guanadrel sulfate	Hylorel	Hypertension	Palpitations, headache, fatigue, nocturia, increased bowel movements, aching limbs, shortness of breath on exertion	10—75 mg/d PO in divided doses
guanethidine sulfate	Ismelin	Hypertension	Dizziness, weakness, fluid retention, diarrhea, syncope	10—50 mg/d PO
guanfacine hydrochloride	Tenex	Hypertension	Dry mouth, sedation, weakness, dizziness, constipation	1—3 mg/d PO at hs (higher doses may be used in some instances)
methyldopa	Aldomet, *generic*	Hypertension	Sedation, bradycardia, vomiting, rash, headache, nausea	250 mg—3 g/d PO in divided doses
prazosin hydrochloride	Minipress	Hypertension	Dizziness, fainting, drowsiness	2—40 mg/d PO in divided doses
reserpine	Serpasil, *generic*	Hypertension	Nausea, vomiting, rash, dry mouth, bradycardia, nasal congestion	0.1—0.5 mg/d PO

(continued)

SUMMARY DRUG TABLE 18–1
(continued)

GENERIC NAME	TRADE NAME*	USES	ADVERSE REACTIONS	DOSE RANGES
BETA-ADRENERGIC BLOCKING AGENTS				
acebutolol hydrochloride	Sectral	Hypertension	Bradycardia, dizziness, vertigo, rash, hyperglycemia, hypotension, agranulocytosis, bronchospasm	200–1200 mg/d PO in divided doses
atenolol	Tenormin	Hypertension	Same as acebutolol	50–100 mg/d PO
metoprolol tartrate	Lopressor	Hypertension	Same as acebutolol	100–450 mg/d PO
nadolol	Corgard	Hypertension	Same as acebutolol	40–320 mg/d PO
pindolol	Visken	Hypertension	Same as acebutolol	5–60 mg/d PO in divided doses
propranolol hydrochloride	Inderal	Hypertension	Same as acebutolol	40–240 mg PO bid, tid or 80–120 mg/d PO
timolol maleate	Blocadren	Hypertension	Same as acebutolol	20–60 mg/d PO in divided doses
VASODILATORS				
hydralazine hydrochloride	Apresoline, *generic*	Hypertension	Headache, anorexia, nausea, vomiting, diarrhea, palpitations	10–50 mg PO bid to qid (up to 300 mg/d may be required for some patients)
minoxidil	Loniten, *generic*	Severe hypertension	Edema, rash, nausea, vomiting, excessive growth of fine body hair	5–100 mg/d PO in single dose or divided doses
CALCIUM-CHANNEL BLOCKING AGENTS				
nicardipine hydrochloride	Cardene	Hypertension	Peripheral edema, palpitations, angina, dizziness, headache, weakness	20–40 mg PO tid
verapamil hydrochloride	Calan, Isoptin, *generic*	Hypertension	Peripheral edema, hypotension, dizziness, headache, nausea, constipation	80 mg PO tid

* The term generic *indicates that the drug is available in a generic form.*

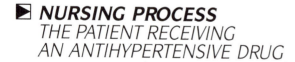

▶ NURSING PROCESS
THE PATIENT RECEIVING AN ANTIHYPERTENSIVE DRUG

ASSESSMENT

Before starting therapy with an antihypertensive drug, the blood pressure and pulse rate are obtained on both arms with the patient in a standing, sitting, and lying position. All readings are properly identified (eg, the readings on each arm and the three positions used to obtain the readings) and recorded on the patient's chart. The patient's weight is also obtained, especially if a diuretic is part of therapy or the physician prescribes a weight loss regimen.

NURSING DIAGNOSIS

Depending on the drug, dose, and the type and severity of hypertension, one or more of the following nursing diagnoses may apply to a person receiving an antihypertensive drug:

▶ Anxiety related to diagnosis, other factors (specify)

▶ High risk for fluid volume deficit related to administration of a diuretic as an antihypertensive drug (when appropriate)

▶ High risk for injury related to dizziness or lightheadedness secondary to postural or orthostatic hypotensive episodes

▶ Noncompliance related to indifference, lack of knowledge, other factors

▶ Knowledge deficit of medication regimen, adverse drug effects, treatment modalities

PLANNING AND IMPLEMENTATION

The major goals of the patient may include a reduction in anxiety and an understanding of and compliance to the prescribed treatment regimen.

The major goals of nursing management may include a reduction in the patient's anxiety, recognition of adverse drug effects, and the development and implementation of an effective teaching plan

ADMINISTRATION. The blood pressure and pulse rate are taken immediately before each administration of an antihypertensive drug and are compared to previous readings. The drug should be withheld and the physician notified if the blood pressure is significantly decreased. The physician is also notified if there is a significant increase in the blood pressure.

Each time the blood pressure is obtained, the same arm is used and the patient is placed in the same position (eg, standing, sitting, or lying down). In some instances, the physician may order the blood pressure taken in one or more positions, such as the standing and lying down positions. The blood pressure and pulse are monitored at every 1 to 4 hours if the patient has severe hypertension, does not respond as expected to drug therapy, or if the patient is critically ill.

Monitoring and recording the blood pressure is an important nursing function, especially early in therapy. The physician may need to adjust the dose of the drug upward or downward, try a different drug, or add another drug to the therapeutic regimen if the patient does not respond adequately to drug therapy.

Daily to weekly weights are obtained on many patients first starting drug therapy for hypertension. Weighing the patient at regular intervals is usually necessary if the patient is placed on a weight-reduction diet to lower the blood pressure, or if the patient is receiving a thiazide or related diuretic as part of antihypertensive therapy.

If the patient is receiving a thiazide or related diuretic, the nursing implications discussed earlier (see Nursing Process, The Patient Receiving a Diuretic) are also considered during antihypertensive therapy.

ADVERSE DRUG REACTIONS. The patient is observed for adverse drug reactions because their occurrence may require a change in the dose or the drug. The physician is informed if any adverse reactions occur. In some instances, the patient may have to tolerate mild adverse reactions, such as dry mouth or mild anorexia.

ANXIETY. Some patients may exhibit anxiety related to their diagnosis or the fact that lifetime therapy for

the control of hypertension is necessary. The patient should be allowed time to ask questions about the treatment and drug regimen prescribed by the physician. The patient should be told that most cases of hypertension can be controlled with drug therapy, thereby eliminating the dangers (stroke, heart attack) associated with hypertension.

HIGH RISK FOR INJURY. If postural hypotension should occur, the patient is advised to rise slowly from a sitting or lying position. When rising from a lying position, sitting on the edge of the bed for 1 or 2 minutes often minimizes these symptoms. Rising slowly from a chair and then standing for 1 to 2 minutes also minimizes the symptoms of postural hypotension. When symptoms of postural hypotension occur, the patient must be assisted in getting out of bed or a chair and with ambulatory activities.

NONCOMPLIANCE AND KNOWLEDGE DEFICIT. To ensure lifetime compliance, the importance of drug therapy in the treatment of hypertension is emphasized.

The adverse reactions that may be seen with a particular antihypertensive agent are explained and the patient is advised to contact the physician if any should occur.

The physician may wish the patient or family to monitor blood pressure during therapy. The technique of taking a blood pressure and pulse rate will need to be taught to the patient or family. Sufficient time for supervised practice must be allowed. The patient is also instructed to keep a record of the blood pressure and bring this to each physician or clinic visit.

The following points are included in a teaching plan for the patient receiving an antihypertensive agent:

▶ Do not discontinue this medication except on the advice of a physician.

▶ Avoid the use any nonprescription drugs (some may contain drugs that are capable of raising the blood pressure) unless use of a specific drug is approved by the physician.

▶ Avoid alcohol unless use has been approved by the physician.

▶ This drug may produce dizziness or light-headedness when rising suddenly from a sitting or lying position. To avoid these effects, rise slowly from a sitting or lying position.

If the patient is receiving a diuretic, the patient and family teaching discussed earlier (see Nursing Process, The Patient Receiving a Diuretic) is also included.

EVALUATION

▶ Anxiety is reduced

▶ Fluid volume deficit is corrected (when appropriate)

▶ No evidence of injury

▶ Patient complies to the prescribed drug regimen

▶ Patient and family demonstrate understanding of drug regimen

▶ Verbalizes importance of complying with the prescribed treatment regimen

19

Central Nervous System Stimulants

On completion of this chapter the student will:

▶ *List the actions and uses of central nervous system stimulants*

▶ *Use the nursing process when administering a central nervous system stimulant*

▶ *Discuss the nursing implications to be considered when administering a central nervous system stimulant*

An *analeptic* is a drug that stimulates the respiratory center of the central nervous system (CNS). Included in this group are doxapram (Dopram) and caffeine. Other CNS stimulants include the amphetamines, the anorexiants, and methylphenidate (Ritalin; Summary Drug Table 19-1). An *anorexiant* is a drug that suppresses the appetite.

▷ Actions of CNS Stimulants

Analeptics

The analeptic doxapram stimulates the respiratory center in the medulla, resulting in an increase in the respiratory rate.

Amphetamines

The amphetamines, for example, amphetamine, dextroamphetamine (Dexedrine), and methamphetamine (Desoxyn), are sympathomimetic (ie, adrenergic) drugs that stimulate the CNS (see chap 6). Their drug action results in an elevation of blood pressure, wakefulness, and an increase or decrease in pulse rate. The ability of these drugs to suppress the appetite is thought to be due to their action on the appetite center in the hypothalamus.

Anorexiants

The action of the anorexiants (eg, phendimetrazine and phentermine) is similar to that of the amphetamines.

SUMMARY DRUG TABLE 19–1
Central Nervous System Stimulants

GENERIC NAME	TRADE NAME*	USES	ADVERSE REACTIONS	DOSE RANGES
amphetamine sulfate	*Generic*	Obesity, narcolepsy, abnormal behavior syndrome in children	Restlessness, insomnia, anorexia, tachycardia, dizziness	Obesity: 5–30 mg/d PO in divided doses; narcolepsy: 5–60 mg/d PO in divided doses; abnormal behavior syndrome: 2.5–40 mg/d (depends on age)
caffeine and sodium benzoate	*Generic*	Prevention of spinal headache; as a stimulant in acute circulatory failure	Nausea, vomiting, restlessness, excitement, tachycardia	200–500 mg IM, IV
dextroamphetamine sulfate	Dexedrine, *generic*	Same as amphetamine	Same as amphetamine	Same as amphetamine
doxapram hydrochloride	Dopram	Drug-induced CNS depression, chronic pulmonary disease associated with acute hypercapnia, stimulation of respirations during postanesthesia	Headache, dizziness, cough, dyspnea, variations in heart rate, disorientation, apprehension	Postanesthesia: 0.5–1 mg/kg IV or 250 mg in 250 mL of dextrose or saline by IV infusion; drug-induced CNS depression: 2 mg/kg IV repeated prn; chronic obstructive pulmonary disease: 400 mg in 180 mL of IV solution and infuse at 1–2 mg/min
methamphetamine hydrochloride	Desoxyn	Exogenous obesity, abnormal behavior syndrome in children	Same as amphetamine	Obesity: 5 mg PO 30 min before each meal; abnormal behavior syndrome: 5 mg PO daily or bid and increased prn
methylphenidate hydrochloride	Ritalin, *generic*	Attention deficit disorders, narcolepsy	Nervousness, insomnia, rash, anorexia, nausea	20–60 mg/d PO in divided doses; children: 5–50 mg/d PO in divided doses
phendimetrazine tartrate	Adphen, *generic*	Exogenous obesity	Palpitation, tachycardia, nervousness, dry mouth, dizziness, anxiety, tremor, mydriasis, cardiac dysrhythmias, euphoria	35 mg PO bid, tid 1 h before the meal; sustained release: 105 mg PO in the morning
phentermine hydrochloride	Phentrol, *generic*	Same as phendimetrazine	Same as phendimetrazine	8 mg PO tid ac or 15–37.5 mg PO in the morning
phenylpropanolamine hydrochloride	Dexatrim, Control, *generic*	Same as phendimetrazine	Same as phendimetrazine	25 mg PO tid ac; sustained release: 75 mg/d PO in the morning

* *The term* generic *indicates that the drug is available in a generic form.*

Caffeine

Caffeine stimulates the CNS at all levels including the cerebral cortex, the medulla, and the spinal cord. Caffeine has mild analeptic (respiratory stimulating) activity. Other actions include cardiac stimulation (which may produce tachycardia) dilatation of coronary and peripheral blood vessels, constriction of cerebral blood vessels, and skeletal muscle stimulation. Caffeine also has mild diuretic activity.

Methylphenidate

Methylphenidate stimulates the cerebral cortex. Its action appears to be similar to the amphetamines (see Actions of CNS Stimulants, Amphetamines) but the exact mode of action of this drug is not fully understood.

▷ Uses of CNS Stimulants

Analeptics

Doxapram is used in the treatment of drug-induced respiratory depression, respiratory depression in chronic pulmonary disease, and acute respiratory insufficiency. This drug may also be used during the postanesthesia period when respiratory depression is due to anesthesia. It is also used to stimulate deep breathing in the postanesthesia patient.

Amphetamines

Amphetamines may be used in the *short-term* treatment of exogenous obesity (obesity due to overeating). Long-term use of these drugs for obesity is not recommended because amphetamines have addiction potential. Amphetamines are also subject to abuse and because of this, their use in treating exogenous obesity has declined. These drugs may also be helpful in the management of narcolepsy, which is a disorder manifested by an uncontrollable desire to sleep during normal waking hours even though the individual has a normal nighttime sleeping pattern. Amphetamines are also used in the management of abnormal behavior syndrome (attention deficit disorder) in children. This disorder is characterized by a short attention span, hyperactivity, impulsiveness, and emotional lability. How the amphetamines, which are CNS stimulants, calm the hyperactive child is unknown.

Anorexiants

Phendimetrazine and phentermine are chemically related to the amphetamines and are used for *short-term* treatment of exogenous obesity. These drugs are available only by prescription and have addiction and abuse potential. Some nonprescription diet aids contain phenylpropanolamine, an adrenergic agent that has actions similar to epinephrine. These diet aids are not true anorexiants, and those containing phenylpropanolamine have limited appetite suppressing ability when compared to the anorexiants. Phenylpropanolamine also has very little abuse potential and has no addiction potential.

Caffeine

Caffeine as caffeine and sodium benzoate is administered intramuscularly (IM) or intravenously (IV) and may be used as a diuretic and as an analeptic in the treatment of poisoning. Because caffeine also has other effects such as constriction of cerebral arteries and stimulation of skeletal muscles, the use of caffeine for this purpose has largely been replaced by narcotic antagonists or other drugs with greater analeptic activity (eg, doxapram). Caffeine may also be used in the treatment of acute circulatory failure but use for this purpose has largely been replaced by other drugs. Given IV, caffeine may be used to relieve headache that follows a lumbar (spinal) puncture. It is also combined with ergotamine for the treatment of migraine headaches. Orally, caffeine, either as a beverage (coffee, tea) or in nonprescription tablet form, may be used by some individuals to relieve fatigue.

Methylphenidate

Methylphenidate is used in the treatment of narcolepsy and attention deficit disorders in children.

▷ Adverse Reactions Associated with the Administration of CNS Stimulants

One of the chief adverse reactions associated with CNS stimulants is overstimulation of the CNS. Overstimulation of the CNS can result in a variety of adverse reactions such as insomnia, tachycardia, nervousness, anorexia, dizziness, and excitement. In some instances, the intensity of these reactions are dose dependent, but some individuals may experience an intense degree of these symptoms even with low doses. Other individuals experience few symptoms of CNS stimulation.

The amphetamines and anorexiants are known to have abuse and addiction potential, and are recommended only for short-term use in selected patients for the treatment of exogenous obesity. When used for treatment of attention deficit disorders in children, long-term use must be followed by gradual withdrawal of the drug.

Long-term use of amphetamines for obesity may result in tolerance to the drug and a tendency to increase the dose. Extreme psychological dependency may also occur.

▶ NURSING PROCESS
THE PATIENT RECEIVING A CNS STIMULANT

ASSESSMENT

Assessment of the patient receiving a CNS stimulant drug depends on the drug, the patient, and the reason for administration.

ANALEPTICS. When a CNS stimulant is prescribed for respiratory depression, initial assessments will include the blood pressure, pulse, and respiratory rate. It is important to note the depth of the respirations and any pattern to the respiratory rate, such as shallow respirations or alternating deep and shallow respirations. A review of recent laboratory tests (if any), such as arterial blood gas studies, is also necessary. Before administration of the drug, an adequate airway is necessary. Oxygen is usually administered before, during, and after drug administration.

AMPHETAMINES. When an amphetamine is prescribed for any reason, the patient is weighed and the blood pressure, pulse, and respiratory rate are taken and recorded before starting drug therapy.

The child with an attention deficit disorder is initially observed for the various patterns of abnormal behavior. A summary of the behavior pattern is recorded in the patient's chart to provide a comparison with future changes that may occur during therapy.

ANOREXIANTS. The anorexiants and amphetamines used in the treatment of obesity are usually prescribed for out-patient use. The blood pressure, pulse, respiratory rate, and weight are taken and recorded before therapy is started.

CAFFEINE. Physical assessments made before the administration of caffeine sodium benzoate, include the blood pressure, pulse, and respiratory rate.

METHYLPHENIDATE. When prescribed for an attention deficit disorder, methylphenidate is usually part of a treatment program that may include psychological, social, and educational measures. Before the start of drug therapy, the blood pressure, pulse, respiratory rate, and weight are obtained. As with administration of an amphetamine for this same disorder, a summary of the behavior pattern is recorded in the patient's chart and provides a comparison to changes that may occur during drug therapy.

NURSING DIAGNOSIS

Depending on the drug, dose, and reason for administration, one or more of the following nursing diagnoses may apply to a person receiving a CNS stimulant:

▶ Anxiety related to diagnosis (some instances), adverse drug reactions

▶ Knowledge deficit of medication regimen, adverse drug effects

PLANNING AND IMPLEMENTATION

The major goals of the patient may include a reduction in anxiety and an understanding of the medication regimen.

The major goals of nursing management may include a reduction in patient or family member anxiety and the development and implementation of an effective teaching plan.

The patient's weight is monitored at intervals depending on the reason for drug use. Those with narcolepsy or an attention deficit disorder may require only monthly weights to monitor weight loss or gain. Those on a weight reduction program may require weekly monitoring of their weight. The blood pressure, pulse, and respiratory rate should be obtained each time the patient visits the physician's office or clinic.

OBSERVATIONS AND NURSING MANAGEMENT. Continued assessment and nursing management depends on the drug used and the reason for use as discussed in later sections.

THE PATIENT WITH RESPIRATORY DEPRESSION. After administration of the drug, the respiratory rate and pattern are closely monitored until the respirations return to normal. The level of consciousness, the blood pressure, and pulse rate are also monitored at 5- to 15-minute intervals or as ordered by the physician. Arterial blood gases may be drawn at intervals to determine the effectiveness of the analeptic, as well as the need for additional drug therapy. The patient is observed for adverse drug reactions, which are immediately reported to the physician.

THE PATIENT WITH ABNORMAL BEHAVIOR SYNDROME. A daily summary of the child's behavior is entered in the patient's record. This provides a record of the results of therapy. During prolonged therapy, behavior summaries may be made on a weekly basis.

THE PATIENT WITH NARCOLEPSY. The patient with narcolepsy requires observation during daytime hours. If periods of sleep are noted, the time of day they occur and their length are recorded. Because most of these individuals are outpatients, the patient and family members are instructed to keep a record of the periods of sleep.

The adverse drug reactions that may occur with the use of an amphetamine, such as insomnia and a significant increase in blood pressure and pulse rate, may be serious enough to require discontinuation of the drug. In some instances, the adverse drug effects are mild and may even disappear during therapy. All adverse reactions are reported to the physician.

ANXIETY. Some patients or family members, for example, the patient with narcolepsy or parents of the child with abnormal behavior syndrome, may have concern over the prescribed drug therapy and the ability of the drug to control symptoms. The patient or family member should be allowed time to ask questions and to discuss the planned treatment regimen.

If anxiety appears to be drug related, the physician is informed because it may be necessary to decrease the dosage or prescribe another drug.

KNOWLEDGE DEFICIT. The treatment regimen and adverse drug reactions are explained to the patient and family. The type of information included in the teaching plan will depend on the drug and the reason for use. The importance of following the recommended dosage schedule should be emphasized. Additional teaching points may include the following.

THE PATIENT WITH ABNORMAL BEHAVIOR SYNDROME. A daily summary should be written of the child's behavior including periods of hyperactivity, general pattern of behavior, socialization with others, attention span, and so on. These are brought to each physician or clinic visit because this record may help the physician determine future drug dosages.

THE PATIENT WITH NARCOLEPSY. A record is kept of the number of times per day that periods of sleepiness occur, and this record is brought to each physician or clinic visit.

THE AMPHETAMINES AND ANOREXIANTS. These drugs are taken early in the day to avoid insomnia. The dose must not be increased or taken more frequently except on the advice of a physician. These drugs may impair the ability to drive or perform hazardous tasks and may mask extreme fatigue. If dizziness, light-headedness, anxiety, nervousness, or tremors occur, the physician should be contacted. The use of coffee, tea, and carbonated beverages containing caffeine should be avoided or taken in small amounts.

CAFFEINE (ORAL, NONPRESCRIPTION). The use of oral caffeine-containing products to stay awake is avoided if there is a history of heart disease, high blood pressure, or stomach ulcers. These products are intended for occasional use and should be discontinued if heart palpitations, dizziness, or light-headedness occurs.

METHYLPHENIDATE. The last daily dose is taken (or given) before 6 PM to avoid insomnia. The physician is notified if nervousness, insomnia, vomiting, fever, palpitations, or skin rash occurs. This drug may impair physical coordination. Caution is necessary when driving (adults) or performing any tasks that may be hazardous (adults and children).

EVALUATION

▶ Anxiety is reduced

▶ Patient complies to the prescribed drug regimen

▶ Patient and family demonstrate understanding of drug regimen

▶ Verbalizes importance of complying with the prescribed treatment regimen

20

Insulin and Oral Hypoglycemic Drugs

On completion of this chapter the student will:

▶ *List the types and uses of the insulins and oral hypoglycemic drugs*

▶ *Discuss the adverse reactions associated with the administration of insulin and oral hypoglycemic drugs*

▶ *Use the nursing process when administering insulin*

▶ *Discuss the nursing implications associated with the administration of insulin*

▶ *List the types and uses of oral hypoglycemic drugs*

▶ *Discuss the adverse reactions associated with the administration of oral hypoglycemic drugs*

▶ *Use the nursing process when administering an oral hypoglycemic agent*

▶ *Discuss the nursing implications associated with the administration of hypoglycemic drugs*

▶ INSULIN

▷ Actions of Insulin

Insulin is a hormone manufactured by the beta cells of the pancreas. It is the principal hormone required for the proper use of glucose by the body. Insulin appears to activate a process that helps glucose molecules enter the cells of striated muscle and adipose tissue. Insulin also stimulates the synthesis of glycogen by the liver and possibly promotes protein synthesis. When the production of insulin by the pancreas is insufficient, the patient has diabetes mellitus.

Diabetes mellitus is a metabolic disorder of the pancreas in which glucose intolerance results from varying degrees of insulin insufficiency. Although no age group is exempt, diabetes is most frequently seen in people between ages 40 and 60.

Onset, peak, and duration are three properties of insulin that are of clinical importance. **Onset** is when insulin first begins to act in the body; **peak** is when the insulin is exerting maximum action; and **duration** is the length of time the insulin remains in effect. To meet the needs of those with diabetes mellitus, various insulin preparations have been developed to delay the onset and prolong the duration of action of insulin. When insulin is combined with protamine (a protein), the absorption of insulin from the injection site is slowed and the duration of action is prolonged. The addition of zinc also modifies the onset and duration of action of insulin.

Insulin is available as purified extracts from beef and pork pancreas and is biologically similar to human insulin. Also available is human insulin, which is derived by two methods. One method is by genetic engineering using stains of *Escherichia coli*, a microorganism found in the gastrointestinal (GI) tract. The other method is by chemical modification of pork insulin. Human insulin appears to cause fewer allergic reactions than insulin obtained from animal sources.

Insulin preparations are classified as rapid-acting, intermediate-acting, or long-acting. Table 20-1 lists the types of insulin preparations and compares their onset, peak, and duration of action.

▷ Uses of Insulin

Insulin is used for the treatment of diabetes mellitus. The two major types of diabetes mellitus are as follows:

Type I—Insulin-dependent diabetes mellitus (IDDM). Former names of this type of diabetes mellitus include juvenile diabetes, juvenile-onset diabetes, and brittle diabetes.

Type II—Non–insulin-dependent diabetes mellitus (NIDDM). Former names of this type of diabetes mellitus include maturity-onset diabetes, adult-onset diabetes, and stable diabetes.

Insulin is necessary for controlling type I diabetes mellitus. Insulin may be necessary for the control of the more severe and complicated forms of type II diabetes mellitus, although some patients with type II diabetes can be controlled on diet alone or diet and an oral hypoglycemic agent (see section on oral hypoglycemic drugs). Insulin may also be used in the treatment of severe diabetic ketoacidosis (DKA) or diabetic coma.

▷ Adverse Reactions Associated with the Administration of Insulin

The two major adverse reactions seen with insulin administration are *hypoglycemia* (low blood glucose or sugar) and *hyperglycemia* (elevated blood glucose or sugar). The signs and symptoms of hypoglycemia and hyperglycemia are listed in Table 20-2.

Hypoglycemia occurs when there is too much insulin in the bloodstream in relation to the available glucose. Hypoglycemia may occur when the patient eats too little food, when the insulin dose is incorrectly measured and is greater than that prescribed, or when the patient drastically increases physical activity. Hyperglycemia may occur if there is too little insulin in the bloodstream in relation to

---

TABLE 20–1
Onset, Peak, and Duration of Action of Various Insulin Preparations*

PREPARATION	ONSET (h)	PEAK (h)	DURATION (h)
RAPID-ACTING INSULINS			
Insulin injection (regular)	½–1	2 ½–5	6–8
Prompt insulin zinc suspension	1–1 ½	5–10	12–16
INTERMEDIATE-ACTING INSULINS			
Isophane insulin suspension (NPH)	1–1 ½	4–12	24
Insulin zinc suspension (lente)	1–2 ½	7–15	24
LONG-ACTING INSULINS			
Protamine zinc insulin (PZI)	4–8	14–24	36
Extended insulin zinc suspension (ultralente)	4–8	10–30	>36

References may vary slightly on these figures.

TABLE 20–2
Signs and Symptoms of Hyperglycemia
and Hypoglycemia

HYPERGLYCEMIA

Polyphagia	Glucosuria
Polydipsia	Ketonuria
Polyuria	Blurred vision
Dehydration	Changes in vision
Weight loss	Hypovolemia
Weakness	Recurrent or persistent infections
Fatigue	Muscle wasting
Muscle cramps	

HYPOGLYCEMIA

Fatigue	Weakness
Confusion	Headache
Diplopia	Psychosis
Personality changes	Rapid, shallow respirations
Hunger	Numbness of the mouth, lips, tongue
Nausea	Pallor
Slurred speech	Staggering gait
Tingling	Tremors
Diaphoresis	Slowed thinking
Lack of coordination	Pulse rate may be normal or abnormal
Dizziness	Convulsions
Coma	

the available glucose. Hyperglycemia also may occur when the patient eats too much food, when too little or no insulin is given, or when the patient experiences emotional stress, infection, surgery, pregnancy, or an acute illness.

On rare occasions, a patient is allergic to the animal (pig or cow) from which insulin is obtained or is allergic to the protein or zinc added to insulin. An individual can also become insulin-resistant (or resistant to insulin) because he or she has developed antibodies against insulin. In these cases, the physician may prescribe human insulin or purified insulin. On rare occasions, some individuals become resistant to the human and purified insulins.

▶ NURSING PROCESS
THE PATIENT RECEIVING INSULIN

ASSESSMENT

If the patient has been recently diagnosed as having diabetes mellitus and has not received insulin or if the patient is a known diabetic, the initial physical assessment before administering the first dose of insulin includes the blood pressure, pulse and respiratory rates, and weight. A general assessment of the skin, mucous membranes, and extremities is made with special attention to any sores or cuts that appear to be infected

or healing poorly, as well as any ulcerations or other skin or mucous membrane changes. The patient history should include dietary habits, a family history of diabetes (if any), and an inquiry into the type and duration of symptoms experienced. The patient's chart is reviewed for recent laboratory and diagnostic tests.

If the patient has diabetes and has been receiving insulin, the history should also include the type and dosage of insulin used, the type of diabetic diet, and the average results of urine testing. Assessment should also include evaluating the patient's past compliance to the prescribed treatment regimen such as diet, weight control, and periodic evaluation by a physician.

NURSING DIAGNOSIS

The nursing diagnoses may depend on the patient's individual needs and are based on the information obtained during assessment.

The extent of the nursing diagnoses depends on factors such as whether the patient is a new diabetic, has had treatment for diabetes, or has not followed the prescribed medical regimen.

▶ Anxiety related to diagnosis, fear of giving own injections, dietary restrictions, other factors (specify)

▶ Ineffective individual coping related to inability to accept diagnosis, other factors (specify)

▶ Fear related to diagnosis, consequences of diabetes

▶ Altered health maintenance related to inability to comprehend drug regimen, lack of equipment to monitor drug effects, lack of knowledge

▶ Noncompliance to treatment regimen related to lack of knowledge, misunderstanding, or complexity of prescribed treatment program, other factors (specify)

▶ Knowledge deficit of insulin administration, urine testing, diet

PLANNING AND IMPLEMENTATION

The major goals of the patient may include a reduction in anxiety and fear, improved ability to cope with the diagnosis, compliance with the prescribed treatment regimen, and an understanding of and compliance to the prescribed treatment regimen.

The major goals of nursing management may include reducing patient fear and anxiety, helping the patient physically and mentally cope with the diagnosis, and developing and implementing an effective teaching plan.

INSULIN ADMINISTRATION. Insulin may be administered in several ways. One method is the use of a needle and syringe. Use of the microfine needles has reduced the discomfort associated with an injection. Another method is the jet injection system, which uses pressure to deliver a fine stream of insulin below the skin. Another method uses a disposable needle and special syringe. The syringe uses a cartridge that is prefilled with a specific type of insulin (regular human insulin, isophane [NPH] insulin, or a mixture of isophane and regular insulin). The number of desired units are then selected by turning a dial and then the locking ring.

Another method of insulin delivery is the insulin pump, which is intended for a select group of individuals, such as the pregnant diabetic with early long-term complications and those with or candidates for renal transplantation. This system attempts to mimic the body's normal pancreatic function, uses only regular insulin, is battery-powered, and requires insertion of a needle into subcutaneous (SC) tissue. The needle is changed every 1 to 3 days. The amount of insulin injected can be adjusted according to blood glucose monitoring, which is usually done four to eight times per day.

The physician may order insulin by trade (brand) name or by the generic name, for example, Ultralente Iletin (trade name) or insulin zinc suspension, extended (generic name; Summary Drug Table 20-1). One brand of insulin is not substituted for another, unless substitution is approved by the physician because some patients may be sensitive to changes in brands of insulin. In addition, one type of insulin is never substituted for another, for example, using insulin zinc suspension instead of the prescribed protamine zinc insulin.

The label of the insulin bottle is read *carefully* for the name, source of insulin (eg, beef, pork, beef and pork, purified beef, and so forth), and the number of units per milliliter (U/mL). The dose of insulin is measured in *units* (U). U40 insulin has 40 U/mL and U100 insulin has 100 U/mL.

If the patient is to receive regular insulin and NPH, or regular and lente insulin, it should be clarified with the physician whether two separate injections are to be given or if the insulins may be mixed in the same syringe. If the two insulins are to be given in the same syringe, the clear insulin (eg, the regular insulin) is drawn into the syringe first.

SUMMARY DRUG TABLE 20–1
Insulin Preparations

TYPE OF INSULIN	TRADE NAME
insulin injection (regular insulin)	*40 U/mL:* Regular Iletin I (beef or pork) *100 U/mL:* Regular Insulin (pork), Beef Regular Iletin II, Pork Regular Iletin II (purified pork), Regular Purified Pork Insulin, Velosulin (purified pork), Humulin R (human insulin, from recombinant DNA), Novolin R, Novolin R Penfill, and Velosulin (human insulin, semisynthetic)
insulin zinc suspension, prompt (semilente)	*40 U/mL:* Semilente Iletin I (beef and pork) *100 U/mL:* Semilente Iletin I (beef and pork), Semilente Insulin (beef), Semilente Purified Pork
isophane insulin suspension (NPH)	*40 U/mL:* NPH Iletin I (beef and pork), NPH Insulin (beef), Beef NPH Iletin II (purified beef), NPH Purified Pork, Pork NPH Iletin II (purified pork), Humulin N (human insulin from recombinant DNA), Novolin N (human insulin, semisynthetic)
isophane insulin suspension and insulin injection (70% isophane insulin and 30% insulin injection)	*100 U/mL:* Mixtard (purified pork), Novolin 70/30 (human insulin, semisynthetic)
insulin zinc suspension (lente) (70% crystalline and 30% amorphous insulin suspension)	*40 U/mL:* Lente Iletin I (beef and pork) *100 U/mL:* Lente Insulin I (beef and pork), Lente Insulin (beef), Lente Iletin II (purified beef or purified pork), Lente Purified Pork Insulin, Humulin L (human insulin from recombinant DNA) Novolin L (human insulin, semisynthetic)
protamine zinc insulin suspension (PZI)	*40 U/mL:* Protamine, Zinc and Iletin I (beef and pork) *100 U/mL:* Protamine, Zinc and Iletin II (purified beef or pork)
insulin zinc suspension, extended (ultralente)	*40 U/mL:* Ultralente Iletin I (beef and pork) *100 U/mL:* Ultralente Insulin (beef), Ultralente Purified Beef

An unexpected response may be obtained when changing from mixed injections to separate injections or vice versa. If the patient had been using insulin mixtures before admission, it also will be important to ask the patient whether the insulins were given separately or together.

The expiration date printed on the label of the insulin bottle is always checked before withdrawing the insulin. Outdated insulin is never used.

Always use an insulin syringe that matches the concentration (eg, U40 or U100) of insulin to be given. A syringe labeled as U40 is used only with insulin labeled as U40; a syringe labeled as U100 is used only with insulin labeled U100.

When insulin is in a suspension, which can be seen when looking at a vial that has been untouched for approximately 1 hour, the vial is *gently* rotated between the palms of the hands and tilted gently end to end *immediately before* withdrawing the insulin. This ensures even distribution of the suspended particles.

The physician's order for the type and dosage of insulin is *carefully* checked immediately before withdrawing the insulin from the vial. All air bubbles must be eliminated from the syringe barrel and hub of the needle before the syringe is withdrawn from the insulin vial. When regular insulin and another insulin are mixed in the same syringe, the insulin must be administered within 5 minutes of withdrawing the two insulins from the two vials.

Insulin injection (regular insulin) is given 15 to 30 minutes before a meal because the onset of action is 30 to 60 minutes. The longer-acting insulins are usually given before breakfast. Insulin is given SC. *Only* insulin injection (regular insulin) may be given intramuscularly (IM) or intravenously (IV), as well as by the SC route.

Insulin may be injected into the arms, thighs, abdomen, or buttocks. Insulin injection sites are rotated to prevent lipodystrophy (atrophy of SC fat), a problem that can interfere with the absorption of insulin from the injection site. The pattern of rotation of the injection sites is carefully planned and then written on the patient's Kardex. Each time insulin is given, the selection of the injection site follows the rotation plan. For example, four rotation sites have been planned for a particular patient, and the rotation sites in order of use are the right arm, left arm, right thigh, left thigh. Before each dose of insulin is given, the nurse checks the patient's chart for the site of the previous injection and uses the next area (according to the rotation plan) for injection. The site used for injection is recorded.

Each time insulin is given, previous injection sites are inspected for signs of inflammation, which may indicate a localized allergic reaction. If inflammation or other skin reactions are noted, the area is not used for injection. Localized allergic reactions, signs of inflammation, or other skin changes are reported to the physician as soon as possible because a different type of insulin may be necessary.

The physician selects the dosage and type of insulin that will most likely meet the requirements of an individual patient. There is no standard dose range of insulin as there is for most other drugs. The dose prescribed for the patient may require changes until the dosage is found that best meets the patient's needs.

Close observation of the diabetic patient is important, especially when the patient is a new diabetic, the insulin dosage is changed, the patient is pregnant, the patient has a medical illness or has had surgery, or the patient failed to adhere to the prescribed diet. The patient is checked at the expected time of onset and peak of action (see Table 20-1) of the insulin given and is observed for signs of hypoglycemia. Hypoglycemia (see Table 20-2), which can develop suddenly, may indicate a need for an adjustment in the insulin dosage or other changes in treatment, such as a change in diet. Signs of hyperglycemia may also occur but are more likely to be less prominent and develop slowly.

HYPOGLYCEMIA. If an episode of hypoglycemia does occur, it must be corrected *as soon as the symptoms are recognized*. Methods of terminating a hypoglycemic reaction include the administration of one or more of the following:

- ► Dilute corn syrup
- ► Orange juice with sugar
- ► A lump of sugar dissolved in the mouth
- ► Commercial glucose products
- ► Glucagon by the SC, IM, or IV route
- ► Glucose 10% or 50% IV

Selection of any one or more of the above methods for terminating a hypoglycemic reaction, as well as other procedures to be followed, such as drawing blood for glucose levels, depends on the written order of the physician or hospital policy. The patient is *never* given an oral fluid or substance to terminate a hypoglycemic reaction unless swallowing and gag reflexes are present. Absence of these reflexes may result in aspiration of the oral fluid or substance into the lungs, which can result in extremely serious consequences and even death. If swallowing and gag reflexes are absent, glucose or glucagon must be given by the parenteral route.

The physician is always notified of any hypoglycemic reaction, the substance and amount used to terminate the reaction, blood samples drawn (if any), the length of time required for the symptoms of hypoglycemia to disappear, and the present status of the patient. After termination of a hypoglycemic reaction, the patient is observed closely for additional hypoglycemic reactions. The length of time close observation is required depends on the peak and duration of the insulin administered.

URINE TESTING. Urine is tested for glucose and ketone (acetone) bodies four times a day: before meals and in the evening before sleep. The results of each urine test are recorded on a flow sheet in the patient's chart. Because of the different brands available for urine testing, the package insert is consulted for directions for using these materials and interpreting the test results. Test results are recorded in percentages, such as 0.1%, 0.25%, 0.5%, 1%, or 2%. The physician is notified when the urine tests positive for ketones or the glucose is above 0.25%.

The patient needs to have the urine collection procedure explained and to know the times of day a specimen is required. The patient is also reminded in advance each time a specimen is needed. When obtaining urine for testing, the second voided specimen is used. The patient is instructed to void and discard the specimen. This is best done about 60 to 90 minutes before the specimen is due for testing. If after 1 hour the patient cannot void the second time, he or she is instructed to drink extra fluids for the next 30 minutes or more. In most cases, the intake of extra fluids helps produce a second voided specimen. If the patient has an indwelling catheter, urine for testing is obtained directly from the catheter and not from the collection bag.

Accuracy in urine testing is extremely important because some patients receive regular insulin based on the results of each urine test. Administration of regular insulin in this manner may be necessary, for example, when the patient is a new diabetic, when the diabetes is difficult to regulate, or when the patient is acutely ill. When regular insulin is given in this manner, the physician writes an order for a specific dose of insulin for each test result. Often, five U of regular insulin is prescribed for each percentage increment (0.1%, 0.25%, 0.5%, 1%, 2%). Thus, a patient with 0.25% glucose would receive 10 U of regular insulin or 15 U of insulin for 0.5% glucose. In some instances, the physician may not prescribe regular insulin if the urine contains 0.1% glucose, but insulin may be necessary when the urine contains 0.25% or more glucose. Each patient is different, and the nurse must carefully check the physician's order for the amount of insulin to be administered for each percentage of glucose in the patient's urine.

ANXIETY AND FEAR. The new diabetic often has many concerns regarding his or her diagnosis. For some, initially coping with diabetes and the methods required for controlling the disorder creates many problems.

Some of the fears and concerns of new diabetics may include having to give themselves an injection, having to follow a diet, weight control, the complications associated with diabetes, and changes in eating times and habits. An effective teaching program helps relieve some of the anxiety seen in the new diabetic. The newly diagnosed diabetic needs time to talk about the disorder, express concerns, and ask questions.

POTENTIAL IMPAIRED ADJUSTMENT, COPING, AND ALTERED HEALTH MAINTENANCE. The new diabetic may have difficulty accepting the diagnosis, and the apparent complexity of the therapeutic regimen can seem overwhelming. Before patients can be expected to carry out treatment, they must accept the fact that they have diabetes, and then deal with their own feelings about having the disorder. The nurse has an important role in helping these patients gradually accept the diagnosis and begin to understand their feelings about it. Understanding diabetes may help patients work with physicians and other medical personnel in managing their diabetes.

NONCOMPLIANCE. Noncompliance is a problem with some diabetics. An occasional lapse in adherence to the prescribed diet occurs in most patients, for example, around holidays or other special occasions. This slip may not cause a problem if it is brief, not excessive, and there is an immediate return to the prescribed regimen. On the other hand, there are those who frequently stray from the prescribed regimen, take extra insulin to cover dietary indiscretions, fast for several days before follow-up blood glucose determinations, and engage in other dangerous behaviors.

Whereas some patients can be convinced that failure to adhere to the prescribed treatment regimen is detrimental to their health, others continue to deviate from the prescribed regimen until a serious complication develops. The nurse must make every effort to stress the importance of adherence to the prescribed treatment during the initial teaching session and during follow-up office or clinic visits.

KNOWLEDGE DEFICIT. A thorough teaching plan is necessary for all new diabetics, for those who have had any change in the management of their diabetes (eg, diet, insulin type, insulin dosage), and for those whose management has changed because of an illness or disability, for example, loss of sight or disabling arthritis. The newly diagnosed diabetic and family must have an explanation of the disease and methods of treatment as soon as the physician has revealed the diagnosis to the patient. The teaching plan is always individualized because the needs of each patient are different.

If the patient is to use a blood glucose monitoring

device, the method of obtaining a small sample of blood from the finger and the use of the device is reviewed with the patient. Printed instructions and illustrations are supplied with the device and reviewed with the patient. The patient is encouraged to purchase the brand recommended by the physician. Time should be allowed for supervised practice.

The following areas may be included in a diabetic teaching plan:

▶ *Urine testing*—the testing material recommended by the physician; a review of the instructions included with the urine testing materials; the technique of urine testing; interpreting test results; how to obtain a specimen; number of times a day or week the urine is tested (as recommended by the physician); keeping a record of test results

▶ *Insulin*—types; how dosage is expressed; calculating the insulin dosage; importance of using only the type, source, and brand name recommended by the physician; importance of not changing brands unless the physician approves; keeping a spare vial on hand; prescription for insulin purchase is not required

▶ *Storage of insulin*—keep insulin in a cool place or in a refrigerator; keep insulin away from heat and direct sunlight

▶ *Needle and syringe*—Purchase requires a prescription; purchasing the same brand and needle size each time; parts of the syringe; reading the syringe scale

▶ *Preparation for administration*—principles of aseptic technique; how to hold the syringe; how to withdraw insulin from the vial; measurement of insulin in the syringe using the syringe scale; mixing insulin in the same syringe (when appropriate); elimination of air in the syringe and needle; what to do if the syringe or needle is contaminated

▶ *Administration of insulin*—sites to be used; rotation of injection sites; angle of injection; administration at the time of day prescribed by the physician; disposal of the needle and syringe

▶ *Diet*—importance of following the prescribed diet; calories allowed; food exchanges; planning daily menus; establishing meal schedules; selecting food from a restaurant menu; reading food labels; using of artificial sweeteners

▶ *Traveling*—importance of carrying an extra supply of insulin and a prescription for needles and syringes; storage of insulin when traveling; protecting needles and syringes from theft; importance of discussing travel plans (especially foreign travel) with the physician

▶ *Hypoglycemia/hyperglycemia*—signs and symptoms of hypoglycemia and hyperglycemia; food or

fluid used to terminate a hypoglycemic reaction; importance of notifying the physician immediately if either reaction occurs

▶ *Personal hygiene*—importance of good skin and foot care, personal cleanliness, frequent dental checkups, and routine eye examinations

▶ *Exercise*—importance of following the physician's recommendations regarding physical activity

▶ *When to notify the physician*—increase in glucose in the urine; urine positive for ketones; if pregnancy occurs (female patient of childbearing age); occurrence of hypoglycemic or hyperglycemic episodes; occurrence of illness, infection, or diarrhea (insulin dosage may require adjustment); appearance of new problems (eg, leg ulcers, numbness of the extremities, significant weight gain or loss)

The diabetic is encouraged to wear identification, such as Medic-Alert, to inform medical personnel and others of the use of insulin to control the disease.

EVALUATION

▶ Anxiety and fear is reduced

▶ Demonstrates beginning ability to cope with the disorder and its required treatment

▶ Patient demonstrates positive outlook and adjustment to diagnosis

▶ Patient verbalizes willingness to comply to the prescribed treatment regimen

▶ Patient and family demonstrate understanding of drug regimen

▶ Patient demonstrates understanding of the information presented in teaching sessions

▶ Patient is able to test own urine, give own insulin injections

▶ THE ORAL HYPOGLYCEMIC DRUGS

The various oral hypoglycemic drugs are listed in Summary Drug Table 20-2.

▷ Actions of the Oral Hypoglycemic Drugs

The oral hypoglycemic drugs appear to lower blood glucose by stimulating the beta-cells of the pancreas

SUMMARY DRUG TABLE 20–2
Oral Hypoglycemic Drugs

GENERIC NAME	TRADE NAME*	DOSE RANGES
acetohexamide	Dymelor, *generic*	250 mg–1 g/d PO (those receiving 1.5 g/d may be on a bid dosing schedule)
chlorpropamide	Diabinese, *generic*	100–700 mg/d PO
glipizide	Glucotrol	5–40 mg/d PO in single dose or divided doses
glyburide	Micronase, DiaBeta	1.25–20 mg/d PO in single dose or divided doses
tolazamide	Tolinase, *generic*	100–1000 mg/d PO (doses over 500 mg are given in divided doses)
tolbutamide	Orinase, Oramide, *generic*	0.25–3 g/d PO

* The term generic *indicates that the drug is available in a generic form.*

to release insulin. Oral hypoglycemic drugs are *not* effective if the beta cells of the pancreas are unable to release a sufficient amount of insulin to meet the individual's needs.

▷ Uses of the Oral Hypoglycemic Drugs

The oral hypoglycemic drugs are of value only in the treatment of patients with type II (non–insulin-dependent or maturity-onset) diabetes mellitus whose condition cannot be controlled by diet alone. These drugs may also be used with insulin in the management of some patients with diabetes mellitus. Use of an oral hypoglycemic agent with insulin may decrease the insulin dosage in some individuals.

▷ Adverse Reactions Associated with the Administration of the Oral Hypoglycemic Drugs

Hypoglycemia may occur with the use of oral hypoglycemic drugs. The elderly, debilitated, or malnourished patient is more likely to experience hypoglycemia; however, this reaction may occur in any individual taking these drugs.

Other adverse reactions seen with these drugs are anorexia, nausea, vomiting, epigastric discomfort, heartburn, and various vague neurologic symptoms such as weakness and numbness of the extremities. Often, these can be eliminated by reducing the dosage or giving the drug in divided doses. If these

reactions become severe, the physician may try another oral hypoglycemic agent or discontinue the use of these drugs. If the drug is discontinued, it may be necessary to control the diabetes with insulin.

Additional adverse reactions include pruritus, urticaria, jaundice, leukopenia, mild anemia, thrombocytopenia, weakness, fatigue, dizziness, and skin rashes.

► NURSING PROCESS
THE PATIENT RECEIVING AN ORAL HYPOGLYCEMIC DRUG

ASSESSMENT

If the patient has been recently diagnosed as having diabetes mellitus and has not received an oral hypoglycemic agent, or if the patient is a known diabetic and has been taking one of these drugs, the initial physical assessment includes weight, blood pressure, pulse, and respiratory rate. A general assessment of the skin, mucous membranes, and extremities is made with special attention to sores or cuts that appear to be healing poorly and ulcerations or other skin or mucous membrane changes. The history should include dietary habits, a family history of diabetes (if any), and an inquiry into the type and duration of symptoms experienced. The patient's chart is reviewed for recent laboratory and diagnostic tests. If the patient has diabetes and has been receiving an oral hypoglycemic drug, the history should also include the name of the drug and the dosage, the type of diabetic diet, the average results of urine testing, and an inquiry into adherence to the dietary and weight control regimen prescribed by the physician.

NURSING DIAGNOSIS

The nursing diagnoses may depend on the patient's individual needs and are based on the information obtained during assessment.

The extent of the nursing diagnoses depends on factors such as whether the patient is a new diabetic, has had treatment for diabetes, or has not followed the prescribed medical regimen.

▶ Anxiety related to diagnosis, dietary restrictions, other factors (specify)

▶ Ineffective individual coping related to inability to accept diagnosis

▶ Altered health maintenance related to inability to comprehend drug regimen, lack of knowledge

▶ Noncompliance to treatment regimen related to lack of knowledge, misunderstanding, or complexity of prescribed treatment program, other factors (specify)

▶ Knowledge deficit of dosage schedule, urine testing, diet

PLANNING AND IMPLEMENTATION

The major goals of the patient may include a reduction in anxiety, improved ability in coping with the diagnosis, compliance with the prescribed treatment regimen, an understanding of and compliance to the prescribed treatment regimen.

The major goals of nursing management may include a reducing patient anxiety, helping the patient to physically and mentally cope with the diagnosis, and developing and implementing an effective teaching plan.

ADMINISTRATION OF ORAL HYPOGLYCEMIC DRUGS. The physician may order an oral hypoglycemic agent given as a single daily dose or in divided doses. Acetohexamide (Dymelor), chlorpropamide (Diabinese), tolazamide (Tolinase), and tolbutamide (Orinase) are given with food to prevent GI upset. Glipizide (Glucotrol) is given 30 minutes before a meal, and glyburide (Micronase) is given with breakfast or with the first main meal of the day. The physician orders the meal with which glyburide is given.

Ongoing assessments conducted daily include monitoring vital signs and observing the patient for adverse drug reactions. The physician may also order daily to weekly weights. The physician is notified if an adverse reaction occurs or if there is a significant weight gain or loss.

HYPOGLYCEMIA. Observing the patient every 2 to 4 hours for episodes of hypoglycemia is especially important during initial therapy or following a change in dos-

age. If both an oral hypoglycemic agent and insulin are given, the patient is observed more frequently for hypoglycemic episodes during the initial period of combination therapy. If the patient is receiving only an oral hypoglycemic agent and a hypoglycemic reaction does occur, it is often (but not always) less intense than one seen with insulin administration.

As discussed under the nursing implications for insulin administration, hypoglycemic reactions must be terminated *immediately*. The method of terminating a hypoglycemic reaction is the same as for a hypoglycemic reaction occurring with insulin administration. The physician is always notified as soon as possible if episodes of hypoglycemia occur because the dosage of the oral hypoglycemic agent (or insulin, when both insulin and an oral hypoglycemic agent are given) may need to be changed.

URINE TESTING. Urine specimens are obtained and tested in the same manner as for insulin (see previous section). The physician is notified if ketones or glucose are present in the urine.

ANXIETY AND COPING. As discussed in the section on insulin, the newly diagnosed diabetic often has many concerns about the management of the disease. Some patients, when learning that management of their diabetes can be achieved by diet and an oral drug, may have a tendency to discount the seriousness of their disorder. Without creating additional anxiety, the nurse must emphasize the importance of following the prescribed treatment regimen.

The newly diagnosed diabetic should be encouraged to talk about the disorder, express concerns, and ask questions. Giving these patients time to talk may also help them begin to cope with their diabetes.

POTENTIAL IMPAIRED ADJUSTMENT AND ALTERED HEALTH MAINTENANCE. In addition to the material regarding impaired adjustment, noncompliance, and altered health maintenance discussed in the previous section on insulin, the patient receiving an oral hypoglycemic drug may also express concern about the possibility of having to take insulin in the future. The nurse should encourage the patient to discuss this and other concerns with the physician.

NONCOMPLIANCE. Failing to comply with the prescribed treatment regimen may be problem with patients taking an oral hypoglycemic drug because of the erroneous belief that not having to take insulin means that their disease is not serious and therefore does not require strict adherence to the recommended dietary plan. It is most important that these patients be informed that control of their diabetes is just as important as for patients requiring insulin and that control is achieved only when they adhere to the treatment regimen prescribed by the physician.

KNOWLEDGE DEFICIT. If the patient is newly diagnosed as having diabetes mellitus, the disease and methods of control are discussed with the patient and family after the physician has revealed the diagnosis to the patient. Although taking an oral hypoglycemic agent is less complicated than self-administration of insulin, the diabetic taking one of these agents needs a thorough explanation of the management of the disease. The teaching plan is individualized because the needs of each patient are different.

► Take the drug exactly as directed on the container (eg, with food, 30 minutes before a meal, and so forth).

► To control diabetes, follow the diet and drug regimen prescribed by the physician *exactly*.

► This drug is not oral insulin and cannot be substituted for insulin.

► Never stop taking this drug or increase or decrease the dose unless told to do so by the physician.

► Take the drug at the same time or times each day.

► Eat meals at approximately the same time each day. Erratic meal hours or skipped meals may result in difficulty in controlling diabetes with this drug.

► Avoid alcohol, dieting, commercial weight loss products, and strenuous exercise programs unless use or participation has been approved by the physician.

► Test urine for glucose and ketones as directed by the physician. Keep a record of test results and bring this record to each physician or clinic visit.

► Maintain good foot and skin care and routine eye and dental examinations for the early detection of the complications that occur in some diabetics.

► Exercise should be moderate: avoid strenuous exercise and erratic periods of exercise.

► Wear identification, such as Medic-Alert, to inform medical personnel and others of diabetes and the drug or drugs currently being used to treat the disease.

► Notify the physician if any of the following occurs: episodes of hypoglycemia, apparent symptoms of hyperglycemia, positive results of urine tests for glucose or ketone bodies, pregnancy (female patient of childbearing age), GI upset, fever, sore throat, unusual bruising or bleeding, diarrhea, rash, yellowing of the skin. Notify the physician also if any serious illness not requiring hospitalization occurs.

The symptoms of hypoglycemia and hyperglycemia are best given to the patient in printed form and then explained. The method recommended by the physician for terminating a hypoglycemic reaction is also explained to the patient.

EVALUATION

► Anxiety is reduced

► Demonstrates beginning ability to cope with the disorder and its required treatment

► Patient demonstrates positive outlook and adjustment to diagnosis

► Patient verbalizes willingness to comply to the prescribed treatment regimen

► Patient and family demonstrate understanding of drug regimen

► Patient and family demonstrate understanding of the information presented in teaching sessions

► Patient is able to test own urine

21

The Sulfonamides

On completion of this chapter the student will:

▶ *List the actions and uses of the sulfonamides*

▶ *List the adverse reactions associated with the administration of the sulfonamides*

▶ *Use the nursing process when administering a sulfonamide*

▶ *Discuss the nursing implications associated with the administration of the sulfonamides*

The sulfonamides ("sulfa") drugs were the first effective agents used in the treatment of infections. The use of sulfonamides began to decline following the introduction of the more effective penicillins and other antibiotics. These drugs still remain important antiinfectives in the treatment of certain types of infections.

acid (PABA), a substance that some, but not all, bacteria need to multiply. Once the rate of bacterial multiplication is slowed, the body's own defense mechanisms (white blood cells) are able to rid the body of the invading microorganisms and therefore control the infection.

▷ Actions of the Sulfonamides

Sulfonamides are **antibacterial** agents, that is, they are active against (anti) bacteria. Another term that may be used to describe the general action of these drugs is **antiinfective** because they are used to treat infections caused by certain bacteria.

The sulfonamides are mostly **bacteriostatic**, which means they slow or retard the multiplication of bacteria. Some antiinfective drugs are **bactericidal**, which means they destroy bacteria.

The sulfonamides have bacteriostatic activity because of their antagonism of para-aminobenzoic

▷ Uses of the Sulfonamides

The sulfonamides are chiefly used to control urinary tract infections caused by certain bacteria such as *Escherichia coli*, *Staphylococcus aureus*, and *Klebsiella-Enterobacter* microorganisms. Sulfasalazine (Alzulfidine) is used solely for the management of ulcerative colitis. Mafenide (Sulfamylon) and silver sulfadiazine (Silvadene) are topical drugs used in the treatment of second-degree and third-degree burns. Additional uses of sulfonamide preparations are given in Summary Drug Table 21-1. Silver sulfadiazine is also discussed in chapter 38.

SUMMARY DRUG TABLE 21–1
Sulfonamide Drugs

GENERIC NAME	TRADE NAME*	USES	ADVERSE REACTIONS	DOSE RANGES
SINGLE AGENTS				
sulfadiazine	*Generic*	Urinary tract infections caused by susceptible microorganisms, chancroid, acute otitis media, *Haemophilus influenzae* and meningococcal meningitis, rheumatic fever	Hematologic changes, Stevens-Johnson syndrome, nausea, vomiting, headache, diarrhea, crystalluria, fever, chills	2–4 g/d PO in 3–6 divided doses
sulfamethizole	Proklar, *generic*	Urinary tract infections caused by susceptible microorganisms	Same as sulfadiazine	0.5–1 g PO tid, qid
sulfamethoxazole	Gantanol, *generic*	Same as sulfadiazine plus chancroid, acute otitis media, meningococcal meningitis	Same as sulfadiazine	Initial dose: 2 g PO; maintenance dose: 1 g PO bid, tid
sulfasalazine	Azulfidine	Ulcerative colitis	Same as sulfadiazine	Initial dose: 3–4 g PO in divided doses; maintenance dose: 500 mg PO qid
sulfisoxazole	Gantrisin, *generic*	Same as sulfadiazine	Same as sulfadiazine	Loading dose: 2–4 g PO; maintenance dose: 4–8 g/d PO in 4–6 divided doses
MULTIPLE PREPARATIONS				
trimethoprim (TMP) and sulfamethoxazole (SMZ)	Septra, Bactrim, *generic*	Urinary tract infections due to susceptible microorganisms, acute otitis media (children), chronic bronchitis (adults) due to *H influenzae* and *S pneumoniae*	Same as sulfadiazine plus rash, epigastric distress, pruritus	160 mg TMP and 800 mg SMZ PO q12h
MISCELLANEOUS SULFONAMIDE PREPARATIONS				
mafenide	Sulfamylon	2nd- and 3rd-degree burns	Pain or burning sensation, rash, itching, facial edema	Applied topically to burned area 1–2 times/d
silver sulfadiazine	Silvadene, *generic*	2nd- and 3rd-degree burns	Burning, itching, rash	Applied topically to burned area 1–2 times/d

* The term generic *indicates that the drug is available in a generic form.*

▷ Adverse Reactions Associated with the Administration of Sulfonamides

The sulfonamides are capable of causing a variety of adverse reactions. Some of these are serious or potentially serious; others are mild. One example of a serious adverse reaction is the hematologic changes that may occur during therapy. Hematologic changes include agranulocytosis, thrombocytopenia, aplastic anemia, and leukopenia. Anorexia is an example of a mild adverse reaction; unless it becomes severe and pronounced weight loss occurs, it may not be necessary to discontinue sulfonamide therapy.

Various types of hypersensitivity (allergic) reactions may be seen during sulfonamide therapy and include the Stevens-Johnson syndrome, urticaria, pruritus, and generalized skin eruptions. The Stevens-Johnson syndrome, also called erythema multiforme, is manifested by fever, cough, muscular aches and pains, headache, and the appearance of lesions on the skin, mucous membranes, eyes, and other organs. The lesions appear as red wheals or blisters, often starting on the face, neck, and extremities. The Stevens-Johnson syndrome, which also may occur with the administration of other types of drugs, can be fatal.

Other adverse reactions that may occur during therapy are nausea, vomiting, diarrhea, abdominal pain, chills, fever, and stomatitis. In some instances, these may be mild, whereas at other times they cause serious problems requiring discontinuation of the drug. Sulfasalazine may cause the urine to be an orange-yellow color; this is not abnormal.

Crystalluria (crystals in the urine) may occur during administration of a sulfonamide, although this problem occurs less frequently with some of the newer sulfonamide preparations. Crystalluria is potentially a serious problem that often can be prevented by increasing the fluid intake during sulfonamide therapy.

The most frequent adverse reaction seen with the application of mafenide is a burning sensation or pain when the drug is applied to the skin. Allergic reactions, such as rash, itching, edema, and urticaria, may also be seen. Burning, rash, and itching may also be seen with the use of silver sulfadiazine. It may be difficult to distinguish between an adverse reaction due to the use of mafenide or silver sulfadiazine and reactions that may occur from the severe burn injury or from other agents used at the same time for the management of the burns.

▶ NURSING PROCESS
THE PATIENT RECEIVING A SULFONAMIDE

ASSESSMENT

The patient receiving a sulfonamide drug almost always has an active infection. However, some patients may be receiving one of these drugs to prevent an infection (prophylaxis) or as part of the management of a disease such as ulcerative colitis.

Before administration of the drug, assessment is focused on the patient's general appearance, the symptoms experienced by the patient, and the length of time these symptoms were present. The vital signs are taken and recorded. Depending on the type and location of the infection or disease, the physician orders laboratory tests such as a urine culture, urinalysis, complete blood count, renal function tests, examination of the stool, and so on.

NURSING DIAGNOSIS

Depending on the drug, dose, and reason for administration, one or more of the following nursing diagnoses may apply to a person receiving a sulfonamide:

▶ Anxiety related to diagnosis, symptoms of infection, other factors (specify)

▶ Noncompliance related to indifference, lack of knowledge, other factors

▶ Knowledge deficit of medication regimen, adverse drug effects

PLANNING AND IMPLEMENTATION

The major goals of the patient may include a reduction in anxiety, absence of adverse drug reactions, and an understanding of and compliance to the prescribed treatment regimen.

The major goals of nursing management may include a reduction in the patient's anxiety, recognition of adverse drug effects, and the development and implementation of an effective teaching plan.

The patient is evaluated for response to the drug, that is, a relief of symptoms and a decrease in temperature (if it was elevated before therapy started). Patients receiving sulfasalazine for ulcerative colitis are closely observed for the relief of symptoms of the disease. All stool samples are inspected and their appearance and number are recorded.

ADMINISTRATION OF SULFONAMIDES. Unless the physician orders otherwise, sulfonamides are given on an empty stomach, that is, 1 hour before or 2 hours after meals. Sulfasalazine may be given with food or immediately after meals if gastrointestinal (GI) irritation occurs. The patient is instructed to drink a full glass of water when taking an oral sulfonamide.

When mafenide or silver sulfadiazine is used in the treatment of burns, the treatment regimen outlined by the physician or the burn treatment unit must be closely followed. There are various burn treatment regimens such as whirlpool baths, special dressings, and cleansing of the burned area. The use of a specific treatment regimen often depends on the extent of the burned area, the degree of the burns, and the physical condition and age of the patient. Other current problems, such as lung damage due to smoke or heat or physical injuries that occurred at the time of the burn injury, may also influence the treatment regimen.

The physician may order cleaning and removal of debris before each application of mafenide or silver sulfadiazine to the burned area. These drugs are applied with a sterile gloved hand. The patient is warned that stinging or burning may be felt during and for a short time after mafenide is applied. Some burning may also be noted with the application of silver sulfadiazine.

It is most important that the burned areas are inspected every 1 to 2 hours because some treatment regimens require keeping the affected areas covered with the mafenide or silver sulfadiazine ointment at all times. It is also important to note any adverse reactions that may occur and to report their occurrence to the physician immediately. Other nursing assessments and evaluations, such as monitoring vital signs, measuring intake and output, and turning and positioning the patient are carried out according to the physician's orders or the burn treatment unit's policies.

ANXIETY. The symptoms of infection, for example, frequent urination or burning on urination in those with a bladder infection, may result in anxiety. The nurse should reassure the patient that symptoms will most likely diminish after a few days of drug therapy.

Mafenide and sometimes silver sulfadiazine causes a stinging or burning sensation, resulting in anxiety before, during, and after application of the drug. While it may not be possible to prevent this discomfort, gentleness in applying the drug may reduce some of the discomfort.

ADVERSE DRUG REACTIONS. The patient is observed for adverse reactions, especially an allergic reaction. If one or more adverse reactions should occur, the next dose of the drug is withheld and the physician is notified.

If the Stevens-Johnson syndrome should occur, lesions on the skin, and mucous membranes may be seen. In addition to notifying the physician of this reaction, care must be exercised to prevent injury to the involved areas.

VITAL SIGNS. The temperature, pulse, respiratory rate, and blood pressure is monitored every 4 hours or as ordered by the physician. If fever is present and the patient's temperature suddenly increases or if the temperature was normal and suddenly increases, the physician is contacted immediately.

FLUIDS. Patients are encouraged to increase their fluid intake to 2000 mL or more a day to prevent crystalluria and stone formation in the genitourinary tract. The intake and output is measured and recorded every 8 hours and the physician is notified if the urinary output decreases or the patient fails to increase his or her oral intake.

PATIENTS WITH DIABETES MELLITUS. Patients who are diabetic and receiving the oral hypoglycemic agent tolbutamide (Orinase) or chlorpropamide (Diabinese) are observed closely for episodes of hypoglycemia (see chap 20). Sulfonamides may inhibit the (hepatic) metabolism of these two oral hypoglycemic drugs and thereby increase the possibility of a hypoglycemic reaction.

NONCOMPLIANCE AND KNOWLEDGE DEFICIT. The importance of completing the prescribed course of therapy must be emphasized.

The following points are included in a teaching plan for the patient and family:

▶ Take the medication as prescribed.
▶ Maintain follow-up care to ensure the infection is controlled.
▶ Take the drug on an empty stomach either 1 hour before or 2 hours after a meal (exception: sulfasalazine which may be taken with food or immediately after a meal if GI upset occurs). Take the medication with a full glass of water.
▶ Do not increase or decrease the time between doses unless directed to do so by the physician.
▶ Complete the full course of therapy. Do not discontinue this medication (unless advised to do so by the physician) even though the symptoms of the infection have disappeared.
▶ Drink *at least* eight to 10 eight-ounce glasses of fluid every day.
▶ Prolonged exposure to sunlight may result in skin reactions (photosensitivity reactions). When going outside, cover exposed areas of the skin or apply a protective sunscreen to exposed areas.
▶ Notify the physician immediately if the following should occur: fever, skin rash or other skin problems, nausea, vomiting, unusual bleeding or bruising, sore throat, or extreme fatigue.
▶ Sulfasalazine: the urine may turn an orange-yellow color. This is not abnormal.

EVALUATION

▶ Anxiety is reduced
▶ No evidence of adverse reactions
▶ Verbalizes importance of complying with the prescribed treatment regimen
▶ Patient and family demonstrate understanding of drug regimen
▶ Verbalizes an understanding of treatment modalities and importance of continued follow-up care

22

The Penicillins and the Cephalosporins

On completion of this chapter the student will:

▶ *List the actions and uses of the penicillins*

▶ *List the adverse reactions associated with the administration of the penicillins*

▶ *List the actions and uses of the cephalosporins*

▶ *List the adverse reactions associated with the administration of the cephalosporins*

▶ *Use the nursing process when administering a penicillin or cephalosporin*

▶ *Discuss the nursing implications associated with the administration of the penicillins or cephalosporins*

▶ THE PENICILLINS

After the introduction of the sulfonamides, newer and more effective drugs were developed for the treatment of infections. The antibacterial properties of penicillin were recognized in 1928, but it was not until 1941 that penicillin was used clinically in the treatment of infections. After the introduction of penicillin, more antibiotics were introduced. Today, there are many antibiotic drugs that can be used in the treatment of infections.

▷ Types of Penicillin

There are two types of penicillin: natural penicillin and the semisynthetic derivatives of penicillin (Summary Drug Table 22-1).

One problem seen with the natural penicillins, for example, penicillin G benzathine (Bicillin), is the increased incidence of **bacterial resistance.** Bacterial resistance is the ability of bacteria to produce the enzyme penicillinase, which inactivates the penicillin. The natural penicillins also have a narrow

SUMMARY DRUG TABLE 22–1
Penicillins

GENERIC NAME	TRADE NAME*	USES	ADVERSE REACTIONS	DOSE RANGES
amoxicillin	Amoxil	Infections due to susceptible microorganisms	Hypersensitivity reactions, superinfections, hematopoietic changes	250–500 mg PO q8h; larger doses may be used in some instances
ampicillin, oral	Polycillin, Amcil, *generic*	Same as amoxicillin	Same as amoxicillin	250–500 mg PO q8h; larger doses may be used in some instances
ampicillin sodium, parenteral	Polycillin-N, Totacillin-N, *generic*	Same as amoxicillin	Same as amoxicillin	25–50 mg/kg/d IM, IV; other dosage ranges may also be used in some instances
azlocillin sodium	Azlin	Same as amoxicillin	Same as amoxicillin	Up to 4 g/dose IV
bacampicillin hydrochloride	Spectrobid	Same as amoxicillin	Same as amoxicillin	400–800 mg PO q12h
carbenicillin disodium	Geopen	Same as amoxicillin	Same as amoxicillin	250–500 mg/kg/d by continuous IV infusion; 50–200 mg/kg/d IM, IV in divided doses
carbenicillin indanyl sodium	Geocillin	Same as amoxicillin	Same as amoxicillin	382–764 mg PO qid
cloxacillin sodium	Cloxapen, Tegopen, *generic*	Same as amoxicillin	Same as amoxicillin	250–500 mg PO q6h
dicloxacillin sodium	Dynapen, *generic*	Same as amoxicillin	Same as amoxicillin	125–250 mg PO q6h
methicillin sodium	Staphcillin	Same as amoxicillin	Same as amoxicillin	4–12 g/d IM, IV in divided doses q4–6h
mezlocillin sodium	Mezlin	Same as amoxicillin	Same as amoxicillin	100–125 mg/kg/d IM in divided doses; 100–350 mg/kg/d IV
nafcillin sodium	Unipen, Nafcil, Nallpen	Same as amoxicillin	Same as amoxicillin	250–500 mg PO q4–6h; 0.5–1 g IV q4h
oxacillin sodium	Bactocill, Prostaphlin	Same as amoxicillin	Same as amoxicillin	0.5–1 g PO q4–6h; 250 mg–1 g (or more) IM, IV, IV infusion
penicillin G (aqueous) parenteral	Pfizerpen, *generic*	Same as amoxicillin	Same as amoxicillin	Up to 30 million U/d IV or up to 2 million U IM
penicillin G benzathine parenteral or oral	Bicillin L-A, Permapen Bicillin	Same as amoxicillin	Same as amoxicillin	1.2–2.4 million U/dose IM or 400,000–600,000 U PO q4–6h
penicillin G potassium, oral	Pentids, *generic*	Same as amoxicillin	Same as amoxicillin	200,000–500,000 U PO q6–12h
penicillin G procaine, aqueous (APPG)	Crysticillin, Wycillin	Same as amoxicillin	Same as amoxicillin	600,000–4.8 million U/d IM
penicillin V (phenoxymethyl)	*Generic*	Same as amoxicillin	Same as amoxicillin	125–500 mg PO q6–12h
penicillin V potassium	Pen-Vee-K, V-Cillin K, Beepen VK, *generic*	Same as amoxicillin	Same as amoxicillin	125–500 mg PO q6–12h

(continued)

SUMMARY DRUG TABLE 22–1
(continued)

GENERIC NAME	TRADE NAME*	USES	ADVERSE REACTIONS	DOSE RANGES
piperacillin sodium	Pipracil	Same as amoxicillin	Same as amoxicillin	3–4 g IV infusion, IM q4–6h
ticarcillin disodium	Ticar	Same as amoxicillin	Same as amoxicillin	200–300 mg/kg/d by IV infusion in divided doses; 1 g IM or direct IV q6h
ticarcillin and clavulanate potassium	Timentin	Same as amoxicillin	Same as amoxicillin	3.1 g by IV infusion q4–6h or 200–300 mg/kg/d IV q4–6h

* The term generic *indicates that the drug is available in a generic form.*

spectrum of activity, which means that they are effective against only a few strains of bacteria.

The semisynthetic penicillins partially solved the problems associated with the natural penicillins. Because of their chemical modifications, they are more slowly excreted by the kidneys and have a somewhat wider spectrum of antibacterial activity.

▷ Actions of the Penicillins

Both the natural and semisynthetic penicillins basically have the same type of action against bacteria. Penicillin prevents bacteria from using a substance (muramic acid peptide) that is necessary for the maintenance of their outer cell wall. Unable to use this substance for cell wall maintenance, the bacteria swell, rupture, assume unusual shapes, and are finally destroyed.

The penicillins may be bactericidal (destroy bacteria) or bacteriostatic (slow or retard the multiplication of bacteria). They are bactericidal against sensitive microorganisms (eg, those microorganisms that will be affected by penicillin) provided there is an adequate concentration of penicillin in the body. An adequate concentration of any drug in the body is referred to as the blood level. An inadequate concentration (or inadequate blood level) of penicillin may produce bacteriostatic activity, which may or may not control the infection.

To determine if a specific type of bacteria is sensitive to penicillin, culture and sensitivity tests are performed. A culture is the placing of the infectious material obtained from areas such as the skin, respiratory tract, and blood on a special growing medium, which is "food" for the bacteria. After a

specified time, the bacteria are examined under a microscope and identified. The sensitivity test involves placing the infectious material on a separate culture plate and then placing small disks, which are impregnated with various antibiotics, over the area. After a specified time, the culture plate is examined. If there is little or no growth around a disk, then the bacteria are considered *sensitive* to the antibiotic that was impregnated in the disk. If there is considerable growth around the disk, then the bacteria are considered *resistant* to the antibiotic impregnated in the disk. After receiving a culture and sensitivity report, the strain of microorganisms causing the infection is known and the antibiotic to which these microorganisms are sensitive and resistant are identified. The physician then selects the antibiotic to which the microorganism is sensitive.

▷ Uses of Penicillin

The natural and semisynthetic penicillins are used in the treatment of infections due to susceptible microorganisms. Culture and sensitivity tests are performed whenever possible to determine which penicillin will best control an infection caused by a specific strain of bacteria. Penicillin is of no value in the treatment of viral or fungal infections.

Penicillin may be prescribed for the treatment of a *potential* infection in certain individuals such as those with a history of rheumatic fever or chronic ear infections. This is called *prophylaxis*. An example of the prophylaxis is the prescribing of penicillin to be taken several days before and after an operative dental procedure, such as an extraction, for the patient with a history of rheumatic fever. A tooth extraction may result in bacteria entering the bloodstream. Because the patient has a history of rheumatic fever, he or she is more susceptible to a repeat episode of rheumatic fever and heart valve damage following a tooth extraction.

▷ Adverse Reactions Associated with the Administration of Penicillin

Hypersensitivity (or allergy) to penicillin occurs in some individuals, especially those with a history of allergy to many substances. Symptoms may include any one or more of the following: skin rash, urticaria, sneezing, wheezing, pruritus, bronchospasm, laryngospasm, angioneurotic edema, hypotension (which can progress to shock), and symptoms resembling serum sickness (chills, fever, edema, joint and muscle pain, malaise). Anaphylactic reactions have also occurred. Once an individual is allergic to one penicillin, he or she is most likely to be allergic to all of the penicillins. This is called *cross-sensitivity* or *cross-allergenicity.*

Another problem associated with penicillin and other antibiotics is **superinfection,** which is a bacterial or fungal overgrowth of microorganisms not susceptible to penicillin. A superinfection may occur because the penicillin not only was bactericidal against pathogenic (disease-causing) microorganisms but may also have affected nonpathogenic microorganisms that normally exist in the body. Bacterial or fungal superinfections result in a new and different infection, which can be potentially serious.

An example of how a superinfection may occur is the yeastlike fungi that usually exist in small numbers in the vagina. The multiplication rate of the microorganisms is slowed and kept under control because of the (normal) presence of a strain of bacteria (*Döderlein's bacillus*) in the vagina. If penicillin therapy destroys the normal microorganisms of the vagina, for example, the *Döderlein's bacillus*, the fungi are now uncontrolled, multiply at a rapid rate, and cause symptoms of a fungal infection called candidiasis (or moniliasis).

Another adverse reaction associated with penicillin administration is hematopoietic changes such as anemia, thrombocytopenia, leukopenia, and bone marrow depression. When given orally, glossitis, stomatitis, dry mouth, gastritis, nausea, vomiting, and abdominal pain may be seen. When penicillin is given intramuscularly (IM), there may be pain at the injection site. Irritation of the vein and phlebitis may be seen with intravenous (IV) administration.

▶ THE CEPHALOSPORINS

The cephalosporins (Summary Drug Table 22-2) are structurally and chemically related to penicillin. Cefoxitin (Mefoxin), moxalactam (Moxam), and cefotetan (Cefotan) are drugs similar to the cephalosporins and have basically the same pharmacologic action.

▷ Types of Cephalosporins

The cephalosporins are divided into three groups: first, second, and third generation agents. They also may be differentiated within each group according to the microorganisms that are sensitive to a specific cephalosporin. Generally, progression from the first to the second, and then to the third generation shows an increase in the sensitivity of gram-negative microorganisms and a decrease in the sensitivity of gram-positive microorganisms. To illustrate this phenomena, a first generation cephalosporin would have more use against gram-positive microorganisms than would a third generation cephalosporin.

Examples of the Cephalosporins

First generation—cephalexin (Keflex), cefazolin (Ancef)

Second generation—cefaclor (Ceclor), cefoxitin (Mefoxin)

Third generation—cefixime (Suprax), moxalactam (Moxam)

▷ Actions of the Cephalosporins

Cephalosporins affect the bacterial cell wall, making it defective and unstable. This action is similar to the action of penicillin. The cephalosporins are usually bactericidal.

▷ Uses of the Cephalosporins

The cephalosporins are used in the treatment of infections due to susceptible microorganisms. Culture and sensitivity tests are performed whenever possible to determine which penicillin will best control an infection caused by a specific strain of bacteria.

SUMMARY DRUG TABLE 22–2
Cephalosporins and Related Antibiotics

GENERIC NAME	TRADE NAME*	USES	ADVERSE REACTIONS	DOSE RANGES
cefaclor	Ceclor	Infections due to susceptible microorganisms	GI disturbances, hypersensitivity, headache, fever	250–500 mg PO q8h
cefadroxil	Duricef, Ultracef, *generic*	Same as cefaclor	Same as cefaclor	1–2 g/d PO in single or divided doses
cefamandole nafate	Mandol	Same as cefaclor	Same as cefaclor	1 g q6–8h IM, IV 1–3 g IV q4–8h
cefazolin	Ancef, Kefzol, *generic*	Same as cefaclor	Same as cefaclor	250 mg–1.5 g IV, IM
cefixime	Suprax	Same as cefaclor	Same as cefaclor	200 mg PO q12h or 400 mg PO once a day
cefonicid sodium	Monocid	Same as cefaclor	Same as cefaclor	0.5–2 g/d IM, IV
cefoperazone sodium	Cefobid	Same as cefaclor	Same as cefaclor	2–4 g/d IM, IV in divided doses q12h; higher doses may also be used
cefotaxime sodium	Claforan	Same as cefaclor	Same as cefaclor	1–12 g/d IM, IV in divided doses
cefotetan disodium	Cefotan	Same as cefaclor	Same as cefaclor	1–2 g IM, IV q12h
cefoxitin sodium	Mefoxin	Same as cefaclor	Same as cefaclor	1–2 g IM, IV q6–8h
ceftriaxone sodium	Rocephin	Same as cefaclor	Same as cefaclor	1–2 g/d IM, IV
cephalexin monohydrate	Keflex, *generic*	Same as cefaclor	Same as cefaclor	1–4 g/d PO in divided doses
cephalothin sodium	Keflin Neutral, *generic*	Same as cefaclor	Same as cefaclor	500 mg–1 g IV, IM q4–6h
cephapirin sodium	Cefadyl, *generic*	Same as cefaclor	Same as cefaclor	500 mg–1 g IM, IV q4–6h
cephradine	Anspor, Velosef, *generic*	Same as cefaclor	Same as cefaclor	250–500 mg q6h PO or 500 mg–1 g q12h PO; 2–4 g/d IM, IV in divided doses
moxalactam disodium	Moxam	Same as cefaclor	Same as cefaclor	2–12 g/d IM, IV in divided doses

* The term generic *indicates that the drug is available in a generic form.*

These drugs also may be used during the preoperative, intraoperative, and postoperative periods to prevent infections in those having surgery on a contaminated or potentially contaminated area such as the gastrointestinal (GI) tract or vagina.

▷ Adverse Reactions Associated with the Administration of the Cephalosporins

The most common adverse reactions seen with administration of the cephalosporins are GI disturbances such as nausea, vomiting, and diarrhea. Hypersensitivity (allergic) reactions may occur, and range from mild to life-threatening. Mild hypersensitivity reactions include pruritus, urticaria, and skin rashes. Anaphylactic reactions, although rare, are life-threatening and require immediate treatment. Because of the close relation of the cephalosporins to penicillin, a patient allergic to penicillin may also be allergic to the cephalosporins.

Other adverse reactions that may be seen with administration of the cephalosporins are hematologic changes, headaches, dizziness, malaise, heartburn, glossitis, and fever.

▶ NURSING PROCESS
THE PATIENT RECEIVING PENICILLIN OR A CEPHALOSPORIN

ASSESSMENT

Before the administration of the first dose of penicillin or a cephalosporin, a general health history is obtained. The health history includes an allergy history, a history of all medical and surgical treatments, a drug history, and the present symptoms of the infection. If the patient has a history of allergy, particularly a drug allergy, this area must be explored to ensure the patient is not allergic to penicillin or a cephalosporin.

Vital signs are taken and recorded. The signs and symptoms of the infection are obtained (when appropriate) from the patient, and an assessment of the infected area (when possible) is recorded on the patient's chart. It is important to describe accurately any signs and symptoms related to the patient's infection, such as color and type of drainage from a wound, pain, redness and inflammation, color of sputum, or presence of an odor. The patient's general appearance is also noted. A culture and sensitivity test is almost always ordered and must be obtained before the first dose of the penicillin or cephalosporin is given.

The results of a culture and sensitivity test take several days because time must be allowed for the bacteria to grow on the culture media. However, infections are treated as soon as possible and therefore the physician selects penicillin, a cephalosporin, or another type of antibiotic based on the location, type of infection, or the appearance of drainage. Once the culture and sensitivity test results are received, the prescribed drug may be continued if the bacteria are sensitive to it. If the bacteria are resistant to the drug, it is discontinued and another drug, to which the bacteria are sensitive, is prescribed.

NURSING DIAGNOSIS

Depending on the drug, dose, and reason for administration, one or more of the following nursing diagnoses may apply to a person receiving a penicillin or cephalosporin:

▶ Anxiety related to diagnosis, route of drug administration (IM,IV), discomfort of injection, other factors (specify)

▶ Noncompliance related to indifference, lack of knowledge, other factors

▶ Knowledge deficit of medication regimen, adverse drug effects

PLANNING AND IMPLEMENTATION

The major goals of the patient may include a reduction in anxiety and an understanding of and compliance to the prescribed treatment regimen.

The major goals of nursing management may include a reduction in the patient's anxiety, correct administration of the prescribed drug, recognition of adverse drug effects, and the development and implementation of an effective teaching plan.

Vital signs are taken every 4 hours or as ordered by the physician. Any increase in temperature is reported to the physician because additional treatment measures, such as administration of an antipyretic drug or change in the drug or dosage, may be necessary. An increase in body temperature several days after the start of therapy may indicate a secondary bacterial infection or failure of the drug to control the original infection.

Patients are evaluated daily for their response to therapy, such as a decrease in temperature, the relief of symptoms caused by the infection (such as pain or discomfort), an increase in appetite, and a change in the appearance or amount of drainage (when originally present). Once an infection is controlled, patients often look better and even state that they feel better. These evaluations are recorded on the patient's chart. The physician is always notified if symptoms of the infection appear to worsen.

Additional culture and sensitivity tests may be performed during therapy because microorganisms causing the infection may become resistant to penicillin or a superinfection may have occurred. A urinalysis, complete blood count (CBC), and renal and hepatic function tests also may be performed at intervals during therapy.

ADMINISTRATION OF PENICILLIN AND THE CEPHALOSPORINS. Penicillin may be ordered in units or milligrams. The cephalosporins are ordered in grams or milligrams.

When preparing a parenteral form of penicillin, the vial is shaken thoroughly before withdrawing the drug to ensure even distribution of the drug in the solution. Some forms of penicillin are in powder or crystalline form and must be made into a liquid (reconstituted) before being withdrawn from the vial. The manufacturer's directions regarding reconstitution are printed on the label or package insert. If no directions for reconstitution are given, the amount of water or saline used depends on the vial size and the dosage to be given. An example of using judgment to determine the amount of fluid (diluent) to be added to the vial that has no manufacturer's recommendation for reconstitution is as follows:

1. Dose in the vial is 1 g.

2. The dose ordered is 0.5 g.

3. The vial will hold up to 4 mL of fluid.

4. *Solution*—2 mL of sterile water or normal saline may be added to the 1 g of powder, mixed thoroughly, and then half of the amount in the vial is withdrawn to give the dose of 0.5 g.

The manufacturer may indicate the type of diluent to be used when reconstituting a specific drug. Some powdered or crystalline drugs, when reconstituted with a given amount of diluent, may yield slightly more or less than the amount of the diluent added to the vial. If there is any question regarding the reconstitution of this or any drug, a pharmacist should be consulted.

Some forms of the cephalosporins are available in premixed vials which are in liquid form and ready for injection. Like the penicillins, some cephalosporins must be reconstituted before use.

To be effective, adequate blood levels of the drug must be maintained. Accidental omission or delay of a dose results in decreased blood levels, which then reduce the effectiveness of the antibiotic. Oral penicillins are best given on an empty stomach, 1 hour before or 2 hours after a meal. Bacampicillin (Spectrobid), penicillin V (Pen-Vee K), and amoxicillin (Amoxil) may be given without regard to meals. The oral cephalosporins are given with food or milk. Cefadroxil (Duricef) and cephradine (Velosef) can be given with or between meals.

The patient should again be questioned about allergy to penicillin or the cephalosporins before administering the first dose, even when an accurate drug history has been taken. Patients should be told that the drug they are receiving is penicillin or a drug similar or related to penicillin (eg, a cephalosporin) because information regarding a drug allergy may have been forgotten at the time the initial drug history was obtained. If a patient states he or she is allergic to penicillin or a cephalosporin, the drug is withheld and the physician is contacted. The cephalosporins are given with great caution, if at all, to those with a history of a penicillin allergy.

The patient should be warned that at the time the drug is injected into the muscle, there may be a stinging or burning sensation. Discomfort at the time of injection occurs because the drug is irritating to the tissues. Previous areas used for injection should be inspected for continued redness, soreness, or other problems, which then should be reported to the physician.

ADVERSE DRUG REACTIONS. After the administration of the first and second doses of penicillin or a cephalosporin, the patient is closely observed for a hypersensitivity reaction. A hypersensitivity reaction may also occur after many doses of any drug, including penicillin or a cephalosporin. The nurse must be constantly aware that a reaction can occur at any time. If a hypersensitivity reaction should occur, the physician is contacted immediately and the drug is withheld until the patient is seen by a physician. Treatment of minor hypersensitivity reactions may include administration of an antihistamine (for a rash or itching). Major hypersensitivity reactions such as bronchospasm, laryngospasm, hypotension, and angioneurotic edema require immediate treatment with drugs such as epinephrine, cortisone, or an IV antihistamine. When respiratory difficulty occurs, a tracheostomy may need to be performed.

The administration of oral penicillin may result in a superinfection in the oral cavity. To detect this problem early, the patient's mouth is inspected daily for signs of glossitis, sore tongue, ulceration, or a black, furry tongue.

When penicillin or a cephalosporin is given, the patient is closely observed for signs of a bacterial or fungal superinfection. Examples of these signs include itching around the anal area, vaginal itching or discharge, diarrhea, chills, fever, sore mouth, and sore throat. Symptoms of a superinfection are reported to the physician before the next dose of the drug is administered. When symptoms are severe, additional treatment measures may be necessary, such as administration of an antipyretic agent for fever or an antifungal agent.

ANXIETY. Patients may have varying degrees of anxiety related to their diagnosis or the fact that the IM injections are uncomfortable or painful. The patient should be reassured that the discomfort or pain is due to the drug but will decrease in a short time. The rotation of IM injection sites helps to reduce discomfort when these drugs are given for a long time.

NONCOMPLIANCE AND KNOWLEDGE DEFICIT. When one of these drugs is prescribed, the patient and family must understand the reason for and the importance of therapy (eg, treatment of an infection or prophylaxis). The dose regimen is carefully reviewed with the patient.

Additional information that may be included in the teaching plan includes the following:

▶ Prophylaxis—Take the drug as prescribed until the physician discontinues therapy.

▶ Infection—Complete the *full* course of therapy. Do not stop the drug even if the symptoms have disappeared unless directed to do so by the physician.

▶ Take the drug at the prescribed times of day because it is important to keep an adequate amount of drug in the body throughout the entire 24 hours of each day.

► Penicillin (oral) — Take the drug on an empty stomach either 1 hour before or 2 hours after meals (*exception* — bacampicillin, penicillin V, amoxicillin).

► Take the cephalosporins (oral) with food or milk. Take cefadroxil (Duricef) and cephradine (Velosef) with or between meals.

► Take each dose with a full glass of water.

► Notify the physician immediately if any one or more of the following should occur: skin rash, hives (urticaria), severe diarrhea, vaginal or anal itching, sore mouth, black furry tongue, sores in the mouth, swelling around the mouth or eyes, breathing difficulty or GI disturbances such as nausea, vomiting, and diarrhea. Do not take the next dose of the drug until the problem is discussed with the physician.

► Oral suspensions — Keep the container refrigerated (if so labeled); shake the drug well before pouring (if so labeled); return the drug to the refrigerator immediately after pouring the dose. Drugs that are kept refrigerated lose their potency when kept at room temperature. A small amount of the drug may be left after the last dose is taken and should be discarded because the drug (in suspension form) begins to lose its potency after a few weeks.

► Never give this drug to another individual even though the symptoms appear to be the same.

► Notify the physician if the symptoms of the infection do not improve or if the condition becomes worse.

EVALUATION

► Anxiety is reduced

► Adverse reactions are identified and reported to the physician

► Patient complies to the prescribed drug regimen

► Patient and family demonstrate understanding of drug regimen

► Verbalizes importance of complying with the prescribed treatment regimen

23

The Broad-Spectrum Antibiotics and Antifungal Drugs

On completion of this chapter the student will:

► *Discuss the types and uses of broad-spectrum antibiotics*
► *List some of the adverse reactions associated with the administration of broad-spectrum antibiotics*
► *Use the nursing process when administering a broad-spectrum antibiotic*
► *Discuss the nursing implications to be considered when administering a broad-spectrum antibiotic*
► *Discuss the uses of antifungal drugs*
► *List some of the adverse reactions associated with the administration of antifungal drugs*
► *Use the nursing process when administering an antifungal drug*
► *Discuss the nursing implications to be considered when administering an antifungal drug*

► BROAD-SPECTRUM ANTIBIOTICS

After penicillin was introduced, it was used for almost every infection. In some patients, penicillin was either partially or totally ineffective; in others, the infection was controlled. Continued use, as well as overuse, of penicillin began to produce penicillin-resistant strains of bacteria, thus making penicillin ineffective for many types of infections. Continued research developed the broad-spectrum antibiotics. Although the penicillins still remain important antibiotics, the physician now has a wide variety of drugs to treat an infection. Summary Drug Table 23-1 lists the various types of broad-spectrum antibiotics.

SUMMARY DRUG TABLE 23–1
Broad-Spectrum Antibiotics

GENERIC NAME	TRADE NAME*	USES	ADVERSE REACTIONS	DOSE RANGES
anikacin sulfate	Amikin	Infections due to susceptible microorganisms	Nephrotoxicity, numbness, tingling, tinnitus, nausea, vomiting, circumoral or peripheral paresthesia, dizziness, vertigo, ototoxicity	15 mg/kg/d IM, IV in 2–3 divided doses
aztreonam	Azactam	Same as amikacin sulfate	Skin rash, abdominal cramps, diarrhea, nausea, vomiting, localized thrombophlebitis or phlebitis	500 mg–1 g IV, IM q6–12h
bacitracin	*Generic*	Infants with pneumonia and empyema	Renal failure	Infants under 2.5 kg: 900 U/kg/24 h IM in 2–3 divided doses; infants over 2.5 kg: 1000 U/kg/24 h IM in 2–3 divided doses
chloramphenicol	Chloromycetin, *generic*	Same as amikacin sulfate	Blood dyscrasias, nausea, vomiting, hypersensitivity reactions	50–100 mg/kg/d PO in divided doses q6h
ciprofloxacin	Cipro	Same as amikacin sulfate	Nausea, diarrhea, headache, abdominal discomfort, rash	250–750 mg PO q12h
clindamycin	Cleocin	Same as amikacin sulfate	Abdominal pain, esophagitis, nausea, vomiting, diarrhea, skin rash, blood dyscrasias	150–450 mg PO q6h; 600 mg–4.8 g/d IV in divided doses; up to 600 mg/dose IM
colistimethate sodium	Coly-Mycin M	Same as amikacin sulfate	Respiratory arrest (IM use), paresthesia, itching, urticaria, tingling of the extremities	2.5–5 mg/kg/d IV, IM in 2–4 divided doses
colistin sulfate	Coly-Mycin S	Same as amikacin sulfate	None reported with recommended doses	5–15 mg/kg/d PO in 3 divided doses
demeclocycline hydrochloride	Declomycin	Same as amikacin sulfate	Nausea, vomiting, diarrhea, epigastric distress, stomatitis, sore throat, rash, photosensitivity reaction	150 mg PO qid or 300 mg PO bid
doxycycline	Vibramycin, *generic*	Same as amikacin sulfate	Same as demeclocycline hydrochloride	100 mg/d PO or 100 mg PO q12h (depending on the type of infection); 100–200 mg IV
erythromycin base	E-Mycin, Eryc, *generic*	Same as amikacin sulfate	Abdominal cramping, nausea, vomiting, diarrhea	250 mg PO q6h, 500 mg PO q12h or 333 mg q8h
erythromycin ethylsuccinate	E.E.S., E-Mycin, *generic*	Same as amikacin sulfate	Same as erythromycin base	400 mg q6h
gentamicin	Garamycin, *generic*	Same as amikacin sulfate	Same as amikacin sulfate	3–5 mg/kg/d IM, IV in 3 divided doses
imipenem cilastatin	Primaxin	Same as amikacin sulfate	Same as aztreonam	250–500 mg IV infusion q6–8h
kanamycin sulfate (parenteral)	Kantrex	Same as amikacin sulfate	Same as amikacin sulfate	7.5 mg/kg IM q12h; 500 mg–1 g IV 2–3 times/d
kanamycin sulfate (oral)	Kantrex	Suppression of intestinal bacteria preoperatively and in hepatic coma	Nausea, vomiting, diarrhea	Preoperative: 1 g/h for 4 h, then 1 g q6h for 36–72 h; hepatic coma: 8–12 g/d in divided doses

(continued)

SUMMARY DRUG TABLE 23–1
(continued)

GENERIC NAME	TRADE NAME*	USES	ADVERSE REACTIONS	DOSE RANGES
lincomycin	Lincocin	Same as amikacin sulfate	Nausea, vomiting, diarrhea, abdominal pain, esophagitis, colitis, skin rash, blood dyscrasias	500 mg PO q6–8h; 600 mg q12–24h IM; up to 8 g/d IV in divided doses
methacycline hydrochloride	Rondomycin	Same as amikacin sulfate	Same as demeclocycline hydrochloride	600 mg/d PO in 2–4 divided doses
metronidazole	Flagyl, *generic*	Same as amikacin sulfate, amebiasis	Seizures, peripheral neuropathy, dizziness, nausea, vomiting, headache, dysuria, urticaria	Initial dose: 15 mg/kg IV infusion followed by 7.5 mg/kg IV infusion q6h (see chap 25 for doses for amebiasis)
minocycline	Minocin	Same as amikacin sulfate	Same as demeclocycline hydrochloride	Oral: initial dose 50–100 mg then 100 mg PO q12h or 50 mg PO qid; IV: initial dose 200 mg then 100 mg q12h
neomycin sulfate (oral)	Mycifradin, *generic*	Same as kanamycin sulfate (oral)	Same as kanamycin sulfate (oral)	Preoperative: 1 g per dose in intervals specified by the physician; hepatic coma: 4–12 g/d PO in divided doses
neomycin sulfate (parenteral)	Mycifradin Sulfate	Same as amikacin sulfate	Same as amikacin sulfate	15 mg/kg/d IM in divided doses q6h
netilmicin sulfate	Netromycin	Same as amikacin sulfate	Same as amikacin sulfate	3–6.5 mg/kg/d IM, IV in divided doses
norfloxacin	Noroxin	Same as amikacin sulfate	Same as ciprofloxacin	400 mg PO bid
novobiocin	Albamycin	Same as amikacin sulfate	Nausea, vomiting, diarrhea, skin rash, urticaria, blood dyscrasias	250 mg PO q6h or 500 mg PO q12h
oxytetracycline	Terramycin, *generic*	Same as amikacin sulfate	Same as demeclocycline hydrochloride	1–2 g/d PO in divided doses; 250 mg daily IM or 150 mg IM every 8 or 12 h
spectinomycin hydrochloride	Trobicin	Same as amikacin sulfate	Soreness at injection site, urticaria, dizziness, nausea, chills, fever	2 g/dose IM
streptomycin sulfate	*Generic*	Same as amikacin sulfate	Same as amikacin sulfate	1–4 g/d IM
tetracycline hydrochloride	Sumycin, Panmycin, *generic*	Same as amikacin sulfate	Same as demeclocycline hydrochloride	Same as oxytetracycline
tobramycin sulfate	Nebcin	Same as amikacin sulfate	Same as amikacin sulfate	3–5 mg/kg/d IM, IV in 3 divided doses
troleandomycin	Tao	Same as amikacin	Abdominal cramping, nausea, vomiting, diarrhea	250–500 mg PO qid
vancomycin	Vancocin	Same as amikacin	Nausea, chills, fever, urticaria, rashes	500 mg PO, IV q6h or 1 g PO q12h

* The term *generic* indicates that the drug is available in a generic form.

▷ Actions of the Broad-Spectrum Antibiotics

Broad-spectrum antibiotics may be bactericidal (destroy bacteria) or bacteriostatic (slow or retard the multiplication of bacteria).

The broad-spectrum antibiotics have different mechanisms by which they affect bacteria. Some act on the bacteria's cell wall; others affect protein synthesis. The ultimate effect of either action is that the bacteria are either destroyed or their multiplication rate is slowed. The mode of action of some antibiotics, for example, metronidazole (Flagyl) is not well understood.

▷ Uses of the Broad-Spectrum Antibiotics

Like penicillin, the broad-spectrum antibiotics are used in the treatment of infections caused by susceptible microorganisms. Culture and sensitivity tests (see chap 22) are performed to determine which antibiotic will best control the infection. These drugs are of no value in the treatment of infections caused by a virus or fungus. There may be times when a secondary bacterial infection has occurred or potentially will occur when the patient has a fungal or viral infection. The physician may then order an antibiotic, but its purpose is for the prevention or treatment of a secondary infection that has followed the primary fungal or viral infection.

Oral kanamycin (Kantrex) and neomycin (Mycifradin) are used preoperatively to reduce the number of bacteria normally present in the intestine. A reduction in intestinal bacteria is thought to lessen the possibility of abdominal infection that may occur after surgery on the bowel. These drugs are also used orally in the management of hepatic coma, where liver failure results in an elevation of blood ammonia levels. By reducing the ammonia-forming bacteria in the intestines, blood ammonia levels may be reduced.

Metronidazole is also used as an amebicide (see chap 25), as well as in the treatment of infections due to susceptible microorganisms. Norfloxacin (Noroxin) is used for urinary tract infections and is discussed in chapter 26.

▷ Adverse Reactions Associated with the Administration of Broad-Spectrum Antibiotics

Superinfections may occur with the use of any antibiotic, especially when these drugs are given for a long time or when repeated courses of therapy are necessary. A superinfection can range from mild to serious and, at times, can become life-threatening. A fungal superinfection often occurs in the mouth, vagina, and around the anal and genital areas. Symptoms include anal or vaginal itching, vaginal discharge, and lesions in the mouth. Bacterial superinfections may vary in location but are often seen in the bowel with diarrhea being the most prominent symptom. See chapter 22 for additional material regarding superinfections.

As with any drug, *hypersensitivity* reactions may be seen when antibiotics are administered. In some instances, these may be mild, and while they require discontinuing the drug, no additional treatment for the allergic reaction may be necessary. Some hypersensitivity reactions are severe and do require immediate treatment.

Some antibiotics are *nephrotoxic*, eg, toxic to the kidney. Symptoms of nephrotoxicity may include protein in the urine (proteinuria), hematuria, increase in the blood urea nitrogen (BUN), decrease in urine output, and an increase in the serum creatinine.

Ototoxicity is an adverse reaction that may be seen with some antibiotics. Symptoms of ototoxicity include tinnitus, dizziness, roaring in the ears, vertigo, and a mild to severe loss of hearing.

Neurotoxicity also may be seen with the administration of some antibiotics. Symptoms of neurotoxicity include numbness, skin tingling, circumoral (around the mouth) paresthesia, peripheral paresthesia, tremors, muscle twitching, convulsions, muscle weakness, and neuromuscular blockade (acute muscular paralysis and apnea).

Tetracyclines

Gastrointestinal reactions that may occur during tetracycline administration include nausea, vomiting, diarrhea, epigastric distress, stomatitis, and sore throat. Skin rashes may also be seen. A photosensitivity (phototoxic) reaction, which is manifested by an exaggerated sunburn reaction when the skin is exposed to sunlight even for brief periods, may be seen with the tetracyclines. Demeclocyline (Declomycin) has been known to cause the most serious photosensitivity reaction. Minocycline (Minocin) is least likely to cause this type of reaction.

The tetracyclines are not given to children under 8 years of age unless their use is absolutely necessary because these drugs may cause permanent yellow-gray-brown discoloration of the teeth.

Chloramphenicol (Chloromycetin)

Serious and sometimes fatal blood dyscrasias are the chief adverse reaction seen with the administration of chloramphenicol (Chloromycetin), and therefore limit its usefulness except in serious infections when less potentially dangerous drugs are ineffective or contraindicated. In addition to blood dyscrasias, nausea and vomiting may also be seen.

Clindamycin (Cleocin) and Lincomycin (Lincocin)

Abdominal pain, esophagitis, nausea, vomiting, diarrhea, skin rash, and blood dyscrasias may be seen with the use of these drugs. These drugs can also cause colitis, which may range from mild to very severe. Discontinuing the drug may relieve the mild form of colitis. The more severe form may require administration of corticosteroids, intravenous (IV) fluids, and electrolytes.

Colistimethate (Coly-Mycin M) and Colistin (Coly-Mycin S)

These two drugs, although chemically related, have different uses and routes of administration. Colistimethate is administered only by the parenteral route. Adverse reactions associated with the administration of this drug include paresthesia, tingling of the extremities, and generalized itching or urticaria. Respiratory arrest has been reported after intramuscular (IM) administration. Colistin is only administered orally and no adverse reactions have been reported when recommended doses are given.

Erythromycins

Abdominal cramping, nausea, vomiting, diarrhea, and allergic reactions have been reported with the administration of the erythromycins. There appears to be a low incidence of adverse reactions with oral use when normal doses are given.

Spectinomycin (Trobicin)

Soreness at the injection site may be seen with the administration of spectinomycin. Other adverse reactions include urticaria, dizziness, nausea, chills, and fever.

Troleandomycin (Tao)

The most frequent adverse reactions seen with troleandomycin are abdominal cramping and discomfort. Nausea, vomiting, and diarrhea, though infrequent, may also be seen.

Vancomycin (Vancocin)

Nausea, chills, fever, urticaria, and skin rashes may be seen with the administration of vancomycin. In addition, ototoxicity and nephrotoxicity have been reported.

Aztreonam (Azactam) and Imipenem-Cilastatin (Primaxin)

Localized thrombophlebitis or phlebitis may be seen after IV administration. Other adverse reactions include skin rash, abdominal cramps, diarrhea, nausea, and vomiting.

Parenteral Aminoglycosides

Amikacin (Amikin), gentamicin (Garamycin), kanamycin (Kantrex), neomycin, netilmicin (Netromycin), streptomycin, and tobramycin (Nebcin) are a group of drugs classified as aminoglycosides. Administration of these drugs can result in ototoxicity and nephrotoxicity. If hearing loss occurs, it is permanent. Symptoms of ototoxicity may occur during drug therapy but may also not occur until after the drug is discontinued. Nephrotoxicity is usually reversible once the drug is discontinued.

Additional adverse reactions may include nausea, vomiting, anorexia, rash, and urticaria. When these agents are given, individual drug references, such as the package insert, should be consulted for more specific adverse reactions.

Oral Aminoglycosides

Kanamycin (Kantrex), and neomycin (Mycifradin) are aminoglycosides that are given orally. Nausea, vomiting, and diarrhea are the most common adverse reactions seen with these drugs.

Novobiocin (Albamycin)

Nausea, vomiting, diarrhea, skin rash, urticaria, and blood dyscrasias may be seen with the administration of this drug.

Bacitracin

The most serious adverse reaction seen with administration of bacitracin is renal failure. The use of this drug is limited to infants with staphylococcal pneumonia and empyema.

Polymixin B (Aerosporin)

This drug is both nephrotoxic and neurotoxic. Occasionally, drug fever, skin rash, and severe pain at the site of injection may be seen.

Metronidazole (Flagyl)

The most common adverse reactions to this drug are related to the GI tract and may include nausea, anorexia, and occasionally vomiting and diarrhea. The most serious adverse reaction is related to the central nervous system (CNS) with seizures and numbness of the extremities.

Fluoroquinolones

Norfloxacin (Noroxin; see chap 26) and ciprofloxacin (Cipro) are synthetic antibiotic agents. The most common adverse effects seen with the administration of these agents include nausea, diarrhea, headache, abdominal discomfort, and skin rash.

▶ NURSING PROCESS
THE PATIENT RECEIVING AN ANTIBIOTIC

ASSESSMENT

Before the administration of any antibiotic, the symptoms of the patient's infection are identified and recorded. Symptoms of an infection may vary and often depend on the organ or system involved and whether the infection is external or internal. Examples of some of the symptoms of an infection in various areas of the body are pain, drainage, redness, changes in the appearance of sputum, general malaise, chills and fever, cough, and swelling.

A thorough allergy history, especially a history of drug allergies, is most important. Some antibiotics have a higher incidence of hypersensitivity reactions in those with a history of allergy to drugs or other substances. If the patient has a history of allergies and has *not* told his or her physician, the first dose of the drug should not be given until this problem is discussed with the physician.

The vital signs are taken and the symptoms of the infection are recorded before the first dose of the antibiotic is given. The physician may order culture and sensitivity tests, and these should also be performed before the first dose of the drug is given. Other laboratory tests such as renal and hepatic function tests, complete blood count (CBC), and urinalysis may also be ordered by the physician.

NURSING DIAGNOSIS

One or more of the following nursing diagnoses may apply to a person receiving an antibiotic. Additional nursing diagnoses, based on the patient's symptoms, may be required.

▶ Anxiety related to infection, seriousness of illness, route of administration, other factors (specify)

▶ Diarrhea related to adverse drug reaction
▶ Potential altered health maintenance related to inability to comprehend drug regimen
▶ Noncompliance related to indifference, lack of knowledge, other factors
▶ Knowledge deficit of medication regimen, adverse drug effects, treatment modalities

PLANNING AND IMPLEMENTATION

The major goals of the patient may include a reduction in anxiety, an absence of adverse drug effects, and an understanding of and compliance to the prescribed treatment regimen.

The major goals of nursing management may include a reduction in the patient's anxiety, recognition of adverse drug effects, the development and implementation of an effective teaching plan.

There are general assessments and evaluations that are common to therapy with any antibiotic. They include the following.

VITAL SIGNS. Vital signs are monitored every 4 hours or as ordered by the physician. The physician is notified if there are changes in the vital signs such as a significant drop in blood pressure, an increase in the pulse or respiratory rate, or a sudden increase in temperature.

OBSERVING FOR ADVERSE REACTIONS. There is a variety of adverse reactions that can be seen with the administration of the antibiotics. The patient is observed at frequent intervals, especially during the first 48 hours of therapy. The occurrence of any adverse reaction is reported to the physician before the next dose of the drug is due. Serious adverse reactions, such as a hypersensitivity reaction, respiratory difficulty, severe diarrhea, or a decided drop in blood pressure, are reported to the physician *immediately.*

ORAL ADMINISTRATION. Some antibiotics, for example, the erythromycins or lincomycin, require taking the drug on an empty stomach, that is, 1 hour before or 2 hours after a meal. The tetracyclines are not to be taken with dairy products and are best taken on an empty stomach. The exceptions are doxycycline (Vibramycin) and minocycline (Minocin), which may be taken with dairy products or food. Many of the antibiotics may be given without regard to food. If there is any doubt about administration of these drugs with or without food, the hospital pharmacist should be consulted.

IM ADMINISTRATION. When an antibiotic is given IM, previous injection sites are inspected for signs of pain or tenderness, redness, and swelling. Some antibiotics may cause temporary local reactions but persistence of a localized reaction should be reported to the physician. Injection sites must be rotated and the site used for injection recorded in the patient's chart.

IV ADMINISTRATION. When an antibiotic is given IV, the needle site and area around the needle are inspected every hour for signs of extravasation of the IV fluid. More frequent assessments may be necessary if the patient is restless or uncooperative. The rate of infusion is checked every 15 minutes and adjusted as needed. The vein for the IV infusion is inspected for signs of tenderness, pain, and redness (which may indicate phlebitis or thrombophlebitis) every 4 hours. If these symptoms are apparent, the IV is restarted in another vein and the problem brought to the attention of the physician. The intake and output are measured and recorded when the patient is receiving these drugs by IV administration.

SUPERINFECTION. A superinfection can occur during therapy with any antibiotic. Symptoms of a superinfection may vary and depend on the microorganism causing the superinfection. Some of the symptoms of a fungal superinfection include sores in the mouth, itching around the anogenital area, and vaginal itching and discharge. Some of the symptoms of a bacterial superinfection include diarrhea, fever, chills, and sore throat. Any new signs and symptoms occurring during antibiotic therapy are reported to the physician, who must then decide if these problems are part of the original infection or if a superinfection has occurred.

EVALUATION OF A RESPONSE TO THERAPY. The initial symptoms of the infection are compared, on a daily basis against the present symptoms and are recorded in the patient's chart. When an antibiotic is ordered for the prevention of an infection (prophylaxis), the patient is observed for symptoms that may indicate the beginning of an infection despite the prophylactic use of the antibiotic. If symptoms of an infection should occur, this is reported to the physician.

ADVERSE DRUG REACTIONS. It is most important to review the adverse reactions associated with the administration of a specific antibiotic before therapy is started. A review of these reactions often determines the assessments and nursing tasks that will be necessary for identification of some of these adverse reactions. For example, if an antibiotic is potentially nephrotoxic, this means that some patients may experience a change in kidney function. Although the physician may order periodic kidney function tests, the patient should also be placed on intake and output. Any changes in the intake and output ratio or in the appearance of the urine may indicate nephrotoxicity and are reported to the physician promptly. Another example is the occurrence of ototoxicity with some antibiotics. Knowing that ototoxicity may occur will result in a care-

ful evaluation of the patient's complaints or comments related to hearing, such as a ringing or buzzing in the ears or an inability to hear. If hearing problems do occur, they are reported to the physician immediately.

All changes in the patient's condition and any new problems that occur, for example, nausea or diarrhea, are brought to the attention of the physician as soon as possible. It is then up to the physician to decide if these changes or problems are a part of the patient's infectious process or due to an adverse drug reaction.

ANXIETY. Patients may exhibit varying degrees of anxiety related to their illness and infection and the necessary drug therapy. When these drugs are given by the parenteral route, anxiety may be experienced because of the discomfort or pain that accompanies an IM injection or IV administration of fluids.

The patient is assured that every effort will be made to reduce pain and discomfort but there are times when this may not be possible. It is best to warn the patient at the time the first IM injection is given that some pain or discomfort may be experienced at the time the drug is injected and for a short time after the drug is given.

NONCOMPLIANCE AND KNOWLEDGE DEFICIT. It is most important that the patient and family understand the prescribed treatment regimen. To decrease the chance of noncompliance, the following points should be emphasized:

► Take the drug at the prescribed time intervals. These time intervals are important because a certain amount of the drug must be in the body at all times in order for the infection to be controlled.

► Do not increase or omit the dose unless advised to do so by the physician.

► Complete the entire course of treatment. Do not stop the drug, except on the advice of a physician, before the course of treatment is completed even though symptoms improve or have disappeared. Failure to complete the prescribed course of treatment may result in a return of the infection.

► Take each dose with a full glass of water.

► Notify the physician if symptoms of the infection become worse or there is no improvement in the original symptoms after about 5 days.

The adverse reactions associated with the specific prescribed antibiotic are explained to the patient. The patient is advised to contact the physician if any of these should occur. Potentially serious adverse reactions such as hypersensitivity reactions, moderate to severe diarrhea, sudden onset of chills and fever, sore throat, sores in the mouth, severe fatigue, or easy bruising are explained, along with the necessity of contacting the physician immediately. Patients should be cautioned against the use of alcoholic beverages during therapy unless use has been approved by the physician.

EVALUATION

▶ Anxiety is reduced

▶ Adverse reactions are identified and reported to the physician

▶ Patient and family demonstrate understanding of drug regimen

▶ Verbalizes importance of complying with the prescribed treatment regimen

▶ ANTIFUNGAL DRUGS

A fungus is a colorless plant lacking chlorophyll. Fungi that cause disease in humans may be yeastlike or moldlike and are called **mycotic infections** or **fungal infections.**

Mycotic infections may be one of two types: (1) superficial mycotic infections or (2) deep (systemic) mycotic infections. The superficial mycotic infections are those occurring on the surface of or just below the skin or nails. Deep mycotic infections are those occurring inside the body, such as in the lungs.

The various antifungal drugs are listed in Summary Drug Table 23-2.

▷ Actions of the Antifungal Drugs

Antifungal drugs may be fungicidal (destroy fungi) or fungistatic (slow or retard the multiplication of fungi).

Amphotericin B (Fungizone Intravenous), miconazole (Monistat IV), nystatin (Mycostatin), and ketoconazole (Nizoral) are thought to have an effect on the cell membrane of the fungus, resulting in a fungicidal or fungistatic effect. The fungicidal or fungistatic effect of these drugs appears to be related to their concentration in body tissues. Fluconazole (Diflucan) has fungistatic activity which appears to result from the depletion of sterols (a group of substances related to fats) in the fungus cells.

Griseofulvin (Grisactin) is deposited in keratin precursor cells, which are then gradually lost (due to the constant shedding of top skin cells), and replaced by new, noninfected cells. The mode of action of flucytosine (Ancobon) is not clearly understood.

Topical antifungals may have both fungistatic of fungicidal activity.

▷ Uses of Antifungal Drugs

Antifungal drugs are used in the treatment of superficial and deep fungal infections. The specific uses of the antifungal agents are given in Summary Drug Table 23-2.

▷ Adverse Reactions Associated with the Administration of Antifungal Drugs

Topical Antifungal Agents

When applied to the skin or mucous membrane, few adverse reactions are seen with these agents. On occasion, a local reaction such as irritation or burning may occur with topical use.

Amphotericin B

Administration often results in serious reactions. The reactions that may be seen include fever, shaking, chills, headache, malaise, anorexia, joint and muscle pain, abnormal renal function, nausea, vomiting, and anemia. This drug is given parenterally usually over several months. Its use is reserved for serious and potentially life-threatening fungal infections. Some of these adverse reactions may be lessened by aspirin, antihistamines, or antiemetics and other types of therapy. Other adverse reactions, such as hearing loss, may have to be tolerated.

Flucytosine

Administration may result in nausea, vomiting, diarrhea, rash, anemia, leukopenia, and thrombocytopenia. Signs of renal impairment include elevated BUN and serum creatinine levels. Periodic renal function tests are usually performed during therapy.

Miconazole

Parenteral administration may result in phlebitis, pruritus, rash, nausea, vomiting, diarrhea, and anorexia. Febrile reactions, drowsiness, and flushing of the skin may also be seen. Vaginal use may result in burning, itching, and irritation. Adverse reactions associated with topical use are rare.

Fluconazole

Administration may result in nausea, vomiting, headache, diarrhea, and skin rash. Abnormal liver

SUMMARY DRUG TABLE 23–2
Antifungal Agents

GENERIC NAME	TRADE NAME*	USES	ADVERSE REACTIONS	DOSE RANGES
amphotericin B	Fungizone Intravenous	Cryptococcosis, blastomycosis, disseminated moniliasis, coccidioidomycosis, histoplasmosis	Fever, headache, anorexia, abnormal renal function, nausea, vomiting, malaise, shaking chills, joint and muscle pain, anemia	0.25–1.5 mg/kg/d IV
fluconazole	Diflucan	Oropharyngeal and esophageal candidiasis, cryptococcal meningitis	Nausea, vomiting, rash, headache	200–400 mg PO, IV first day followed by 100–200 mg/d PO, IV
flucytosine	Ancobon	Infections caused by susceptible strains of *Candida* or *Cryptococcus*	Nausea, vomiting, diarrhea, rash, anemia, leukopenia, thrombocytopenia	50–150 mg/kg/d PO in divided doses q6h
griseofulvin microsize, ultramicrosize	Grisactin, Grisactin Ultra, Fulvicin-U/F, Fulvicin-P/G, *generic*	Ringworm infections	Rash, urticaria, oral thrush, nausea, vomiting, headache, diarrhea	Microsize: 500 mg–1 g/d PO; ultramicrosize: 330–750 mg/d PO
ketoconazole	Nizoral	Candidiasis, oral thrush, blastomycosis, histoplasmosis, coccidioidomycosis, chronic mucocutaneous candidiasis	Nausea, vomiting, headache, dizziness, abdominal pain, pruritus	200–400 mg/d PO
miconazole nitrate	Monistat 3 or 7, Micatin, Monistat-Derm	Vulvovaginal candidiasis, topical fungal infections (ringworm, athlete's foot, topical candidiasis)	Vaginal use: burning, itching, irritation; topical: irritation, burning	Vaginal cream: 1 applicatorful daily at hs; vaginal suppository: 1 daily at hs; topical cream, powder, lotion: cover affected areas bid
miconazole (parenteral)	Monistat i.v.	Coccidioidomycosis, candidiasis, cryptococcosis	Phlebitis, pruritus, rash, nausea, vomiting, diarrhea, anorexia, febrile reactions, drowsiness, flushing of the skin	200–3600 mg/d IV infusion
nystatin (oral)	Mycostatin, *generic*	Intestinal candidiasis	Rare	500,000–1 million U PO tid
nystatin (topical)	Nilstat, Mycostatin	Cutaneous or mucocutaneous infections caused by *Candida*	Rare	Apply 2–3 times/d
nystatin (vaginal)	Nilstat, Mycostatin, *generic*	Vulvovaginal candidiasis	Rare	1 tablet/d intravaginally

* The term generic indicates that the drug is available in a generic form.

function tests may be seen and may require follow-up tests to determine if liver function has been affected.

Griseofulvin

Administration may result in a hypersensitivity-type reaction that includes rash and urticaria. Nausea, vomiting, oral thrush, diarrhea, and headache may also be seen.

Ketoconazole

This drug is usually well-tolerated, but nausea, vomiting, headache, dizziness, abdominal pain, and pruritus may be seen. Most adverse reactions are mild and transient. On rare occasions, hepatic toxicity may be seen and the drug must be discontinued immediately. Monthly hepatic function tests are recommended.

Nystatin

This drug is usually well tolerated, with few reported adverse reactions. Large oral doses have caused diarrhea, GI distress, nausea, and vomiting.

▶ NURSING PROCESS
THE PATIENT RECEIVING AN ANTIFUNGAL AGENT

ASSESSMENT

Before administration of the first dose of an antifungal drug, the patient is assessed for signs of the infection. Superficial fungus infections of the skin or skin structures (hair, nails) are inspected and described on the patient's record. For other superficial and deep fungus infections, the patient's signs and symptoms are recorded. Information gathered before the administration of the first dose establishes a data base for comparison during therapy. The vital signs are taken and recorded. If the patient is scheduled to receive amphotericin or flucytosine, he or she must be weighed because the dosage of the drug is determined according to the patient's weight.

NURSING DIAGNOSIS

Depending on the drug, dose, and reason for administration, one or more of the following nursing diagnoses may apply to a person receiving an antifungal drug:

▶ Anxiety related to diagnosis, symptoms, treatment modalities, other factors (specify)

▶ Noncompliance related to indifference, lack of knowledge, length of treatment, other factors

▶ Knowledge deficit of medication regimen, adverse drug effects, treatment modalities

PLANNING AND IMPLEMENTATION

The major goals of the patient may include a reduction in anxiety and an understanding of and compliance to the prescribed treatment regimen.

The major goals of nursing management may include a reduction in the patient's anxiety, recognition of adverse drug effects, and the development and implementation of an effective teaching plan

OBSERVATIONS AND NURSING MANAGEMENT. The patient is observed every 2 to 4 hours for adverse drug reactions when an antifungal agent is given by the oral or parenteral route. When these drugs are applied topically to the skin, the area is inspected at the time of each application for localized skin reactions. When

used vaginally, the patient is questioned regarding any discomfort or other sensations experienced after insertion of the antifungal preparation. The response to therapy is evaluated daily and noted in the patient's chart. Additional assessments and specific areas of nursing management for some of the antifungal drugs are discussed below.

AMPHOTERICIN B. This drug is administered daily or every other day over several months. The patient is often acutely ill with a life-threatening deep fungus infection. Vital signs are monitored every 2 to 4 hours depending on the patient's condition. The IV infusion is normally given over 6 or more hours. The manufacturer recommends administration immediately after reconstitution and protection of the IV solution from exposure to light. A brown paper bag or aluminum foil may be wrapped around the infusion bottle after reconstitution of the powder and during administration of the solution. Some authorities believe that this maneuver is not necessary because the solution decomposes slowly. The physician or hospital pharmacist should be consulted regarding the need to use or not use a protective covering for the infusion container.

The IV infusion rate and the infusion site are checked frequently during administration of the drug. This is especially important if the patient is restless or confused. The intake and output are monitored closely because this drug may be nephrotoxic. In some instances, hourly measurements of the urinary output may be necessary. Periodic laboratory tests are usually ordered to monitor the patient's response to therapy and to detect toxic drug reactions.

FLUCYTOSINE. Flucytosine is given orally. The prescribed dose may range from two to six capsules per dose. To reduce the incidence of GI distress, the capsules may be given one or two at a time over a 15-minute period. If GI distress still occurs, the physician is notified.

MICONAZOLE. Miconazole may be given by IV infusion over 30 to 60 minutes. Fungal infections of the bladder are treated with IV administration of this drug and instillation of the IV form into the bladder. Fungal meningitis is also treated with an IV infusion of the drug and instillation of the drug into the subarachnoid space by means of a lumbar, cervical, or cisternal puncture.

The vital signs are monitored every 2 to 4 hours depending on the patient's condition. The intake and output are measured and the physician is notified if the oral intake is inadequate or there is a change in the intake and output ratio. If nausea and vomiting occurs, the physician is notified because additional measures, such as giving the infusion over a longer time or administering an antiemetic, may be necessary.

FLUCONAZOLE. When administered IV, the manufacturer's directions regarding removal of the wrapping around the container must be followed. The overwrap must not be removed until the unit is ready for use.

ANXIETY. Superficial and deep fungal infections respond slowly to antifungal therapy. Many patients experience anxiety and depression over the fact that therapy must continue for a prolonged time. Depending on the method of treatment, patients may be faced with many problems during therapy and therefore need time to talk about their problems as they arise. Examples of problems are the cost of treatment, hospitalization (when required), the failure of treatment to adequately control the infection, and loss of income.

NONCOMPLIANCE AND KNOWLEDGE DEFICIT. It is most important that the patient and family understand that therapy must be continued until the infection is under control. This may, in some instances, take weeks or months. The following points may be included in a patient teaching plan:

Topical Antifungal Drugs
▶ Clean the involved area and apply the ointment or cream to the skin as directed by the physician.
▶ Do not increase or decrease the amount used or number of times the ointment or cream should be applied unless directed to do so by the physician.
▶ If the drug (cream or tablet) is to be inserted vaginally, insert the drug high in the vagina using the applicator provided with the product.
▶ If the patient is being treated for a ringworm infection, the following points may be included:
  ▶ Keep towels and facecloths used for bathing separate from those of other family members to avoid the spread of the infection.
  ▶ Keep the infected area clean and dry.

Flucytosine
▶ Nausea and vomiting may occur with this drug and may be reduced or eliminated by taking a few capsules at a time over a 15-minute period. If nausea, vomiting, or diarrhea persists, notify the physician as soon as possible.

Griseofulvin
▶ Beneficial effects may not be noticed for some time; therefore, take the drug for the full course of therapy.
▶ Avoid exposure to sunlight and sunlamps because an exaggerated skin reaction (which is similar to a severe sunburn) may occur even after a brief exposure to ultraviolet light.

Ketoconazole
▶ Complete the full course of therapy as prescribed by the physician.
▶ Do not take this drug with an antacid.
▶ Avoid the use of nonprescription drugs unless use of a specific drug is approved by the physician.
▶ This drug may produce headache, dizziness, and drowsiness. If drowsiness or dizziness should occur, observe caution while driving or performing other hazardous tasks.
▶ Notify the physician if abdominal pain, fever, or diarrhea become pronounced.

Miconazole
▶ When a vaginal cream is prescribed, wear a sanitary napkin after insertion of the drug to prevent staining of the clothing and bed linen.

Nystatin
▶ Oral candidiasis—keep the liquid drug in the mouth as long as possible before swallowing. Avoid the use of commercial mouthwashes. Brush teeth immediately after eating.

EVALUATION
▶ Anxiety is reduced
▶ Adverse reactions are identified and reported to the physician
▶ Patient and family demonstrate understanding of drug regimen
▶ Verbalizes importance of complying with the prescribed treatment regimen

24

Antitubercular and Leprostatic Agents

On completion of this chapter the student will:

▶ *Discuss the drugs used in the treatment of tuberculosis*

▶ *Discuss the adverse reactions associated with the administration of drugs used in the treatment of tuberculosis*

▶ *Use the nursing process when administering an antitubercular agent*

▶ *Discuss the nursing implications to be considered when administering an antitubercular agent*

▶ *Discuss the drugs used in the treatment of leprosy*

▶ *Discuss the adverse reactions associated with the administration of drugs used in the treatment of leprosy*

▶ *Use the nursing process when administering a leprostatic agent*

▶ *Discuss the nursing implications to be considered when administering a leprostatic drug*

▶ ANTITUBERCULAR AGENTS

Tuberculosis is caused by the *Mycobacterium tuberculosis* bacillus and infects both animals and humans. The drugs used in the treatment of tuberculosis do not "cure" the disease, but they contain it and render the patient noninfectious to others.

The various drugs used in the treatment of tuberculosis, usually referred to as antitubercular drugs, are listed in Summary Drug Table 24-1.

▷ Actions of the Antitubercular Drugs

The antitubercular drugs are bacteriostatic against the *M tuberculosis* bacillus. The bacteriostatic activity of these drugs is usually due to an inhibition of bacterial cell wall synthesis, which slows the multiplication rate of the bacteria.

SUMMARY DRUG TABLE 24–1
Antitubercular and Leprostatic Agents

GENERIC NAME	TRADE NAME*	USES	ADVERSE REACTIONS	DOSE RANGES
ANTITUBERCULAR DRUGS				
aminosalicylate sodium (PAS)	Teebacin, *generic*	Tuberculosis	Nausea, vomiting, diarrhea, abdominal pain	14–16 g/d PO in 2–3 divided doses
capreomycin sulfate	Capastat	Same as aminosalicylate	Nephrotoxicity, ototoxicity, leukocytosis, leukopenia	1 g/d IM
cycloserine	Seromycin	Same as aminosalicylate	Convulsions, drowsiness, skin rash, headache	500 mg–1 g/d PO in divided doses
ethambutol hydrochloride	Myambutol	Same as aminosalicylate	Decrease in visual acuity, dermatitis, anaphylactoid reactions, pruritus	15–25 mg/kg/d PO
ethionamide	Trecator-SC	Same as aminosalicylate	GI upset, peripheral neuritis, psychic disturbances	0.5–1 g/d PO in divided doses
isoniazid (INH)	Laniazid, *generic*	Same as aminosalicylate; preventive therapy for specific situations	Peripheral neuropathy, fever, skin eruptions, agranulocytosis, anemia, jaundice, nausea, vomiting, hypersensitivity reactions	Treatment of tuberculosis: up to 300 mg/d PO; preventive treatment: 300 mg/d PO
pyrazinamide	*Generic*	Same as aminosalicylate	Hepatotoxicity, nausea, vomiting, diarrhea	20–35 mg/kg/d PO in 3–4 divided doses
rifampin	Rifadin, Rimactane	Same as aminosalicylate	Heartburn, epigastric distress, anorexia, nausea, vomiting, hypersensitivity reactions	600 mg/d PO, IV
streptomycin sulfate	*Generic*	Same as aminosalicylate, nontuberculous infections due to susceptible microorganisms	Nephrotoxicity, numbness, tingling, tinnitus, nausea, vomiting, circumoral or peripheral paresthesia, dizziness, vertigo	1 g/d IM
LEPROSTATIC AGENTS				
clofazimine	Lamprene	Leprosy	Skin pigmentation, abdominal pain, diarrhea, nausea, vomiting	100–200 mg/d PO
dapsone	*Generic*	Leprosy, dermatitis herpetiformis	Blood cell hemolysis, nausea, vomiting, anorexia, blurred vision	Leprosy: 50–100 mg/d PO; dermatitis herpetiformis: 50–300 mg/d PO

* The term generic *indicates that the drug is available in a generic form.*

▷ Uses of the Antitubercular Drugs

Antitubercular drugs are used in the treatment of active tuberculosis. Treatment of tuberculosis usually involves the use of two or more drugs at the same time.

Isoniazid is used for the treatment of tuberculosis, as well as for preventive therapy (prophylaxis) in the following:

▷ Household members and other close associates

of those recently diagnosed as having tuberculosis

▷ Those whose tuberculin skin test has become positive in the last 2 years

▷ Those with positive skin tests whose radiographic findings indicate nonprogressive, healed, or quiescent tubercular lesions

▷ Those at risk of developing tuberculosis (eg, those with Hodgkin's disease, severe diabetes mellitus, leukemia, and other serious illnesses and those receiving corticosteroids or drug therapy for a malignancy)

▷ Any positive skin test in a patient under age 35 and primarily in children up to age 7

▷ Persons with acquired immunodeficiency syndrome (AIDS) or AIDS-related complex or who are positive for the human immunodeficiency virus who have a positive tuberculosis skin test, or a negative tuberculosis skin test but a history of a prior significant reaction to purified protein derivative (a skin test for tuberculosis).

Bacterial resistance develops, sometimes rapidly, with the use of antitubercular drugs. To slow the development of bacterial resistance, the physician may use two or more drugs even with initial therapy. Using a combination of drugs appears to slow the development of bacterial resistance.

▷ Adverse Reactions Associated with the Administration of Antitubercular Drugs

The following adverse reactions may be seen during administration of antitubercular drugs.

Aminosalicylate (PAS). The most common adverse reactions associated with aminosalicylate are related to the gastrointestinal (GI) tract and include nausea, vomiting, diarrhea, and abdominal pain. Hypersensitivity reactions have also been reported.

Capreomycin (Capastat). The two major adverse reactions associated with capreomycin are ototoxicity and nephrotoxicity. Leukocytosis and leukopenia have also occurred. The physician may order a complete blood count (CBC) and renal function tests at periodic intervals. Hearing testing may also be done periodically.

Cycloserine (Seromycin). Doses of cycloserine larger than 500 mg/d have been reported to cause headache, drowsiness, and convulsions in some patients. A skin rash, which is not related to the size of the dosage, may also occur.

Ethambutol (Myambutol). A decrease in visual acuity, which appears to be related to the dose given and the duration of treatment, has occurred in some patients receiving ethambutol. Usually, this adverse reaction disappears when the drug is discontinued. Other adverse reactions are dermatitis, pruritus, anaphylactoid reactions, joint pain, anorexia, nausea, and vomiting.

Ethionamide (Trecator S.C.). GI intolerance, peripheral neuritis, and psychic disturbances may be seen with the administration of ethionamide. Pa-

tients with diabetes mellitus who are taking this drug may require adjustments of their insulin or oral hypoglycemic dosages.

Isoniazid. The incidence of adverse reactions appears to be higher when larger doses of isoniazid are prescribed. Adverse reactions include hypersensitivity reactions, hematologic changes, peripheral neuropathy, jaundice, fever, skin eruptions, nausea, vomiting, and epigastric distress. Severe, and sometimes fatal, hepatitis has been associated with isoniazid therapy and may appear after many months of treatment.

Pyrazinamide. Hepatotoxicity is the principal adverse reaction seen with pyrazinamide use. Symptoms of hepatotoxicity may range from none (except for slightly abnormal hepatic function tests) to a more severe reaction such as jaundice. Nausea, vomiting, and diarrhea may also be seen.

Rifampin (Rifadin). Nausea, vomiting, epigastric distress, heartburn, and diarrhea may be seen with administration of rifampin.

Streptomycin. Nephrotoxicity, ototoxicity, numbness, tingling, tinnitus, nausea, vomiting, dizziness, vertigo, and circumoral (around the mouth) paresthesia may be noted with the administration of streptomycin. Soreness at the injection site may also be noted, especially when the drug is given for a long time.

▶ NURSING PROCESS
THE PATIENT RECEIVING AN ANTITUBERCULAR AGENT

ASSESSMENT

Once the diagnosis of tuberculosis is confirmed, the physician selects the drug that will best control the spread of the disease and make the patient noninfectious to others. Many laboratory and diagnostic tests may be necessary before starting drug therapy, for example, radiographic studies, culture and sensitivity tests, and various types of laboratory tests such as CBC.

Assessment may also include a family history and a history of contacts if the patient has active tuberculosis.

Immediately before drug therapy is started, the patient's vital signs and weight are obtained. Depending on the severity of the disease, patients may be treated initially in the hospital and then discharged to their home for supervised follow-up care, or they may have all treatment instituted on an outpatient basis.

NURSING DIAGNOSIS

Depending on the individual and the methods of treatment, one or more of the following nursing diagnoses may apply to the patient receiving an antitubercular drug:

▶ Anxiety related to diagnosis, long-term treatment regimen, other factors (specify)

▶ Noncompliance related to indifference, lack of knowledge, other factors

▶ Knowledge deficit of medication regimen, adverse drug effects, treatment modalities

PLANNING AND IMPLEMENTATION

The major goals of the patient may include a reduction in anxiety and an understanding of and compliance to the prescribed treatment regimen.

The major goals of nursing management may include a reduction in the patient's anxiety, recognition of adverse drug effects, and the development and implementation of an effective teaching plan.

ADMINISTRATION. If the antitubercular drug is given by the parenteral route, injection sites are rotated. At the time of each injection, previous injection sites are inspected for signs of swelling, redness, and tenderness. If a localized reaction persists or if the area appears to be infected, the physician is notified.

Aminosalicylate, ethambutol, ethionamide are given with food or meals to prevent GI side effects such as nausea, vomiting, and abdominal pain or discomfort. If GI side effects do occur, this problem is discussed with the physician.

Isoniazid is best given on an empty stomach either 1 hour before or 2 hours after a meal as a single daily dose. If GI upset does occur, isoniazid may then be given with food.

ADVERSE DRUG REACTIONS. When patients are receiving this drug, they are observed daily for the appearance of adverse drug reactions. These observations are especially important when a drug is known to be nephrotoxic or ototoxic. If adverse reactions occur, they are reported to the physician. The vital signs are monitored daily or as frequently as every 4 hours when the patient is hospitalized.

Psychic disturbances may occur with the administration of ethambutol. If the patient appears depressed, withdrawn, noncommunicative, or has other personality changes, the problem is brought to the attention of the physician.

Hepatitis may occur with the use of isoniazid and pyrazinamide. The patient is observed for early signs of hepatitis, such as fever, anorexia, nausea, vomiting, fatigue, malaise, and weakness. Periodic liver function tests may be ordered by the physician.

ANXIETY. The diagnosis, as well as the necessity of long-term treatment and follow-up, are often distressing to the patient. Patients diagnosed as having tuberculosis may have many questions about the disease and its treatment. The nurse must allow time for the patient and family members to ask questions. In some instances, it may be necessary to refer the patient to other health care workers such as a social service worker or the dietitian.

NONCOMPLIANCE AND KNOWLEDGE DEFICIT. Antitubercular drugs are given for a long time, and careful patient and family instruction and close medical supervision are necessary. The patient and family are also given an explanation of the importance of a long period of drug therapy and told that short-term therapy is of *no value* in treating this disease. This should be stressed because noncompliance can be a problem whenever a disease or disorder requires long-term treatment.

The dosage schedule and adverse effects associated with the prescribed drug are reviewed with the patient and family.

Information applying to all patients taking these drugs includes the following:

▶ The results of drug therapy will be monitored at periodic intervals. Laboratory and diagnostic tests and visits to the physician's office or clinic are necessary.

▶ Take the drug exactly as directed on the prescription container. Do not omit, increase, or decrease a dose unless advised to do so by the physician.

▶ Avoid the use of nonprescription drugs, especially those containing aspirin, unless use has been approved by the physician.

▶ Discuss the drinking of alcoholic beverages with the physician. A limited amount of alcohol may be allowed, but excessive intake usually is to be avoided.

The following information is also included when a specific antitubercular drug is prescribed:

▶ Aminosalicylate, ethambutol, ethionamide—Take these drugs with food or meals.

▶ Aminosalicylate—If aftertaste occurs, experiment with methods to eliminate this problem, for example, use sugarless gum, juice, or mouthwash.

▶ Cycloserine—This drug may cause drowsiness. Do not drive or perform other hazardous tasks if drowsiness occurs.

► Isoniazid—Take this drug 1 hour before or 2 hours after meals. If GI upset occurs, take the drug with food.

► Ethionamide—This drug may cause GI upset (nausea, vomiting, diarrhea), loss of appetite, a metallic taste in the mouth, or salivation. If these become bothersome or increase in severity, notify the physician. Diabetic patient—Test urine at least daily or as recommended by the physician. Notify the physician if the urine test is positive for glucose or ketones.

► Ethambutol—Take this drug once a day at the same time each day. If a dose is missed, do *not* double the dose the next day. Notify the physician if any changes in vision occur or if a skin rash occurs.

► Pyrazinamide—Notify the physician if any of the following occurs: nausea, vomiting, loss of appetite, fever, malaise, visual changes, yellowish discoloration of the skin, or severe pain in the knees, feet, or wrists. (*Note:* Pain in these area may be signs of active gout.)

EVALUATION

► Anxiety is reduced

► Adverse reactions are identified and reported to the physician

► Verbalizes an understanding of treatment modalities and importance of continued follow-up care

► Patient and family demonstrate understanding of drug regimen

► Patient complies to the prescribed drug regimen

► THE LEPROSTATICS

Dapsone and clofazimine (Lamprene) are the two drugs currently being used to treat leprosy (Hansen's disease). Although rare in the colder climates, this disease may be seen in tropical and subtropical zones.

▷ Actions of the Leprostatics

Dapsone is bactericidal and bacteriostatic against the microorganism causing leprosy (*Mycobacterium leprae*). Clofazimine is primarily bactericidal. The mode of action of these drugs is unknown.

▷ Uses of the Leprostatics

These drugs are used in the treatment of leprosy. Dapsone also may be used in the treatment of dermatitis herpetiformis, a chronic, inflammatory skin disease. The leprostatics are listed in Summary Drug Table 24-1.

▷ Adverse Reactions Associated with the Administration of the Leprostatics

Dapsone administration may result in hemolysis (destruction of red blood cells), nausea, vomiting, anorexia, and blurred vision. Clofazimine may cause pigmentation of the skin, abdominal pain, diarrhea, nausea, and vomiting.

► NURSING PROCESS
THE PATIENT RECEIVING A LEPROSTATIC

ASSESSMENT

A complete physical examination and history is performed before the institution of therapy. The involved areas are examined and described in detail on the patient's record to provide a database for comparison during therapy.

NURSING DIAGNOSIS

Depending on the individual, one or more of the following nursing diagnoses may apply to the patient receiving a leprostatic:

► Anxiety related to diagnosis, long-term treatment regimen, other factors (specify)

► Noncompliance related to indifference, lack of knowledge, other factors

► Knowledge deficit of medication regimen, adverse drug effects, treatment modalities

PLANNING AND IMPLEMENTATION

The major goals of the patient may include a reduction in anxiety and an understanding of and compliance to the prescribed treatment regimen.

The major goals of nursing management may include a reduction in the patient's anxiety, and the development and implementation of an effective teaching plan.

These drugs are often given on an outpatient basis. Each time the patient is seen in the clinic or physician's office, a general physical examination is performed, with particular attention to the affected areas.

ADMINISTRATION. Leprostatics are given orally and are taken with food to minimize GI upset. Antitubercular drugs, such as rifampin, may be given concurrently during initial therapy to minimize bacterial resistance to the leprostatic drug.

ANXIETY. Treatment with a leprostatic drug may require many years. These patients are faced with long-term medical and drug therapy and possibly severe disfigurement. The nurse must spend time with these patients, allowing them to verbalize their anxieties, problems, and fears.

NONCOMPLIANCE AND KNOWLEDGE DEFICIT. To ensure compliance to the treatment regimen, the dosage schedule, possible adverse effects, and scheduled follow-up visits are explained to the patient and family members. It is important to emphasize the importance of adhering to the prescribed dosage schedule.

EVALUATION

► Anxiety is reduced

► Adverse reactions are identified and reported to the physician

► Verbalizes an understanding of treatment modalities and importance of continued follow-up care

► Patient and family demonstrate understanding of drug regimen

► Patient complies to the prescribed drug regimen

25

Drugs Used in the Treatment of Parasitic Infections

On completion of this chapter the student will:

▶ *Discuss the use and major adverse effects of the drugs used in the prevention and treatment of malaria*

▶ *Use the nursing process when administering a drug used in the prevention or treatment of malaria*

▶ *Discuss the use and major adverse effects of the drugs used in the treatment of helminthic infections*

▶ *Use the nursing process when administering a drug used in the treatment of helminthic infections*

▶ *Discuss the use and major adverse effects of the drugs used in the treatment of amebiasis*

▶ *Use the nursing process when administering a drug used in the treatment of amebiasis*

▶ *Discuss the nursing implications to be considered when administering drugs used in the treatment of malaria, helminthic infections, or amebiasis*

Malaria, helminthiasis (invasion by helminths), and amebiasis (invasion of the body by the ameba, *Entamoeba histolytica*) are worldwide health problems. Because of the range and ease of travel to other countries, individuals coming from areas where these diseases are not prevalent may contract a parasitic disease.

▶ ANTIMALARIAL DRUGS

Malaria is rare in the United States but this disease may be seen by health care professionals practicing in countries where this problem exists. Malaria may also be seen in the United States in those who have

SUMMARY DRUG TABLE 25–1
Drugs Used for Parasitic Infections

GENERIC NAME	TRADE NAME*	USES	ADVERSE REACTIONS	DOSE RANGES
ANTIMALARIAL DRUGS				
chloroquine hydrochloride	Aralen HCl	Suppression and treatment of acute attacks when oral therapy is not feasible	Hypotension, headache, nausea, vomiting, ECG changes, diarrhea, anorexia, abdominal cramps	4–5 mL IM initially and repeat in 6 h if needed; begin oral therapy as soon as possible
chloroquine phosphate	Aralen Phosphate, *generic*	Suppression and treatment of acute attacks of malaria	Same as chloroquine hydrochloride	Suppression: 500 mg/wk PO; treatment: initial dose 600 mg PO, second dose 300 mg PO in 6 h, then 300 mg/d PO for 2 d
hydroxychloroquine sulfate	Plaquenil Sulfate	Same as chloroquine phosphate; lupus erythematosus and rheumatoid arthritis	Same as chloroquine hydrochloride	Malaria: 400 mg/wk PO; lupus erythematosus: see Summary Drug Table 42-1; rheumatoid arthritis: see Summary Drug Table 42-1
mefloquine hydrochloride	Lariam	Prevention and treament of malaria	Vomiting, fever, nausea, dizziness, headache, GI complaints	Treatment: 5 tablets as a single dose; prevention: 1 tablet weekly for 4 wk then 1 tablet every other week
primaquine phosphate	*Generic*	Malaria	Nausea, vomiting, epigastric distress, abdominal cramps	26.3 mg/d PO for 14 d or 79 mg once a week for 8 wk
pyrimethamine	Daraprim	Prevention of malaria	Nausea, vomiting, anorexia	25 mg PO once a week
quinacrine hydrochloride	Atabrine HCl	Treatment and suppression of malaria	Headache, dizziness, nausea, anorexia, abdominal cramps, diarrhea	200 mg with 1 g of sodium bicarbonate PO q6h × 5 doses then 100 mg PO q8h for 6 d; malaria suppression: 100 mg/d PO
quinine sulfate	Quine, *generic*	Malaria, nocturnal leg cramps	Symptoms of cinchonism (see text), vertigo, skin rash, visual disturbances	Malaria: 650 mg PO q8h; nocturnal leg cramps: 260–300 mg PO hs
ANTHELMINTIC AGENTS				
mebendazole	Vermox	Pinworm, roundworm, hookworm, whipworm	Abdominal pain, diarrhea	1 tablet morning and evening for 3 d
niclosamide	Niclocide	Tapeworm	Nausea, vomiting, abdominal discomfort	2 g PO as a single dose or daily for 7 d depending on type of tapeworm
piperazine	*Generic*	Pinworm, roundworm	Nausea, vomiting, abdominal cramps, headache, vertigo	Pinworm: up to 2.5 g/d PO for 7 d; roundworm: 3.5 g/d PO for 2 d
pyrantel	Antiminth	Roundworm, pinworm	Anorexia, nausea, abdominal cramps, vomiting	Up to 1 g PO as a single dose
quinacrine hydrochloride	Atabrine HCl	Tapeworm	See quinacrine hydrochloride (above)	See package insert for instructions regarding special diet, enemas, and dosage schedules
thiabendazole	Mintezol	Threadworm, whipworm, hookworm, pinworm, roundworm	Anorexia, nausea, vomiting, dizziness	Patients weighing less than 150 lb: 10 mg/lb PO; patients weighing more than 150 lb: 1.5 g PO with length of treatment depending on helminth being eradicated

(continued)

SUMMARY DRUG TABLE 25–1
(continued)

GENERIC NAME	TRADE NAME*	USES	ADVERSE REACTIONS	DOSE RANGES
AMEBICIDES				
chloroquine hydrochloride	Aralen Hydrochloride	Extraintestinal amebiasis	See chloroquine hydrochloride (above)	4–5 mL IM daily for 10–12 d
chloroquine phosphate	Aralen Phosphate, *generic*	Extraintestinal amebiasis	See chloroquine phosphate (above)	1 g/d PO for 2 d, then 500 mg/d PO 2–3 wk
iodoquinol	Yodoxin, *generic*	Intestinal amebiasis	Skin eruptions, nausea, vomiting, fever, chills	650 mg PO tid pc
metronidazole	Flagyl, *generic*	Acute intestinal amebiasis	Convulsive seizures, neuropathy, nausea, headache	750 mg PO tid for 5–10 d
paromomycin sulfate	Humatin	Intestinal amebiasis	Nausea, vomiting, diarrhea	25–35 mg/kg/d PO in divided doses for 5–10 d

* The term generic *indicates that the drug is available in a generic form.*

traveled to or lived in areas where this disease is a health problem.

Malaria is transmitted by a certain species of the *Anopheles* mosquito. The four different protozoans causing malaria are *Plasmodium falciparum*, *Plasmodium malariae*, *Plasmodium ovale*, and *Plasmodium vivax*.

Drugs that are used in treating or preventing malaria are called antimalarial drugs. Examples of antimalarial drugs in use today are listed in Summary Drug Table 25-1.

ter the individual's red blood cells, the symptoms of malaria (shaking chills and fever) appear.

Antimalarial drugs interfere with or are active against the life cycle of the plasmodium, primarily when it is present in the red blood cells. Destruction at this stage of the plasmodium life cycle prevents the development of the male and female forms of the plasmodium, which must then enter the mosquito (when the mosquito bites an infected individual) to begin its life cycle.

▷ Actions of Antimalarial Drugs

The plasmodium causing malaria must enter the mosquito to develop and reproduce. When the mosquito bites a person infected with malaria, it ingests the male and female forms of the plasmodium (gametocytes). These mate in the mosquito's stomach and ultimately form sporozoites (an animal reproductive cell) that make their way to the salivary glands of the mosquito. When the mosquito bites an individual, the sporozoites enter the individual's bloodstream and lodge in the liver and other tissues. These sporozoites undergo asexual cell division and reproduction, forming merozoites (cells formed as a result of asexual reproduction). The merozoites then divide asexually and enter the red blood cells of the individual where they form the male and female forms of the plasmodium. When the merozoites en-

▷ Uses of Antimalarial Drugs

There are two terms used when discussing the use of antimalarial drugs: (1) *suppression*, the prevention of malaria, and (2) *treatment*, the management of a malarial attack.

Not all antimalarial drugs are effective in preventing (suppressing) or treating all four of the plasmodium causing malaria. In addition, resistant plasmodium strains have developed and some antimalarial drugs are no longer effective against some of these strains. The physician must select the antimalarial drug that reportedly is effective, at present, for the type of malaria the individual either has (treatment) or could contract (prevention) in a specific area of the world.

Additional uses of some of the antimalarial drugs are given in Summary Drug Table 25-1.

▷ Adverse Reactions Associated with the Administration of Antimalarial Drugs

Chloroquine (Aralen) and Hydroxychloroquine (Plaquenil). The adverse reactions associated with the administration of chloroquine and hydroxychloroquine include hypotension, electrocardiographic (ECG) changes, headache, nausea, vomiting, anorexia, diarrhea, and abdominal cramps. Long-term use has caused damage to the retina of the eye in some patients.

Quinicrine (Atabrine). The most frequent adverse reactions seen with quinacrine include headache, dizziness, and gastrointestinal (GI) complaints. Long-term therapy can result in aplastic anemia, hepatitis, and skin eruptions.

Quinine. Quinine is chemically related to the cardiac depressant quinidine. The use of quinine can cause *cinchonism* at full therapeutic doses. Symptoms of cinchonism include tinnitus, dizziness, headache, GI disturbances, and visual disturbances. These symptoms usually disappear when the dosage is reduced. Other adverse reactions include hematologic changes, vertigo, and skin rash.

Mefloquine (Lariam). Administration of mefloquine may result in vomiting, dizziness, nausea, fever, headache, and visual disturbances. The administration of primaquine may result in nausea, vomiting, epigastric distress, and abdominal cramps. Pyrimethamine (Daraprim) administration may result in nausea, vomiting, and anorexia.

▶ NURSING PROCESS
THE PATIENT RECEIVING AN ANTIMALARIAL DRUG

ASSESSMENT

When an antimalarial drug is given to a hospitalized patient with malaria, the initial assessment includes vital signs and a summary of the nature and duration of the symptoms. Laboratory tests may be ordered for the diagnosis of malaria. Additional laboratory tests, such as a complete blood count (CBC), may be ordered to determine the patient's general health status.

NURSING DIAGNOSIS

Depending on the reason for administration (prophylaxis or treatment), one or more of the following nursing diagnoses may apply to a person receiving an antimalarial drug:

- ▶ Noncompliance related to indifference, lack of knowledge, other factors
- ▶ Knowledge deficit of medication regimen, adverse drug effects, treatment modalities, importance of adhering to the medication regimen

PLANNING AND IMPLEMENTATION

The major goal of the patient may include an understanding of and compliance to the prescribed treatment or prophylaxis regimen.

The major goal of nursing management may include the development and implementation of an effective teaching plan.

If the patient is hospitalized with malaria, vital signs are taken every 4 hours or as ordered by the physician. The patient is observed every 1 to 2 hours for the symptoms of malaria. Antipyretics may be ordered for fever. If the patient is acutely ill, intake and output measurements may be necessary. In some instances, intravenous (IV) fluids may be required.

ADMINISTRATION. These drugs are given with food or meals. The exception is quinacrine which is given after meals with a full glass of water, tea, or fruit juice.

NONCOMPLIANCE AND KNOWLEDGE DEFICIT. When an antimalarial drug is used for prophylaxis and taken once a week, the drug must be taken on the same day each week. Prophylaxis is usually started 1 week before departure to an area where malaria is prevalent.

The patient must have a complete understanding of the treatment regimen. The drug dosage schedule should be reviewed with the patient. The importance of adhering to the prescribed dosage schedule for the prevention or treatment of malaria should be stressed.

The following additional information is relevant to specific antimalarial drugs:

- ▶ Chloroquine and hydroxychloroquine—Take these drugs with food or milk. These drugs may cause diarrhea, loss of appetite, nausea, stomach pain, or vomiting. Notify the physician if these become pronounced. Also notify the physician if any of the following occur: visual changes, ringing in the ears, difficulty in hearing, fever, sore throat, unusual bleeding or bruising, unusual color (blue-black) of the skin, skin rash, or unusual muscle weakness.
- ▶ Quinacrine—Take this drug with food or meals. A yellow color to the skin or urine may be seen. Contact the physician promptly if any visual changes occur.
- ▶ Quinine—Take this drug with food or immediately

after a meal. Do not drive or perform other hazardous tasks requiring alertness if blurred vision or dizziness occurs. If the tablet or capsule is difficult to swallow, do *not* chew the tablet or open the capsule because the drug is irritating to the stomach.

EVALUATION

▶ Verbalizes importance of complying with the prescribed treatment or prophylaxis regimen

▶ Verbalizes an understanding of the prophylaxis or treatment schedule

▶ ANTHELMINTIC DRUGS

Anthelmintic (against helminths) drugs are used to treat **helminthiasis,** which is an invasion of the body by **helminths** or worms. Roundworms, pinworms, whipworms, hookworms, and tapeworms are examples of helminths.

Drugs that are used in treating a helminthic infection are called anthelmintics. Examples of anthelmintic drugs and their uses are listed in Summary Drug Table 25-1.

▷ Actions of the Anthelmintic Drugs

The various anthelmintic drugs act in a variety of ways.

Mebendazole (Vermox). Mebendazole blocks the uptake of glucose by the helminth, resulting in a depletion of the helminth's own glycogen. Glycogen depletion results in a decreased formation of adenosine triphosphate (ATP), which is required by the helminth for reproduction and survival.

Niclosamide (Niclocide). The head (scolex) and proximal segments of the helminth are killed on contact with niclosamide. The head then becomes loosened from the intestinal wall and is passed in the feces. This results in death of the helminth.

Piperazine. The action of piperazine against pinworms (*Enterobius* species) is unknown. When roundworms (*Ascaris* species) are present, this drug paralyzes the helminth, causing it to dislodge from the intestinal wall and be excreted in the feces.

Pyrantel (Antiminth). The activity of pyrantel is probably due to its ability to paralyze the helminth, which then releases its grip on the intestinal wall and is excreted in the feces.

Quinacrine (Atabrine). Quinacrine decreases protein synthesis, which then results in the death of the helminth.

Thiabendazole (Mintezol). The exact mechanism of action of thiabendazole is unknown. Thiabendazole appears to suppress egg or larval production and therefore may interrupt the life cycle of the helminth.

▷ Uses of Anthelmintic Drugs

The helminth must first be identified by examination of the stool for the ova (eggs) and the parasite. Once the type of helminth is identified, the physician selects the drug most likely to eradicate it.

▷ Adverse Reactions Associated with the Administration of Anthelmintic Drugs

Adverse reactions associated with the anthelmintic drugs are usually mild when the drug is used in the recommended dosage. Some patients receiving niclosamide, piperazine, and pyrantel may experience GI side effects such as nausea, vomiting, abdominal cramps, or diarrhea. The same adverse reactions as seen with the use of quinacrine in the treatment of malaria (see previous section) may also be seen when this drug is used for the treatment of helminthic infections.

▶ NURSING PROCESS
THE PATIENT RECEIVING AN ANTHELMINTIC DRUG

ASSESSMENT

The diagnosis of a helminthic infection is made by examination of the stool for ova and all or part of the helminth. Several stool specimens may be necessary before the helminth is seen and identified. The patient history may also lead to a suspicion of a helminthic infection, but some patients have no symptoms.

When a pinworm infection is suspected, diagnosis is made by examining and taking a specimen from the anal area, preferably early in the morning before the patient gets out of bed.

Patients with massive helminthic infections may or may not be acutely ill. The acutely ill patient requires hospitalization, but many individuals with helminthic infections may be treated on an outpatient basis.

The vital signs are obtained before the anthelmintic drug is given. Weighing the patient may also be necessary if the drug's dosage is determined by weight or if the patient is acutely ill.

NURSING DIAGNOSIS

Depending on the individual and the type of helminthic infection, one or more of the following nursing diagnoses may apply to a patient receiving an anthelmintic drug:

▶ Anxiety related to diagnosis, treatment regimen

▶ Noncompliance related to lack of knowledge, other factors

▶ Knowledge deficit of medication regimen, adverse drug effects, treatment modalities

PLANNING AND IMPLEMENTATION

The major goals of the patient may include a reduction in anxiety and an understanding of and compliance to the prescribed treatment regimen.

The major goals of nursing management may include a reduction in the patient's anxiety and the development and implementation of an effective teaching plan.

Unless ordered otherwise, all stools of patients with tapeworm, roundworm, hookworm, or whipworm that are passed following administration of the drug are saved and visually inspected for passage of the helminth. The physician may also order stool specimens sent to the laboratory for examination.

If the patient is acutely ill or has a massive infection, vital signs are monitored every 4 hours. Intake and output measurements may also be necessary in these patients.

The patient is observed for adverse drug reactions, as well as severe episodes of diarrhea, both of which are reported to the physician if they occur.

Depending on hospital policy, as well as the type of helminthic infection, linen precautions may be necessary. Gloves should be worn by all personnel when changing bed linens, emptying bedpans, or obtaining or handling stool specimens. The hands are washed thoroughly after removing the gloves. Patients are also instructed to wash their hands thoroughly following personal care and use of the bedpan.

ADMINISTRATION. Because these patients have a parasite living in their intestine, the method of administration of an anthelmintic drug may vary somewhat from the administration of other drugs.

▶ Mebendazole—Tablets may be crushed, mixed with food, chewed, or swallowed whole.

▶ Niclosamide—The tablet must be chewed thoroughly before swallowing. Only a small amount of water is to be used in swallowing the drug. If the patient is uncooperative, the tablet is crushed and then mixed with a small amount of water and spoon-fed to the patient.

▶ Piperazine and pyrantel—These drugs may be given with food to minimize gastric distress.

▶ Quinacrine—The package insert or the physician's orders must be reviewed carefully for the directions regarding a special diet and enemas that usually are necessary before the drug is given for a helminthic infection. When necessary, the tablets may be pulverized for ease in administration. Honey or jam may be used to disguise the bitter taste of the pulverized tablet.

▶ Thiabendazole—This drug is given with food to minimize GI upset and distress.

ANXIETY. The diagnosis of a helminthic infection is often distressing to patients and their family. The nurse should take time to explain the treatment and future preventive measures, as well as allow the patient or family members time to discuss their concerns or ask questions.

NONCOMPLIANCE AND KNOWLEDGE DEFICIT. When an anthelmintic is prescribed on an outpatient basis, the patient or a family member must receive complete instructions about taking the drug, as well as household precautions that should be followed until the helminth is eliminated from the intestine.

The following information may be included in a teaching plan for the patient and family:

▶ Follow the dosage schedule exactly as printed on the prescription container. (See earlier section on administration for the directions specific for each drug.) Follow the directions for taking the drug to eradicate the helminth.

▶ Follow-up stool specimens are absolutely necessary because this is the only way to determine the success of drug therapy.

▶ To prevent reinfection and the infection of others in the household, change and launder bed linens and undergarments daily, separate from those of other members of the family.

▶ Daily bathing (showering is best) is recommended. Disinfect toilet facilities and the bathtub daily.

▶ Wash the hands thoroughly after urinating or defecating and before preparing and eating food. It is important to clean under the fingernails daily and avoid putting fingers in the mouth and nailbiting.

EVALUATION

▶ Anxiety is reduced

▶ Verbalizes an understanding of treatment regimen modalities and importance of continued follow-up testing

▶ Describes or lists measures used to prevent the spread of infection to others

▶ Verbalizes importance of complying with the prescribed treatment regimen and preventive measures

▶ AMEBICIDES

Amebicides (drugs that kill amebas) are used for the treatment of amebiasis caused by the parasite *Entamoeba histolytica*. This infection is seen throughout the world but is less common in developed countries where sanitary facilities prevent the spread of this microorganism. Examples of amebicides are listed in Summary Drug Table 25-1.

▷ Actions of the Amebicides

These drugs are amebicidal (ie, they kill amebas). The two types of amebiasis are intestinal and extraintestinal. In the intestinal form, amebas are confined to the intestine, and a drug effective for this form of amebiasis is selected. The extraintestinal form is present when ameba are found outside of the intestine, such as in the liver. The extraintestinal form of amebiasis is more difficult to treat.

▷ Uses of the Amebicides

Chloroquine (Aralen) is used in the treatment of extraintestinal amebiasis. Iodoquinol (Yodoxin), metronidazole (Flagyl), and paromomycin (Humatin) are used to treat intestinal amebiasis.

▷ Adverse Reactions Associated with the Administration of the Amebicides

Chloroquine. Hypotension, ECG changes, headache, nausea, vomiting, anorexia, diarrhea, abdominal cramps, and psychic stimulation can occur with the use of chloroquine.

Iodoquinol. Various types of skin eruptions, nausea, vomiting, fever, chills, abdominal cramps, ver-

tigo, and diarrhea may occur with administration of iodoquinol.

Metronidazole. Convulsive seizures, headache, nausea, and peripheral neuropathy (numbness and tingling of the extremities) have been reported with the use of metronidazole.

Paromomycin. Nausea, vomiting, and diarrhea are the most common reactions seen with administration of paromomycin.

▶ NURSING PROCESS
THE PATIENT RECEIVING AN AMEBICIDE

ASSESSMENT

Diagnosis of amebiasis is made by examination of the stool as well as by the symptoms. Once the patient is diagnosed as having amebiasis, local health department regulations often require investigation into the source of infection. A thorough foreign travel history is necessary. If the patient has not traveled to a foreign country, further investigation of local travel, use of restaurants, the local water supply (especially well water), and so on may be necessary to identify the source of the infection. Immediate family members are usually tested for possible amebiasis.

Before administration of the first dose of an amebicide, the vital signs and weight are obtained. The general physical status of the patient is evaluated, and the patient is examined for evidence of dehydration, especially if severe vomiting and diarrhea have occurred.

NURSING DIAGNOSIS

Depending on the type of amebiasis and the condition of the patient, one or more of the following nursing diagnoses may apply to a person receiving an amebicide:

▶ Anxiety related to diagnosis, treatment regimen, other factors (specify)

▶ Noncompliance related to lack of knowledge, other factors

▶ Diarrhea related to amebiasis

▶ High risk for fluid volume deficit related to amebiasis

▶ Knowledge deficit of medication regimen, adverse drug effects, treatment modalities

PLANNING AND IMPLEMENTATION

The major goals of the patient may include a reduction in anxiety, an absence of diarrhea, maintenance of an adequate intake of fluids, an understanding of the treatment regimen (hospitalized patients), and an understanding of and compliance to the prescribed treatment regimen (outpatients).

The major goals of nursing management may include a reduction in patient anxiety, control of diarrhea, absence of a fluid volume deficit, and the development and implementation of an effective teaching plan.

The patient with amebiasis may or may not be acutely ill. Nursing management depends on the condition of the patient and the information obtained during the initial assessment.

If the patient is acutely ill or has vomiting and diarrhea, the intake and output is measured and the patient is closely observed for signs of dehydration. If dehydration is apparent, the physician is notified. If the patient is or becomes dehydrated, oral or IV fluid and electrolyte replacement may be necessary. Vital signs are taken every 4 hours or as ordered by the physician.

Isolation is usually not necessary but hospital policy may require isolation procedures. Stool precautions are usually necessary. The hands must be thoroughly washed after all patient care and the handling of stool specimens.

DIARRHEA, FLUID VOLUME DEFICIT. The number, character, and color of stools passed are recorded. Daily stool specimens may be ordered to be sent to the laboratory for examination. All stool specimens saved for examination are delivered to the laboratory *immediately* because the ameba dies (and therefore cannot be seen microscopically) when the specimen cools. The laboratory must be told that the patient has amebiasis because the specimen must be kept at or near body temperature until examined under a microscope.

The patient with severe or frequent episodes of diarrhea is observed for symptoms of a fluid volume deficit. The physician is informed if signs of dehydration be apparent because IV fluids may be necessary.

ANXIETY. The patient should have the treatment measures and the necessary laboratory examination of stool specimens explained. The patient and family members should be allowed time to discuss this problem and ask questions about the treatment and future preventive measures. It is most important that the nurse explain preventive measures in detail.

NONCOMPLIANCE AND KNOWLEDGE DEFICIT. The importance of completing the full course of treatment must be stressed. Patients receiving an amebicide on an outpatient basis may be given the following information:

► Take the drug exactly as prescribed. Complete the *full* course of therapy to eradicate the helminth. Failure to complete treatment may result in a return of the infection.

► Prevention—Follow measures to control the spread of infection. Wash hands immediately before eating or preparing food and after defecation.

► Food handlers—Do not resume work until a full course of treatment is completed and stools are negative for the ameba.

► Chloroquine—Notify the physician if any of the following occurs: ringing in the ears, difficulty hearing, visual changes, fever, sore throat, unusual bleeding or bruising.

► Iodoquinol—Notify the physician if nausea, vomiting, or other GI distress becomes severe.

► Metronidazole—This drug may cause GI upset. Take this drug with food or meals. The use of alcohol, in any form, must be avoided until the course of treatment is completed. The ingestion of alcohol may cause a mild to severe reaction with symptoms of severe vomiting, headache, nausea, abdominal cramps, flushing, and sweating. These symptoms may be so severe that hospitalization may be required.

► Paromomycin—Notify the physician if any of the following occurs: vaginal or rectal itching, soreness of the mouth or tongue, fever, cough, or a black furry tongue.

EVALUATION

► Anxiety is reduced

► Bowel elimination is normal

► Verbalizes an understanding of treatment modalities and importance of continued follow-up care

► Verbalizes importance of complying with the prescribed treatment regimen

26

Miscellaneous Antiinfective Drugs

On completion of this chapter the student will:

▶ *Discuss the antiviral agents, urinary antiinfectives, pentamidine isethionate, furazolidone, topical antiseptics and germicides, and ophthalmic and otic preparations covered in this chapter*

▶ *List some of the major adverse effects associated with the administration of the miscellaneous antiinfective drugs covered in this chapter*

▶ *Use the nursing process when administering one of the miscellaneous antiinfective drugs covered in this chapter*

▶ *Discuss the nursing implications to be considered when administering the miscellaneous antiinfective drugs covered in this chapter*

An antiinfective drug, as the name indicates, is used in the treatment of infection. Antibiotics, such as tetracycline and penicillin, are antiinfective drugs. Not all antiinfectives are antibiotics; some antiinfectives are chemicals not belonging to the antibiotic class that are successful in controlling an infection.

This chapter covers various types of antiinfective drugs, namely the antiviral agents, urinary antiinfectives, pentamidine isethionate, furazolidone, topical antiseptics and germicides, and ophthalmic and otic preparations.

▶ ANTIVIRAL AGENTS

Although viral infections are common, few drugs are available for the treatment of some types of viral infections.

Acyclovir (Zovirax), amantadine (Symmetrel), ganciclovir (Cytovene), ribavirin (Virazole), vidarabine (Vira-A), and zidovudine (AZT, Retrovir) are the antiviral agents presently in use.

▷ Actions of Antiviral Agents

Acyclovir, ganciclovir, ribavirin, and zidovudine appear to inhibit the replication of some viruses. The exact mode of action of amantadine and vidarabine is not completely understood.

▷ Uses of Antiviral Agents

Although infections caused by a virus are common, antiviral agents have limited use since they are only effective in a small number of specific viral infections.

Unlabeled uses are included for some drugs. Although documentation of their effectiveness is lacking, the physician may decide to prescribe the drug since there are very few effective antiviral agents.

Acyclovir.   Acyclovir is used for the initial and recurrent treatment of the herpes simplex virus (HSV-1 and HSV-2) and for the treatment of herpes zoster (shingles). Examples of the unlabeled uses of this drug include the treatment of infectious mononucleosis and varicella (chickenpox) pneumonia.

Amantadine.   Amantadine is used for the prevention or treatment of influenza A virus respiratory tract illness in high risk patients. This drug is also used in the treatment of Parkinson's disease.

Ganciclovir.   Ganciclovir is used in the treatment of retinitis (inflammation of the retina of the eye) caused by the cytomegalovirus (CMV) in immunocompromised individuals such as those with acquired immunodeficiency syndrome (AIDS) or those who have recently undergone bone marrow transplantation.

Ribavirin.   Ribavirin is used to treat infants and young children with severe lower respiratory tract infections due to the respiratory syncytial virus. Unlabeled uses of this drug include treatment of influenza A and B (aerosol form), acute and chronic hepatitis, herpes genitalis, and measles (oral form).

Vidarabine.   Vidarabine drug may be used in the treatment of herpes simplex virus encephalitis. An unlabeled use of this drug is the early treatment of herpes zoster in immunocompromised patients.

Zidovudine.   Commonly known as AZT, zidovudine is used orally for the treatment of patients with a human immunodeficiency virus infection (AIDS) and impaired immunity. It is also given intravenously (IV) to patients with symptomatic AIDS or advanced AIDS-related complex.

▷ Adverse Reactions Associated with the Administration of Antiviral Agents

The more common adverse reactions associated with the administration of these drugs are listed in Summary Drug Table 26-1.

▶ NURSING PROCESS
THE PATIENT RECEIVING AN ANTIVIRAL AGENT

ASSESSMENT

Assessment of the patient receiving an antiviral agent depends on the patient's symptoms or diagnosis. The patient's symptoms are recorded and vital signs are taken. Additional assessments may be necessary in certain types of viral infections or in patients who are acutely ill.

NURSING DIAGNOSIS

Depending on the reason for administration, one or more of the following nursing diagnoses may apply to a person receiving an antiviral agent:

▶ Anxiety related to diagnosis, symptoms of illness
▶ Knowledge deficit of medication regimen, adverse drug effects

PLANNING AND IMPLEMENTATION

The major goals of the patient may include a reduction in anxiety and an understanding of and compliance to the prescribed treatment regimen.

The major goals of nursing management may include a reduction in the patient's anxiety and the development and implementation of an effective teaching plan.

Depending on the patient's symptoms, vital signs may be monitored every 4 hours or as ordered by the physician. The patient is also observed for adverse drug reactions, which are brought to the attention of the physician.

ADMINISTRATION. Acyclovir, ganciclovir, vidarabine, and zidovudine may be given IV. These drugs are never given intramuscularly (IM) or subcutaneously (SC). These drugs are prepared according to the manufacturer's directions. The administration rate is ordered by the physician. Ribavirin is given by aerosol with a small particle aerosol generator.

ANXIETY. Because these drugs may be used in the treatment of certain types of severe and sometimes life-threatening viral infections, the patient may be concerned over her or his diagnosis and prognosis. The nurse must allow the patient time to talk and ask questions about methods of treatment, especially when the drug is given IV. In these instances, the prescribed treatment methods are explained to the patient and family members.

SUMMARY DRUG TABLE 26–1
Miscellaneous Antinfective Drugs

GENERIC NAME	TRADE NAME*	USES	ADVERSE REACTIONS	DOSE RANGES
ANTIVIRAL DRUGS				
acyclovir	Zovirax	Herpes simplex, herpes zoster	Nausea, vomiting, diarrhea, headache	Oral: 200 mg q4h while awake for a total of 5 capsules/d for 10 d; parenteral: 5 mg/kg IV q8h for 7 d
amantadine	Symmetrel, *generic*	Prevention or treatment of influenza A	Nausea, dizziness, light-headedness, blurred vision	200 mg/d PO or 100 mg PO bid
ganciclovir sodium	Cytovene	Retinitis caused by cy-tomegalovirus	Hematologic changes, fever, rash	5 mg/kg IV, IM, SC q12h for 14–21 d, then qd
ribavirin	Virazole	Severe lower respiratory tract infection (infants, young children)	Worsening of pulmonary status, bacterial pneumonia, hypotension, cardiac arrest	Administered by aerosol with special aerosol generator
vidarabine	Vira-A	Herpes simplex encephalitis	Anorexia, nausea, vomiting	15 mg/kg/d IV
zidovudine (AZT)	Retrovir	HIV infection	Asthenia, diaphoresis, anorexia, diarrhea, nausea, GI pain, paresthesias	100–200 mg PO q4h; 1–2 mg/kg IV q4h
URINARY ANTIINFECTIVES				
cinoxacin	Cinobac Pul-vules	Infections caused by susceptible microorganisms	Nausea, abdominal pain, anorexia, vomiting, diarrhea, perineal burning, headache, dizziness	1 g/d PO in 2–4 divided doses; smaller doses may be used when renal function is impaired
methenamine mandelate	Mandelamine, *generic*	Same as cinoxacin	GI disturbances, dysuria, bladder irritation	1 g PO qid
nalidixic acid	NegGram	Same as cinoxacin	Drowsiness, weakness, abdominal pain, nausea, vomiting, diarrhea, rash, anorexia, dizziness, headache, visual disturbances	2–4 g/d PO in divided doses
nitrofurantoin	Furadantin, *generic*	Same as cinoxacin	Anorexia, nausea, vomiting, rash, peripheral neuropathy, hyersensitivity reactions, headache	50–100 mg PO qid
norfloxacin	Noroxin	Same as cinoxacin	Nausea, abdominal pain, headache, dizziness	400 mg PO bid
trimethoprim (TMP)	Trimpex, *generic*	Same as cinoxacin	Rash, pruritus, epigastric distress, nausea, vomiting	100 mg PO q12h or 200 mg PO q24h
trimethoprim and sulfa-methoxazole (TMP-SMZ)	Septra, Bactrim, *generic*	Same as cinoxacin	See trimethoprim (above) and sulfamethoxazole in Summary Drug Table 21-1	160 mg TMP/800 mg SMZ PO q12h
OTHER				
pentamidine isethionate	Pentam 300, NebuPent	*Pneumocystis carinii* pneumonia	Leukopenia, hypoglycemia, thrombocytopenia, hypotension	4 mg/kg IM, IV daily for 14 d; aerosol: 300 mg once every 4 wk using the Respirgard II nebulizer
furazolidone	Furoxone	Diarrhea caused by susceptible microorganisms	Nausea, anorexia, hypoglycemia, orthostatic hypotension, headache, drug fever, urticaria	100 mg PO qid

* The term generic *indicates that the drug is available in a generic form.*

KNOWLEDGE DEFICIT. When an antiviral agent is given orally, the patient and family must have the dosage regimen explained. When prescribed for herpes, the patient is instructed to avoid sexual intercourse when visible lesions are present.

EVALUATION

▶ Anxiety is reduced

▶ Verbalizes an understanding of treatment modalities and importance of continued follow-up care

▶ Patient and family demonstrate understanding of drug regimen

▶ Verbalizes importance of complying with the prescribed treatment regimen

▶ URINARY ANTIINFECTIVES

Urinary antiinfectives do not belong to the antibiotic or sulfonamide group of drugs, but they have an effect on bacteria. Although administered systemically, that is, by the oral or parenteral route, they do not achieve significant levels in the bloodstream and are of no value in the treatment of systemic infections. They are primarily excreted by the kidneys and exert their major antibacterial effects in the urine.

▷ Actions of Urinary Antiinfectives

As a result of their high concentration in the urine, these drugs appear to interfere, in some manner, with bacterial multiplication.

▷ Uses of Urinary Antiinfectives

Like the sulfonamides (see chap 21), the systemic antiinfectives are used for urinary tract infections (UTIs) that are due to susceptible microorganisms.

▷ Adverse Reactions Associated with the Administration of the Urinary Antiinfectives

Cinoxacin (Cinobac). Nausea, abdominal pain, vomiting, anorexia, diarrhea, perineal burning, headache, and dizziness may be seen with the administration of cinoxacin.

Methenamine Mandelate (Mandelamine). Mandelamine administration may result in gastrointestinal (GI) disturbances, such as anorexia, nausea, vomiting, stomatitis, and cramps. Large doses may result in burning on urination and bladder irritation.

Nalidixic Acid (NegGram). Abdominal pain, nausea, vomiting, anorexia, diarrhea, rash, drowsiness, dizziness, blurred vision, weakness, and headache may occur with the administration of nalidixic acid. Visual disturbances, when they do occur, are noted after each dose and often disappear after a few days of therapy.

Nitrofurantoin (Furadantin). Nitrofurantoin administration may result in nausea, vomiting, anorexia, rash, peripheral neuropathy, headache, and hypersensitivity reactions which may range from mild to severe. Acute or chronic pulmonary reactions manifested by dyspnea, chest pain, cough, and malaise have been seen. When a pulmonary reaction occurs, the drug is discontinued immediately because the reaction can become serious and fatalities have occurred.

Norfloxacin (Noroxin). Nausea, abdominal pain, headache, and dizziness may occur with the administration of norfloxacin.

Trimethoprim (Trimpex). Trimethoprim administration may result in rash, pruritus, epigastric distress, nausea, and vomiting. When trimethoprim is combined with sulfamethoxazole (Septra), the adverse effects associated with a sulfonamide may also occur.

▶ NURSING PROCESS
THE PATIENT RECEIVING A URINARY ANTIINFECTIVE

ASSESSMENT

When a UTI has been diagnosed, sensitivity tests are performed to determine bacterial sensitivity to the drugs (antibiotics and urinary antiinfectives) that will control the infection. The symptoms before starting therapy are included in the patient history. Vital signs are taken and a urine sample for culture and sensitivity is obtained before the first dose of the drug is given.

NURSING DIAGNOSIS

Depending on the patient and the severity of the UTI, one or more of the following nursing diagnoses may apply to a person receiving a urinary antiinfective:

▶ Anxiety related to symptoms

▶ Noncompliance related to indifference, lack of knowledge, other factors

▶ Knowledge deficit of medication regimen, adverse drug effects

PLANNING AND IMPLEMENTATION

The major goals of the patient may include a reduction in anxiety and an understanding of and compliance to the prescribed treatment regimen.

The major goals of nursing management may include a reduction in the patient's anxiety, recognition of adverse drug effects, and the development and implementation of an effective teaching plan.

The vital signs are monitored every 4 hours or as ordered by the physician. Any significant rise in the temperature is reported to the physician because methods of reducing the fever or repeat culture and sensitivity tests may be necessary.

The intake and output are measured especially when the physician orders an increase in fluid intake or a kidney infection is being treated. The physician may also order daily urinary pH levels when methenamine or nitrofurantoin is administered. These drugs work best in acid urine; failure of the urine to remain acidic may require administration of a urinary acidifier such as ascorbic acid.

The patient's response to therapy is monitored daily. If after several days the symptoms of the UTI have not improved or if they become worse, the physician is notified as soon as possible. Periodic urinalysis and urine culture and sensitivity tests may be ordered to monitor the effects of drug therapy.

ADMINISTRATION. Systemic antiinfective drugs may be given with food to prevent GI upset. Nitrofurantoin must be given with food, meals, or milk because this drug is irritating to the stomach.

ADVERSE DRUG REACTIONS. The patient is observed for adverse drug reactions, which are reported to the physician before the next dose is due. Patients receiving nitrofurantoin are observed for signs of a pulmonary reaction (see earlier discussion of adverse reactions), which can be serious. Any symptoms believed to be related to the respiratory system are reported to the physician immediately.

ANXIETY. The symptoms of a UTI, for example, burning and pain on urination and frequent urination, often are distressing to the patient. The patient should be assured that symptoms most likely will decrease or disappear in a few days.

NONCOMPLIANCE AND KNOWLEDGE DEFICIT. Many times, systemic antiinfective drugs are prescribed on an outpatient basis because mild UTIs rarely require hospitalization. Completing the full course of therapy should be emphasized during patient and family teaching because even though symptoms may disappear after a few days of therapy, a full course of treatment must be completed to eradicate the infection.

The following points may be included in a patient and family teaching plan:

▶ Take the drug with food or meals (nitrofurantoin *must* be taken with food or milk). If GI upset occurs despite taking the drug with food, contact the physician.

▶ Take the drug at the intervals prescribed by the physician. Complete the full course of therapy and do *not* discontinue taking the medication even though the symptoms have disappeared, unless directed to do so by the physician.

▶ During therapy with this drug, do not take any nonprescription drug unless its use has been approved by the physician.

▶ Notify the physician immediately if symptoms do not improve after 3 or 4 days.

▶ When taking nitrofurantoin, notify the physician immediately if any of the following occur: fever, chills, cough, shortness of breath, chest pain, or difficulty breathing. Do not take the next dose of the drug until the physician has been contacted.

EVALUATION

▶ Anxiety is reduced

▶ Verbalizes an understanding of treatment modalities

▶ Patient and family demonstrate understanding of drug regimen

▶ Verbalizes importance of complying with the prescribed treatment regimen

▶ PENTAMIDINE ISETHIONATE

Pentamidine isethionate (Pentam 300, NebuPent) is used in the treatment (injectable form) or prevention (aerosol form) of *Pneumocystis carinii* pneumonia, a pneumonia seen in those with AIDS. The mode of action of this drug is not fully understood.

▷ Adverse Reactions Associated with the Administration of Pentamidine Isethionate

More than half of the patients receiving this drug by the parenteral route experience some adverse reaction. Severe and sometimes life-threatening reactions include leukopenia, hypoglycemia, thrombocytopenia, and hypotension. Moderate or less severe reactions include changes in some laboratory tests, such as the serum creatinine and liver function tests. Nausea and anorexia may also be seen.

Aerosol administration may result in fatigue, a metallic taste in the mouth, dyspnea, and anorexia.

▶ NURSING PROCESS
THE PATIENT RECEIVING PENTAMIDINE ISETHIONATE

ASSESSMENT

Assessment of the AIDS patient receiving this drug depends on the degree of illness, as well as the protocol established by the hospital, clinic, or hospice. The patient's vital signs and weight should be obtained and present symptoms documented.

NURSING DIAGNOSIS

Depending on the patient, route of administration, and other factors, one or more of the following nursing diagnoses may apply to a person receiving pentamidine isethionate:

▶ Anxiety related to diagnosis, prognosis
▶ Knowledge deficit of the treatment regimen

PLANNING AND IMPLEMENTATION

The major goals of the patient may include a reduction in anxiety and an understanding of the treatment regimen.

The major goals of nursing management may include a reduction in the patient's anxiety, a recognition of adverse drug reactions, and a complete explanation of the treatment regimen.

ADMINISTRATION. This drug may be given deep IM or IV. The drug is prepared according to the manufacturer's directions. When given by the IV route, the drug is allowed to infuse over 1 hour. When given by aerosol, a special nebulizer (Respirgard II) must be used and the drug delivered until the chamber is empty.

ANXIETY. The use of the nebulizer is demonstrated or explained to the patient. When IV or IM administration is prescribed, the method of administration is explained to the patient.

EVALUATION

▶ Anxiety is reduced
▶ Verbalizes understanding of treatment regimen

▶ FURAZOLIDONE

Furazolidone (Furoxone) is used in the treatment of diarrhea due to certain strains of bacteria or protozoa, and enteritis caused by susceptible microorganisms. This drug has bactericidal activity but does not affect the normal bacterial flora of the intestine.

▷ Adverse Reactions Associated with the Administration of Furazolidone

The most common adverse reactions are nausea and anorexia. Additional adverse reactions may include hypoglycemia, orthostatic hypotension, urticaria, drug fever, and headache.

▶ NURSING PROCESS
THE PATIENT RECEIVING FURAZOLIDONE

ASSESSMENT

A history of the type (or appearance) and daily number of bowel movements is obtained. The patient should also be assessed for signs of dehydration and electrolyte imbalance.

NURSING DIAGNOSIS

Depending on the degree and severity of the infection and the condition of the patient, one or more of the following nursing diagnoses may apply to the patient receiving furazolidone:

▶ Anxiety related to symptoms
▶ Knowledge deficit of dosage regimen

PLANNING AND IMPLEMENTATION

The major goals of the patient may include a reduction in anxiety, absence of frequent loose stools, and an understanding of the dosage regimen.

The major goals of nursing management may include a reduction in the patient's anxiety and the development and implementation of an effective teaching plan.

The appearance and approximate amount of each stool passed are recorded in the patient's record. Vital signs are monitored every 4 hours or as ordered by the physician.

ANXIETY. The patient is reassured that the drug will most likely eliminate the cause of diarrhea.

KNOWLEDGE DEFICIT. A complete explanation of the dosage regimen and possible adverse reactions are given to the patient and family. If therapy extends beyond 5 days, foods containing tyramine should be avoided. The patient must be given a list of foods containing this substance, for example, unpasteurized cheese, wine, beer, fermented products, and broad beans.

Additional points that may be included in a teaching plan are the following:

▶ *Avoid* the use of alcohol during and for 4 days after completing a course of treatment. If alcohol is used, a moderate to severe disulfiram-like reaction (throbbing headache, flushing, respiratory difficulty, chest pains, dyspnea, severe nausea, vomiting) may occur.
▶ The urine may appear brown. This is not abnormal.
▶ Avoid the use of over-the-counter prescriptions unless use of a specific drug is approved by the physician.
▶ Notify the physician if symptoms are not relieved in 5 days or become worse.
▶ Diabetic patient—Hypoglycemia may occur during the use of this drug. The physician may need to monitor blood glucose levels and adjust the dose of insulin or an oral hypoglycemic drug. Contact the physician immediately if episodes of hypoglycemia occur.

EVALUATION

▶ Anxiety is reduced
▶ Bowel elimination is normal
▶ Verbalizes an understanding of dosage regimen
▶ Patient and family demonstrate understanding of drug regimen

▶ TOPICAL ANTISEPTICS AND GERMICIDES

An **antiseptic** is an agent that stops, slows, or prevents the growth of microorganisms. A **germicide** is an agent that kills bacteria.

▷ Actions of Topical Antiseptics and Germicides

The exact mechanism of action of topical antiseptics and germicides is not well understood. These agents affect a variety of microorganisms. Some of these drugs have a short duration of action, whereas others have a long duration of action. The action of these agents may depend on the strength used and the time the drug is in contact with the skin or mucous membrane.

Benzalkonium (Zephiran). Benzalkonium is a rapid-acting preparation with a moderately long duration of action. It is active against bacteria and some viruses, fungi, and protozoa. Solutions are bacteriostatic or bactericidal depending on their concentration.

Chlorhexidine (Hibiclens). Chlorhexidine affects a wide range of microorganisms, including gram-positive and gram-negative bacteria.

Hexachlorophene (pHisoHex). Hexachlorophene is a bacteriostatic cleansing agent. It has activity against staphylococci and other gram-positive bacteria. Cumulative action occurs with repeated use. The antibacterial residue left by this agent is resistant to removal by many soaps, solvents, and detergents. Its activity may last for many days.

Iodine. Iodine has antiinfective action against many bacteria, fungi, viruses, yeasts, and protozoa. **Povidone-iodine** (Betadine) is a combination of iodine and povidone, which liberates free iodine. Povidone-iodine is often preferred over iodine solution or tincture because it is less irritating to the skin and does not stain the skin or clothing. Unlike iodine, treated areas may be bandaged or taped.

Nitrofurazone (Furacin). Nitrofurazone has a broad spectrum of activity and is bactericidal against most bacteria commonly causing skin infections, including many that have become resistant to antibiotics.

Merbromin (Mercurochrome). Merbromin contains 25% mercury. It has only fair antiseptic activity.

Thimerosal (Merthiolate). Thimerosal contains 49% mercury. This product has sustained bacteriostatic and fungistatic activity.

▷ Uses of Topical Antiseptics and Germicides

Topical antiseptics and germicides are primarily used to reduce the number of bacteria on skin surfaces. Some of these agents may also be used on mucous membranes. Nitrofurazone is frequently used in the treatment of burns.

▷ Adverse Reactions Associated with the Use of Topical Antiseptics and Germicides

Topical antiseptics and germicides have few adverse reactions. Occasionally, an individual may be allergic to the drug and a skin rash or itching may occur. If an allergic reaction is noted, use of the topical agent should be discontinued.

▶ *NURSING PROCESS* *USING TOPICAL ANTISEPTICS AND GERMICIDES*

ASSESSMENT

The involved area is visually inspected and findings are recorded on the patient's record.

NURSING DIAGNOSIS

▶ Anxiety related to symptoms, injury, infection, other factors

▶ Knowledge deficit of use of product

PLANNING AND IMPLEMENTATION

The major goals of the patient may include an understanding of the application and use of an antiseptic or germicide.

The major goals of nursing management are the development and implementation of an effective patient teaching plan.

Topical antiseptics and germicides are *not* a substitute for clean or aseptic techniques. They must be used as directed to obtain maximum effectiveness.

ADMINISTRATION. Topical antiseptics and germicides are used, instilled, or applied as directed by the physician or the label of the product. Antiseptic and germicidal agents kept at the patient's bedside must be *clearly* labeled with the name of the product, the strength, and, when applicable, the date of preparation of the solution. Hard-to-read or soiled, stained labels are replaced as needed. These solutions are not kept at the bedside of any patient who is confused or disoriented because the solution may be mistaken for water or another beverage and ingested.

BENZALKONIUM. An occlusive dressing is not recommended following the use of benzalkonium.

IODINE SOLUTION OR TINCTURE. Iodine permanently stains clothing and temporarily stains the skin. The patient's personal clothing should be removed or protected when iodine solution or tincture is applied. Occlusive dressings should not be used after application of these products unless a dressing is specifically ordered by the physician. Povidone-iodine does not stain the skin and will wash out of clothing with soap and water.

KNOWLEDGE DEFICIT. If the physician has prescribed or recommended the use of a topical germicide or antiseptic, the following may be included in a patient and family teaching plan:

▶ Follow the directions on the label or use as directed by the physician.

▶ Do not apply to areas other than those specified by the physician.

▶ Keep this product away from the eyes (unless use in or around the eye has been recommended or prescribed). If the product is accidentally spilled or splashed in the eye, wash the eye immediately with copious amounts of running water. Contact the physician *immediately* if burning, pain, redness, discomfort, or blurred vision persists for more than a few minutes.

▶ Discontinue use if rash, burning, itching, or other skin problems occur.

EVALUATION

▶ Anxiety is reduced

▶ Patient or family member demonstrates understanding of use and application

▶ OPHTHALMIC AND OTIC PREPARATIONS

Various types of preparations are used for the treatment of eye and ear disorders. Examples of ophthalmic and otic preparations are given in Summary Drug Table 26-2.

▷ Uses of Ophthalmic and Otic Preparations

Examples of uses of ophthalmic preparations include eye infections, treatment of glaucoma, preparation for eye surgery, and eye pain or inflammation. Examples of uses of otic preparations include pain, infection, and inflammation of the external auditory canal.

▷ Adverse Reactions Associated with the Administration of an Otic or Ophthalmic Preparation

The incidence of adverse reactions is usually small. Since some ophthalmic preparations may be absorbed systemically, some of the adverse effects associated with systemic administration of the particular drug may be noted. When antibiotics are prescribed, a superinfection may be seen with prolonged or repeated use.

▶ NURSING PROCESS
THE PATIENT RECEIVING AN OPHTHALMIC PREPARATION

ASSESSMENT

The physician examines the eye and external structures surrounding the eye and prescribes the drug that are indicated for treatment of the disorder.

NURSING DIAGNOSIS

Depending on the physician's diagnosis and the patient's symptoms, one or more of the following may apply to the patient receiving an ophthalmic preparation:

- ▶ Anxiety related to eye pain or discomfort, diagnosis, other factors
- ▶ Knowledge deficit of instillation of eye medication, treatment regimen

PLANNING AND IMPLEMENTATION

The major goals of the patient may include a reduction in anxiety and an understanding of the application and use of an ophthalmic preparation.

The major goals of nursing management are a reduction in the patient's anxiety and the development and implementation of an effective patient teaching plan.

ADMINISTRATION. Only preparations labeled as *ophthalmic* are instilled in the eye. The label of the preparation must be checked *carefully* for the name of the drug, the percentage of the preparation, and a statement indicating that the preparation is for ophthalmic use. Ophthalmic ointments are applied to the eyelids or dropped into the lower conjunctival sac; ophthalmic solutions are dropped into the lower conjunctival sac.

When a patient is scheduled for eye surgery, it is most important that the eye drops ordered by the physician are instilled at the correct time. This is especially important when the purpose of the drug is to change the size of the pupil.

ANXIETY. Eye injuries and some eye infections are very painful. Other eye conditions may result in discomfort or a loss of or change in vision. The patient with an eye disorder or injury usually has great concern over the effect the problem will have on his or her vision. Patients need to be reassured that every effort is being made to treat the disorder.

KNOWLEDGE DEFICIT. The patient or a family member will require instruction in the technique of instilling an ophthalmic preparation. The following information may be given to the patient and family member when an eye ointment or solution is prescribed:

- ▶ Wash the hands thoroughly before cleansing the eyelids, instilling eye drops, or applying an eye ointment.
- ▶ Instill the prescribed number of drops or amount of ointment in the eye. If more than one type of ophthalmic preparation is being instilled, wait the recommended time interval before instilling the second medication (usually 5 minutes for a solution and 10–15 minutes for an ointment).
- ▶ Complete a full course of treatment with the prescribed drug to achieve satisfactory results.
- ▶ Do not rub the eyes and keep hands away from the eyes.
- ▶ Do not use nonprescription eye products during or after treatment unless use has been approved by the physician.
- ▶ Replace the cap of the eye medication immediately after instilling the eye drops or ointment. Do not touch the tip of the container or tube.

SUMMARY DRUG TABLE 26–2
Ophthalmic and Otic Preparations

GENERIC NAME	TRADE NAME*	USES	DOSAGE
OPHTHALMIC PREPARATIONS			
bacitracin	AK-Tracin	Eye infections	0.5 inch 2–8 times/d
betaxolol hydrochloride	Betoptic	Ocular hypertension, chronic open-angle glaucoma	1 drop bid
carbachol, topical	Isopto Carba-chol	Glaucoma	1–2 drops in affected eye 1–4 times/d
cromolyn sodium	Opticrom 4%	Allergic disorders of the eye	1–2 drops in each eye 4–6 times/d
dipivefrin hydrochloride	Propine	Chronic open-angle glaucoma	1 drop into affected eye q12h
epinephrine hydrochloride	Epifrin, *generic*	Same as dipivefrin	1–2 drops into affected eye 1–2 times/d
erythromycin	AK-Mycin *generic*	Eye infections	0.5 inch 2–8 times/d
gentamicin	Genoptic, Garamycin Ophthalmic, *generic*	Eye infections	Ointment or solution applied or instilled 2–8 times/d
doxuridine	Stoxil, Herplex Liquifilm	Herpes simplex keratitis	Ointment: 5 applications qd; solution: 1 drop q1–2h
levobunolol hydrochloride	Betagan Liquifilm	Same as betaxolol hydrochloride	1 drop in affected eye 1–2 times/d
metipranolol hydrochloride	OptiPranolol	Same as betaxolol hydrochloride	1 drop in affected eye 2 times/d
natamycin	Natacyn	Fungal blepharitis, conjunctivitis, keratitis	1 drop per dose
phenylephrine hydrochloride	Isopto Frin, *generic*	Uveitis, wide-angle glaucoma	1–2 drops per dose
pilocarpine hydrochloride	Isopto-Carpine	Chronic simple glaucoma, Chronic angle-closure glaucoma, acute glaucoma, to counteract the effect of cycloplegics and mydriatics	1–2 drops in affected eye up to 6 times/d
prednisolone acetate	AK-Tate, *generic*	Inflammatory conditions of the eye	1–2 drops per dose
sodium sulfacetamide	Sodium Sulamyd, *generic*	Conjunctivitis, corneal ulcer, superficial eye infections	1–3 drops instilled every 2–3 h
timolol maleate	Timoptic	Chronic open-angle glaucoma, aphakic patients with glaucoma, elevated intraocular pressure, secondary glaucoma	1 drop in affected eye 1–2 times/d
tobramycin	Tobrex	Eye infections	Ointment or solution applied or instilled 2–8 times/d
vidarabine	Vita-A	Acute keratoconjunctivitis and recurrent epithelial keratitis due to herpes simplex virus types 1 and 2	0.5 inch of ointment instilled into the conjunctival sac 5 times/d

(continued)

SUMMARY DRUG TABLE 26-2
(continued)

GENERIC NAME	TRADE NAME*	USES	DOSAGE
OTIC PREPARATIONS			
chloramphenicol	Chloromycetin Otic	Superficial infections of the external auditory canal	2–3 drops into the ear 3 times/d
hydrocortisone, neomycin sulfate, polymixin B	AK-Spore H.C. Otic, Drotic	Same as chloramphenicol	4 drops into the ear 3–4 times/d

* The term generic *indicates that the drug is available in a generic form.*

▶ Temporary blurring of vision may occur. Avoid activities requiring visual acuity until vision returns to normal.

▶ Notify the physician if symptoms do not improve or become worse.

EVALUATION

▶ Anxiety is reduced

▶ Demonstrates ability to instill ophthalmic preparation in eye

▶ Patient and family demonstrate understanding of drug regimen

▶ Verbalizes knowledge and importance of treatment regimen

▶ NURSING PROCESS
THE PATIENT RECEIVING AN OTIC PREPARATION

ASSESSMENT

The physician examines the ear and external structures surrounding the ear and prescribes the drug that is indicated for treatment of the disorder.

NURSING DIAGNOSIS

Depending on the physician's diagnosis and the patient's symptoms, one or more of the following may apply to the patient receiving an otic preparation:

▶ Anxiety related to ear pain or discomfort, changes in hearing, diagnosis, other factors

▶ Knowledge deficit of instillation of ear medication, treatment regimen

PLANNING AND IMPLEMENTATION

The major goals of the patient may include a reduction in anxiety and an understanding of the application and use of an otic preparation.

The major goals of nursing management are a reduction in the patient's anxiety and the development and implementation of an effective patient teaching plan.

ADMINISTRATION. Only preparations label as *otic* are instilled in the ear. The label of the preparation must be checked *carefully* for the name of the drug and a statement indicating that the preparation is for otic use.

The container may be held in the hand for a few minutes to warm to body temperature. Cold and warm (above body temperature) preparations may cause dizziness or other sensations following instillation into the ear.

When instilling ear drops, the patient should lie on his or her side with the ear toward the ceiling. In the adult, the earlobe is pulled up and back. In children, the earlobe is pulled down and back.

ANXIETY. Ear disorders may result in symptoms such as pain, a feeling of fullness in the ear, tinnitus, dizziness, or a change in hearing. The patient with an ear disorder or injury usually has great concern over the effect the problem will have on his or her hearing. Patients need to be reassured that every effort is being made to treat the disorder and relieve symptoms.

KNOWLEDGE DEFICIT. The patient or a family member requires instruction in the instillation technique of an otic preparation. The following information may be given to the patient when an ear ointment or solution is prescribed:

▶ Wash the hands thoroughly before cleansing the area around the ear (when necessary) and instilling ear drops or ointment.

► Instill the prescribed number of drops or amount of ointment in the ear.

► Complete a full course of treatment with the prescribed drug to achieve satisfactory results.

► Do not use nonprescription ear products during or after treatment unless use has been approved by the physician.

► Replace the cap of the medication immediately after instilling the ear drops or ointment.

► Temporary changes in hearing or a feeling of fullness in the ear may occur for a short time after the medication has been instilled.

► Do not insert anything into the ear canal before or after applying the prescribed medication unless advised to do so by the physician.

► Notify the physician if symptoms do not improve or become worse.

EVALUATION

► Anxiety is reduced

► Demonstrates ability to instill otic preparation in ear

► Verbalizes knowledge and importance of treatment regimen

► Patient and family demonstrate understanding of drug regimen

27

Pituitary and Adrenocortical Hormones

On completion of this chapter the student will:

▶ *List the hormones produced by the pituitary gland and the adrenal cortex*

▶ *State the functions of the pituitary and adrenocortical hormones*

▶ *List the actions, uses, and adverse reactions of pituitary and adrenocortical hormones*

▶ *Discuss the major adverse reactions associated with the administration of the pituitary and adrenocortical hormones*

▶ *Use the nursing process when administering a gonadotropin, growth hormone, adrenocorticotropic hormone, vasopressin, or a glucocorticoid or mineralocorticoid*

▶ *Discuss the nursing implications to be considered when administering a pituitary or adrenocortical hormone*

The pituitary gland lies deep within the cranial vault, connected to the brain by a stalk and protected by an indentation of the sphenoid bone called the sella turcica. There are two parts to the pituitary gland: the **anterior** pituitary or **adenohypophysis** and the **posterior** pituitary or **neurohypophysis.** The hormones of the pituitary and the organs or structures influenced by these hormones are shown in Figure 27-1.

Pituitary hormones regulate growth, metabolism, the reproductive cycle, electrolyte balance, and water retention or loss. Anterior and posterior pituitary hormones are summarized in Summary Drug Table 27-1.

▶ ANTERIOR PITUITARY HORMONES

The hormones of the anterior pituitary include growth hormone, adrenocorticotropic hormone (ACTH), thyroid-stimulating hormone (TSH), follicle-stimulating hormone (FSH), luteinizing hor-

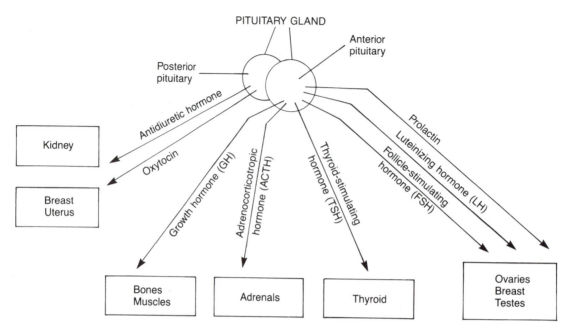

PITUITARY GLAND

FIGURE 27–1. Hormones of the anterior and posterior pituitary gland.

mone (LH), and prolactin. All but prolactin are used medically.

▷ The Gonadotropins

Follicle-stimulating hormone and **leutinizing hormone** are called **gonadotropins** because they influence the gonads (the organs of reproduction). In both sexes, FSH and LH influence the secretion of sex hormones, development of secondary sex characteristics, and the reproductive cycle. **Prolactin,** which is also secreted by the anterior pituitary, stimulates the production of breast milk in the postpartum patient. Additional functions of prolactin are not well understood.

Actions and Uses of Gonadotropins

Menotropins (Pergonal) and urofollitropin (Metrodin) are purified preparations of the gonadotropins (FSH and LH) extracted from the urine of postmenopausal women. Menotropins is used to induce ovulation and pregnancy in the anovulatory (failure to produce an ovum or failure to ovulate) female. In the male, it is used to induce the production of sperm (spermatogenesis). Urofollitropin is used to induce ovulation in women with polycystic ovarian disease.

Clomiphene (Clomid) is a synthetic nonsteroidal compound used to induce ovulation and pregnancy in the anovulatory female. Chorionic gonadotropin (human chorionic gonadotropin, or HCC) is extracted from human placentas and contains FSH and LH. It is used to induce ovulation and pregnancy in the anovulatory female. This drug is also used for the treatment of prepubertal cryptorchism (failure of the testes to descend into the scrotum).

Adverse Reactions Associated with Administration of Gonadotropins

The adverse reactions associated with menotropins include ovarian enlargement, hemoperitoneum (blood in the peritoneal cavity), and febrile reactions. Multiple births and birth defects have been reported with the use of this drug. Administration of clomiphene may result in vasomotor flushes (which are like the hot flashes of menopause), abdominal discomfort, ovarian enlargement, blurred vision, nausea, vomiting, and nervousness. Chorionic gonadotropin administration may result in headache, irritability, restlessness, fatigue, edema, and precocious puberty (when given for cryptorchism). Urofollitropin administration may result in mild to moderate ovarian enlargement, nausea, vomiting, breast tenderness, and ectopic pregnancy.

▶ NURSING PROCESS
THE PATIENT RECEIVING A GONADOTROPIN

ASSESSMENT

These drugs are almost always administered on an outpatient basis. Before prescribing any one of these drugs, a thorough medical history is taken and a phy-

SUMMARY DRUG TABLE 27–1
Anterior and Posterior Pituitary Hormones

GENERIC NAME	TRADE NAME*	USES	ADVERSE REACTIONS	DOSE RANGES
ANTERIOR PITUITARY HORMONES				
adrenocortico-tropic hormone (cortico-trotropin, ACTH)	Acthar, *generic*	Diagnostic testing of adreno-cortical function, acute exacerbation of multiple sclerosis, nonsuppurative thyroiditis, hypercalcemia associated with malignancies	Same as for glucocorticoids (see Table 27-2)	Diagnostic: 10–25 U in 500 mL 5% dextrose IV infused over 8-h period; other uses: 80–120 U/d IM
chorionic gonadotropin (HCG)	GLukor, A.P.L., *generic*	Ovulatory failure, prepubertal cryptorchism	Headache, irritability, nervousness, edema, fatigue, restlessness, precocious puberty	Dosage, frequency, length of treatment is individualized; ranges are 500–10,000 U/dose
clomiphene citrate	Clomid, Serophene	Ovulatory failure	Vasomotor flushes, abdominal discomfort, blurred vision, ovarian enlargement, nausea, vomiting, nervousness	First course: 50 mg/d PO for 5 d; second and third course (if necessary) 100 mg/d PO for 5 d
menotropins	Pergonal	Ovulatory failure, stimulation of spermatogenesis	Ovarian enlargement, hemoperitoneum, febrile reactions	75–150 IU IM
somatrem	Protropin	Growth failure due to deficiency of pituitary growth hormone in children	Failure to respond to therapy due to development of antibodies	Up to 0.1 mg/kg SC, IM 3 times/wk
somatropin	Humatrope	Same as somatrem	Same as somatrem	Up to 0.06 mg/kg SC, IM 3 times/wk
urofollitropin	Metrodin	Induction of ovulation	Ovarian enlargement, nausea, vomiting, breast tenderness, ectopic pregnancy	Dose range: 75–100 IU IM
POSTERIOR PITUITARY HORMONES				
desmopressin acetate	DDAVP	Replacement therapy in management of diabetes insipidus	Headache, nausea, nasal congestion	0.1–0.4 mL/d as a nasal solution (dosage may be divided); 0.5–1 mL/d SC, IV
lypressin	Diapid	Same as desmopressin	Rhinorrhea, nasal congestion, irritation of nasal passages	1–2 sprays in each nostril qid
oxytocin	Pitocin	Induction of labor	See Summary Drug Table 30-1	See Summary Drug Table 30-1
vasopressin	Pitressin Synthetic	Diabetes insipidus, prevention and treatment of postoperative abdominal distention	Tremor, sweating, vertigo, nausea, vomiting, abdominal cramps, hypersensitivity reactions	Diabetes insipidus: 5–10 U SC, IM; abdominal distention: 5–10 U IM

* The term generic indicates that the drug is available in a generic form.

sical examination is performed by the physician. Additional laboratory and diagnostic tests for ovarian function and tubal patency may also be performed.

Vital signs and weight are taken and recorded before therapy is instituted.

NURSING DIAGNOSIS

Depending on the individual, one or more of the following nursing diagnoses may apply to the patient receiving a gonadotropin:

▶ Anxiety related to inability to conceive, treatment outcome, other factors

▶ Knowledge deficit of treatment regimen, adverse drug reactions

PLANNING AND IMPLEMENTATION

The major goals of the patient may include a reduction in anxiety and an understanding of the treatment regimen.

The major goals of nursing management may include a reduction in the patient's anxiety and the development and implementation of an effective teaching plan.

Menotropins and chorionic gonadotropin injections are given in the physician's office or clinic. Clomiphene is an oral tablet and is prescribed for self-administration. At the time of each office or clinic visit, the patient is questioned regarding the occurrence of adverse reactions. Vital signs and weight may also be taken at this time.

ANXIETY. Patients wishing to become pregnant often experience a great deal of anxiety. The success rate of these drugs varies and depends on many factors. The physician usually discusses the value of this, as well as other approaches, with the patient and her sexual partner. The nurse may help relieve anxiety by offering encouragement and allowing the patient time to talk about her problems or concerns about the proposed treatment program.

KNOWLEDGE DEFICIT. When the patient is receiving menotropins, chorionic gonadotropin, or both of these drugs, she is encouraged to keep all physician appointments. The physician explains the possible risks associated with therapy for ovulatory failure. Symptoms that require notification of the physician are explained to the patient.

The following information may be given when clomiphene is prescribed for ovulatory failure:

▶ Take the drug as prescribed (5 days); do not stop taking the drug before the course of therapy is finished unless told to do so by the physician.

▶ Notify the physician if bloating, stomach or pelvic pain, jaundice, blurred vision, hot flashes, breast discomfort, headache, nausea, or vomiting occurs.

▶ This drug may cause dizziness or light-headedness. If these occur, do not drive or perform other tasks requiring alertness.

EVALUATION

▶ Anxiety is reduced

▶ Demonstrates knowledge of treatment and dosage

regimen, adverse drug reactions, involved risks of treatment, and importance of complying with the physician's recommendations

▷ Growth Hormone

Growth hormone, also called somatotrophic hormone, is secreted by the anterior pituitary. This hormone regulates the growth of the individual until somewhere around early adulthood or the time when the person no longer gains height. Other hormones, such as insulin and thyroid hormone, are also concerned with growth.

Growth hormone is available as the synthetic products somatrem (Protropin) and somatropin (Humatrope). Both are of recombinant DNA origin and are identical to human growth hormone. These drugs are administered to children who have failed to grow because of a deficiency of pituitary growth hormone. These drugs are used only before closure of bone epiphyses (the ends of bones, separated from the main bone but joined to its cartilage, that allow for growth or lengthening of the bone) and is ineffective in those with closed epiphyses. When the epiphyses close, growth (in height) can no longer occur.

Adverse Reactions Associated with Administration of Growth Hormone

Antibodies to somatropin and somatrem may develop in a small number of patients, resulting in a failure to respond to therapy, namely, failure of the drug to produce growth in the child.

▶ NURSING PROCESS
THE PATIENT RECEIVING GROWTH HORMONE

ASSESSMENT

A thorough physical examination and laboratory and diagnostic tests are performed before a child is accepted in a growth program. Before starting therapy, vital signs and the height and weight are obtained and recorded.

NURSING DIAGNOSIS

▶ Anxiety related to failure to grow (parents and child)

▶ Knowledge deficit of the treatment program

PLANNING AND IMPLEMENTATION

The major goals of the patient and parents may include a reduction in anxiety and an understanding of the treatment program.

The major goals of nursing management may include a reduction in the patient's and parents' anxiety and the development and implementation of an effective teaching plan.

Each time the child visits the physician's office or clinic, various height and weight measurements are taken and recorded to evaluate the response to therapy. Periodic laboratory tests and yearly bone surveys may be performed. The bone surveys check bone growth, as well as detects epiphyseal closure, at which time therapy must be stopped.

ANXIETY. The parents, and sometimes the children, may be concerned over a failure to grow, as well as the success or possible failure of treatment with a growth hormone. The parents and children should be allowed time to ask questions not only before therapy is started but also during the months of growth hormone treatment.

KNOWLEDGE DEFICIT. When the patient is receiving growth hormone, the physician discusses in detail the therapeutic regimen for increasing growth (height) with the child's parents or guardians. The parents are encouraged to keep all clinic or physician's office visits.

EVALUATION

► Anxiety is reduced
► Parents verbalize understanding of treatment program

▷ Adrenocorticotropic Hormone

ACTH (corticotropin) is an anterior pituitary hormone that stimulates the adrenal cortex to produce and secrete adrenocortical hormones, primarily the glucocorticoids. ACTH is used for diagnostic testing of adrenocortical function. This drug may also be used for the management of acute exacerbations of multiple sclerosis, nonsuppurative thyroiditis, and hypercalcemia associated with cancer.

Adverse Reactions Associated with the Administration of Adrenocorticotropic Hormone

Because ACTH stimulates the release of glucocorticoids from the adrenal gland, adverse reactions seen with the administration of this hormone are the same as for the glucocorticoids (see section on the adrenocortical hormones).

► NURSING PROCESS
THE PATIENT RECEIVING ADRENOCORTICOTROPIC HORMONE

ASSESSMENT

The patient's chart is reviewed for the diagnosis, laboratory tests, and other pertinent information. Vital signs are taken. Additional assessments depend on the patient's condition and diagnosis.

NURSING DIAGNOSIS

Depending on the patient's condition and reason for administration, one or more of the following may apply to the patient receiving ACTH:

► Anxiety related to diagnosis, treatment regimen, other factors
► Knowledge deficit of treatment regimen

PLANNING AND IMPLEMENTATION

The major goals of the patient may include a reduction in anxiety and an understanding of the treatment regimen.

The major goals of nursing management may include a reduction in the patient's anxiety and the development and implementation of an effective teaching plan.

Nursing management depends on the patient's diagnosis, physical status, and the reason for use of the drug and may include vital signs every 4 hours, and observation for the adverse reactions seen with glucocorticoid administration (see section on the adrenocortical hormones).

ADMINISTRATION. During intravenous (IV) administration of adrenocorticotropic hormone, the patient is observed for hypersensitivity reactions; symptoms may include a rash, urticaria, hypotension, tachycardia, or difficulty in breathing. If the drug is given intramuscularly (IM), the patient is observed for hypersensitivity reactions immediately and for about 2 hours after the drug is given. If a hypersensitivity reaction occurs after IM or IV administration, the physician is notified immediately. If the patient has multiple sclerosis, an evaluation of the patient's response to the drug is made daily, and current symptoms are compared with those present before treatment was started.

ANXIETY, KNOWLEDGE DEFICIT. The treatment regimen and method of administration (IM, IV, subcutaneous [SC]) is explained to the patient. Occasionally, this drug may be given in the physician's office or clinic. The patient is instructed to avoid contact with those who have an infection because resistance to infection may be decreased. In addition, the diabetic patient is advised to monitor his or her blood glucose (if self-monitoring is being done) or urine closely and notify the physician if glucose appears in the urine or the blood glucose shows a significant rise. The patient is also instructed to notify the physician if a marked weight gain, swelling in the extremities, muscle weakness, or persistent headache occurs.

EVALUATION

▶ Anxiety is reduced
▶ Patient verbalizes understanding of treatment regimen, adverse effects requiring notification of the physician

▶ POSTERIOR PITUITARY HORMONES

The posterior pituitary gland produces two hormones: **vasopressin (antidiuretic hormone, ADH)** and **oxytocin.** Oxytocin is discussed in chapter 30. Posterior pituitary hormones are summarized in Summary Drug Table 27-1.

▷ Vasopressin

Vasopressin (Pitressin Synthetic) and its derivatives, namely lypressin (Diapid) and desmopressin (DDAVP), regulate the reabsorption of water by the kidneys. Vasopressin is secreted by the pituitary when body fluids must be conserved. An example of this mechanism may be seen when an individual has severe vomiting and diarrhea with little or no fluid intake. When this and similar conditions are present, the posterior pituitary releases the hormone vasopressin, water in the kidneys is reabsorbed into the blood (ie, conserved), and the urine becomes concentrated. Vasopressin also has some vasopressor activity.

Vasopressin and its derivatives are used in the treatment of diabetes insipidus, a disease due to the failure of the pituitary to secrete vasopressin or due to surgical removal of the pituitary. Vasopressin

may also be used for the prevention and treatment of postoperative abdominal distention.

Adverse Reactions Associated with Administration of Vasopressin

Local or systemic hypersensitivity reactions may occur in some patients receiving vasopressin. Tremor, sweating, vertigo, nausea, vomiting, and abdominal cramps may also be seen.

▶ NURSING PROCESS
THE PATIENT RECEIVING VASOPRESSIN

ASSESSMENT

Before the administration of the first dose of vasopressin for the management of diabetes insipidus, the blood pressure, pulse, and respiratory rate are taken. The patient is also weighed. The physician may order serum electrolyte levels and other laboratory tests.

Before administration of vasopressin to relieve abdominal distention, the blood pressure, pulse, and respiratory rate are obtained. The abdomen is auscultated and the findings are recorded. The abdominal girth is also measured and recorded.

NURSING DIAGNOSIS

Depending on the route of administration and the patient's diagnosis, one or more of the following nursing diagnoses may apply to a person receiving vasopressin:

▶ Anxiety related to symptoms of diabetes insipidus, methods of treatment, pain or discomfort due to abdominal distention, other factors
▶ Fluid volume deficit related to inadequate fluid intake, need to increase dose of drug, failure to recognize symptoms of dehydration (diabetes insipidus)
▶ Noncompliance related to lack of knowledge (diabetes insipidus)
▶ Knowledge deficit of treatment regimen, use of nasal spray, dosage adjustment, adverse drug reactions (diabetes insipidus)

PLANNING AND IMPLEMENTATION

The major goals of the patient may include a reduction in anxiety, correction of a fluid volume deficit, and an understanding of and compliance to the prescribed treatment regimen.

The major goals of nursing management may in-

clude a reduction in the patient's anxiety, recognition of signs of dehydration, recognition of adverse drug effects, and the development and implementation of an effective teaching plan.

OBSERVATIONS AND NURSING MANAGEMENT. The nursing management of the patient receiving vasopressin depends on the reason for the use of the drug, as discussed later.

ABDOMINAL DISTENTION. Only vasopressin is used for the management of abdominal distention. After administration of vasopressin for abdominal distention, a rectal tube may be ordered. The lubricated end of the tube is inserted past the anal sphincter and taped in place. Usually the tube is left in place for 1 hour. The abdomen is auscultated every 15 to 30 minutes and the abdominal girth is measured every hour or as ordered by the physician.

DIABETES INSIPIDUS. Vasopressin may be given IM or SC. Vasopressin tannate is given IM. Lypressin is given intranasally and desmopressin may be given intranasally, SC, or IV. When the drug is to be administered intranasally, the physician orders the method of administration.

Vasopressin tannate, which is given IM, is suspended in peanut oil. Because the fluid in the ampule is thick, the ampule is warmed to body temperature before withdrawing the drug.

The blood pressure, pulse, and respiratory rate are monitored every 4 hours or as ordered by the physician. The physician is notified if there are any significant changes in these vital signs because a dosage adjustment may be necessary.

The dosage of vasopressin or its derivatives may require periodic adjustments. After administration of the drug, the patient is observed every 10 to 15 minutes for signs of an excessive dosage (eg, blanching of the skin, abdominal cramps, and nausea). If these occur, the patient is reassured that recovery from these effects will occur in a few minutes. If signs of excessive dosage occur, the physician must be notified before the next dose of the drug is due because a change in the dosage may be necessary. Administration of one or two glasses of water at the time the drug is administered may reduce the incidence or severity of the excessive dosage effects. The physician is also notified immediately if a hypersensitivity reaction occurs.

The administration of vasopressin conserves body water; therefore, the patient is observed frequently for signs of fluid overload (or water intoxication). Signs of fluid overload include drowsiness, restlessness, confusion, and headache. If these occur, the physician is notified immediately because a dosage adjustment, the restriction of oral or IV fluids, and the administration of a diuretic may be necessary.

ANXIETY. The symptoms of diabetes insipidus include the voiding of a large volume of urine at frequent intervals during the day and throughout the night. Accompanied by frequent urination is the need to drink large volumes of fluid because these patients are continually thirsty. Until controlled by medication, these symptoms cause a great deal of anxiety. The patient should be reassured that with medication these symptoms will most likely be reduced or eliminated.

If the patient is receiving vasopressin for abdominal distention, the method of treating this problem and the necessary monitoring of drug effectiveness (auscultation of the abdomen for bowel sounds, insertion of a rectal tube, measurement of the abdomen) is explained in detail to the patient.

FLUID VOLUME DEFICIT. When the patient has diabetes insipidus, the intake and output must be measured accurately and the patient observed for signs of dehydration. This is especially important early in treatment and until such time as the optimum dosage is determined and symptoms have diminished. If the patient's output greatly exceeds his or her intake, the physician must be notified. In some instances, the physician may order specific gravity and volume measurements of each voiding or at hourly intervals. These results are recorded on a flow sheet and aid the physician in adjusting the dosage to the patient's needs.

It is most important that these patients be supplied with large amounts of drinking water. The water container must be refilled at frequent intervals. This is especially important when the patient has limited ambulatory activities.

NONCOMPLIANCE AND KNOWLEDGE DEFICIT. If lypressin or desmopressin is to be used in the form of a nasal spray for the patient with diabetes insipidus, the technique of instillation is demonstrated. Illustrated patient instructions are included with the drug and should be reviewed with the patient.

On occasion, it may be necessary for the patient to self-administer vasopressin by the parenteral route. The patient or a family member requires instruction in the preparation and administration of the drug and measurement of the specific gravity of the urine.

The importance of adhering to the prescribed treatment program to control symptoms is stressed. In addition to instruction in administration, the following may be included in a patient and family teaching plan:

▶ Drink one or two glasses of water immediately before taking the drug.
▶ Measure the amount of fluids taken each day.
▶ Measure the amount of urine passed at each voiding, and then total the amount for each 24-hour period.

► Rotate injection sites.

► Contact the physician immediately if any of the following occur: a significant increase or decrease in urinary output, abdominal cramps, blanching of the skin, nausea, signs of inflammation or infection at the injection sites, confusion, headache, or drowsiness.

EVALUATION

► Anxiety is reduced

► Signs of a fluid volume deficit are absent (diabetes insipidus)

► Verbalizes an understanding of treatment modalities and importance of continued follow-up care (diabetes insipidus)

► Patient and family demonstrate understanding of drug regimen

► Adverse reactions are identified and reported to the physician (diabetes insipidus)

► Verbalizes importance of complying with the prescribed treatment regimen (diabetes insipidus)

► THE ADRENOCORTICAL HORMONES

The adrenal cortex manufacturers the **glucocorticoids,** the **mineralocorticoids,** and small amounts of **sex hormones.** The glucocorticoids and mineralocorticoids are essential to life and influence many organs and structures of the body. The glu-

SUMMARY DRUG TABLE 27–2
Glucocorticoids and Mineralocorticoids

GENERIC NAME	TRADE NAME*	USES	ADVERSE REACTIONS	DOSE RANGES
GLUCOCORTICOIDS				
cortisone	Cortone Acetate, *generic*	See Table 27-1	See Table 27-2	25–300 mg/d PO or 20–300 mg/d IM
dexamethasone	Decadron, *generic*	See Table 27-1	See Table 27-2	Initial dosage: 0.75–9 mg/d PO; further doses depend on disease being treated
dexamethasone acetate	Decadron-LA, *generic*	See Table 27-1	See Table 27-2	8–16 mg IM; may be repeated in 1–3 wk
hydrocortisone (cortisol)	Cortef, *generic*	See Table 27-1	See Table 27-2	Initial dosage: 20–240 mg/d PO; ⅓–½ oral dosage IM
methylprednisolone	Medrol, *generic*	See Table 27-1	See Table 27-2	Initial dosage: 4–48 mg/d PO; maintenance dose based on response to therapy
methylprednisolone acetate	Depo-Medrol, *generic*	See Table 27-1	See Table 27-2	40–120 mg IM
prednisolone	Delta-Cortef, *generic*	See Table 27-1	See Table 27-2	5–60 mg/d PO
prednisone	Meticorten, *generic*	See Table 27-1	See Table 27-2	Initial dosage: 5–60 mg/d PO
triamcinolone	Aristocort, *generic*	See Table 27-1	See Table 27-2	Initial dosage: 4–60 mg/d PO
triamcinolone diacetate	Aristocort L.A., *generic*	See Table 27-1	See Table 27-2	40 mg/wk IM (average dose)
MINERALOCORTICOIDS				
fludrocortisone acetate (has both glucocorticoid and mineralocorticoid activity)	Florinef Acetate	Partial replacement therapy for Addison's disease, salt-losing adrenogenital syndrome	See Table 27–2	Addison's disease: 0.05–0.2 mg/d PO; adrenogenital syndrome: 0.1–0.2 mg/d

* The term generic *indicates that the drug is available in a generic form.*

cocorticoids and mineralocorticoids are collectively called **corticosteroids.** Their uses and dose ranges are given in Summary Drug Table 27-2.

▷ Actions of the Adrenocortical Hormones

The Glucocorticoids. Although there are several glucocorticoids produced by the adrenal cortex, the two most prominent are hydrocortisone and cortisone. The glucocorticoids influence or regulate functions, such as the immune response system, the regulation of glucose, fat and protein metabolism, and control of the antiinflammatory response. Examples of the glucocorticoids include cortisone, hydrocortisone (Cortef), prednisone, prednisolone, and triamcinolone.

The Mineralocorticoids. The mineralocorticoids consist of **aldosterone** and **desoxycorticosterone** and play an important role in conserving sodium and increasing the excretion of potassium. Because of these activities, the mineralocorticoids play an important role in controlling salt and water balance. Of these two hormones, aldosterone is the more potent. Deficiencies of the mineralocorticoids results in a loss of sodium and water and a retention of potassium.

Fludrocortisone (Florinef) is a drug that has both glucocorticoid and mineralocorticoid activity and is the only presently available mineralocorticoid drug.

▷ Uses of the Adrenocortical Hormones

Glucocorticoids. The uses of the glucocorticoids are given in Table 27-1.

Mineralocorticoids. Fludrocortisone is used for replacement therapy for primary and secondary adrenocortical deficiency because this drug has *both* mineralocorticoid and glucocorticoid activity.

▷ Adverse Reactions Associated with Administration of the Adrenocortical Hormones

Glucocorticoids. The adverse reactions that may be seen with the administration of the glucocorticoids are given in Table 27-2. Long- or short-term high-dose therapy may also produce many of the signs and symptoms seen with Cushing's syndrome, a disease due to the overproduction of endogenous glucocorticoids. Some of the signs and symptoms of this Cushing's-like (or cushingoid) state include a "buffalo" hump (a hump on the back of the neck), moon face, oily skin and acne, osteoporosis, purple striae on the abdomen and hips, skin pigmentation, and weight gain. When a serious disease or disorder is being treated, it is often necessary to allow these effects to occur since therapy with these drugs is absolutely necessary.

Mineralocorticoids. Fludrocortisone has the same adverse reactions as the glucocorticoids (see Table 27-2).

▶ NURSING PROCESS
THE PATIENT RECEIVING A GLUCOCORTICOID OR MINERALOCORTICOID

ASSESSMENT

Before the administration of a glucocorticoid or mineralocorticoid, the blood pressure, pulse, and respiratory rate are taken. Additional physical assessments depend on the reason for use and the general condition of the patient. When feasible, an assessment of the area of disease involvement, such as the respiratory tract or skin, is performed and the findings are recorded in the patient's record. These findings provide baseline data for the evaluation of the patient's response to drug therapy. Patients who are acutely ill or have a serious systemic disease should be weighed before starting therapy.

NURSING DIAGNOSIS

Depending on the drug, dose, and reason for administration, one or more of the following nursing diagnoses may apply to a person receiving a glucocorticoid or mineralocorticoid:

▶ Anxiety related to symptoms of disorder, diagnosis, other factors
▶ Noncompliance related to indifference, lack of knowledge, other factors
▶ Knowledge deficit of medication regimen, adverse drug effects, treatment modalities

PLANNING AND IMPLEMENTATION

The major goals of the patient may include a reduction in anxiety and an understanding of and compliance to the prescribed treatment regimen.

TABLE 27–1
Uses of Glucocorticoids

ENDOCRINE DISORDERS

Primary or secondary adrenal cortical insufficiency, congenital adrenal hyperplasia, nonsuppressive thyroiditis, hypercalcemia associated with cancer

RHEUMATIC DISORDERS

Short-term management of acute ankylosing spondylitis, acute and subacute bursitis, acute nonspecific tenosynovitis, acute gouty arthritis, psoriatic arthritis, rheumatoid arthritis, posttraumatic osteoarthritis, synovitis of osteoarthritis, epicondylitis

COLLAGEN DISEASES

Lupus erythematosus, acute rheumatic carditis, systemic dermatomyositis

DERMATOLOGIC DISEASES

Pemphigus, bullous dermatitis herpetiformis, severe erythema multiforme (Stevens-Johnson syndrome), exfoliative dermatitis, mycosis fungoides, severe psoriasis, severe seborrheic dermatitis, angioedema, urticaria, various skin disorders such as lichen planus or keloids

ALLERGIC STATES

Control of severe or incapacitating allergic conditions not controlled by other methods, bronchial asthma (including status asthmaticus), contact dermatitis, atopic dermatitis, serum sickness, drug hypersensitivity reactions

OPHTHALMIC DISEASES

Severe acute and chronic allergic and inflammatory processes, keratitis, allergic corneal marginal ulcers, herpes zoster of the eye, iritis, iridocyclitis, chorioretinitis, diffuse posterior uveitis, optic neuritis, sympathetic ophthalmia, anterior segment inflammation

RESPIRATORY DISEASES

Sarcoidosis, berylliosis, fulminating or disseminated pulmonary tuberculosis, aspiration pneumonia

HEMATOLOGIC DISORDERS

Idiopathic or secondary thrombocytopenic purpura, hemolytic anemia, red blood cell anemia, congenital hypoplastic anemia

NEOPLASTIC DISEASES

Leukemias, lymphomas

EDEMATOUS STATES

To induce diuresis or remission of proteinuria in the nephrotic state

GASTROINTESTINAL DISEASES

During critical period of ulcerative colitis, regional enteritis, intractable sprue

NERVOUS SYSTEM

Acute exacerbations of multiple sclerosis

TABLE 27–2
Adverse Effects of Glucocorticoids

FLUID AND ELECTROLYTE DISTURBANCES

Sodium and fluid retention, congestive heart failure in susceptible patients, potassium loss, hypokalemic alkalosis, hypertension, hypocalcemia, hypotension or shock-like reactions

MUSCULOSKELETAL

Muscle weakness, loss of muscle mass, tendon rupture, osteoporosis, aseptic necrosis of femoral and humoral heads, spontaneous fractures

CARDIOVASCULAR

Thromboembolism or fat embolism, thrombophlebitis, necrotizing angiitis, syncopal episodes

GASTROINTESTINAL

Pancreatitis, abdominal distention, ulcerative esophagitis, nausea, increased appetite and weight gain, possible peptic ulcer with perforation

DERMATOLOGIC

Impaired wound healing, thin fragile skin, petechiae, ecchymoses, erythema, increased sweating, suppression of skin test reactions, subcutaneous fat atrophy, purpura, striae, hyperpigmentation, hirsutism, acneiform eruptions, urticaria

NEUROLOGIC

Convulsions, steroid-induced catatonia, increased intracranial pressure with papilledema (usually after treatment is discontinued), vertigo, headache, neuritis or paresthesias, steroid psychosis, insomnia

ENDOCRINE

Amenorrhea, other menstrual irregularities, development of cushingoid state, suppression of growth in children, secondary adrenocortical and pituitary unresponsiveness (particularly in times of stress), decreased carbohydrate tolerance, manifestation of latent diabetes mellitus, increased requirements for insulin or oral hypoglycemic agents (in diabetics)

OPHTHALMIC

Posterior subcapsular cataracts, increased intraocular pressure, glaucoma, exophthalmos

METABOLIC

Negative nitrogen balance (due to protein catabolism)

OTHER

Anaphylactoid or hypersensitivity reactions, aggravation of existing infections, malaise, increase or decrease in sperm motility and number

The major goals of nursing management may include a reduction in the patient's anxiety and the development and implementation of an effective teaching plan.

ADMINISTRATION. The glucocorticoids may be ordered to be given orally, IM, SC, or IV. The label of the parenteral container must be checked to be sure the drug can be given by the prescribed route.

The physician may also inject the drug into a joint (intraarticular), a lesion (intralesional), soft tissue, or bursa.

ALTERNATE-DAY THERAPY. The alternate-day therapy approach to glucocorticoid administration may be ordered in the treatment of some diseases and disorders, especially the arthritic disorders. This regimen involves giving twice the daily dose of the glucocorticoid every other day. The drug is given only once on the alternate day and *before 9 AM.* The purpose of alternate-day administration is to provide the patient requiring long-term glucocorticoid therapy with the beneficial effects of the drug while minimizing certain undesirable reactions (see Table 27-2).

Plasma levels of the endogenous adrenocortical hormones vary throughout the day and nighttime hours. They are normally *higher* between 2 AM and about 8 AM, and *lower* between 4 PM and midnight. When plasma levels are lower, the anterior pituitary releases ACTH, which, in turn, stimulates the adrenal cortex to manufacture and release glucocorticoids. When plasma levels are high, the pituitary gland does not release ACTH. The response of the pituitary to high or low plasma levels of glucocorticoids and the resulting release or nonrelease of ACTH is an example of the *feedback mechanism,* which may also be seen in other glands of the body, such as the thyroid gland.

Administration of glucocorticoids several times a day and over a short time (as little as 5–10 days) results in shutting off the pituitary release of ACTH because there are always high levels of the glucocorticoids in the plasma (which is due to the body's own glucocorticoid production plus the administration of a glucocorticoid drug). Ultimately, the pituitary atrophies and creases to release ACTH. Without ACTH, the adrenals fail to manufacture and release (endogenous) glucocorticoids. When this happens, the patient has acute adrenal insufficiency, which is a life-threatening situation until corrected with the administration of an exogenous glucocorticoid.

Administration of a short-acting glucocorticoid on alternate days and before 9 AM, when glucocorticoid plasma levels are still relatively high, does *not* affect the release of ACTH later on in the day, yet gives the patient the benefit of exogenous glucocorticoid therapy.

DAILY ASSESSMENTS. Daily assessments of the patient receiving a glucocorticoid or mineralocorticoid and the frequency of these assessments depend largely on the disease being treated. Areas to be included in the patient care plan must be based on nursing judgment, as well as specific orders written by the physician.

▶ Vital signs should be monitored vital signs every 4 to 8 hours.

▶ The patient's response to the drug is evaluated daily; evaluations are made more frequently if a glucocorticoid is used for emergency situations. Because these drugs are used to treat a great many diseases and conditions, an evaluation of drug response is based on the patient's diagnosis and the signs and symptoms of his or her disease.

▶ The patient is weighed daily to weekly.

▶ The patient is observed for signs of electrolyte imbalance, especially hypocalcemia, hypokalemia, and hypernatremia (see chap 17).

▶ The patient is observed daily for signs of adverse effects of the mineralocorticoid or glucocorticoid.

▶ The patient is observed receiving a glucocorticoid for mental changes, especially if there is a history of depression or other psychiatric problems or if high doses of the drug are being given. Mental changes are documented accurately and the physician is informed of their occurrence. Patients that appear extremely depressed are closely observed at frequent intervals.

▶ The patient is observed for signs of an infection, which may be masked by glucocorticoid therapy. Any slight rise in temperature, sore throat, or other signs of infection is reported to the physician as soon as possible.

▶ Because of a possible decreased resistance to infection during glucocorticoid therapy, nursing personnel and visitors with any type of infection or recent exposure to an infectious disease should avoid patient contact.

▶ Diabetic patients receiving a glucocorticoid may require frequent adjustment of their insulin or oral hypoglycemic drug dosage. If the urine is positive for glucose or ketones, the physician is notified.

▶ The urine of the nondiabetic patient is checked weekly for glucose and ketone bodies because glucocorticoids may aggravate latent diabetes.

▶ Dietary adjustment for the increased loss of potassium and the retention of sodium may be necessary.

▶ Patients on long-term glucocorticoid therapy, especially those allowed limited activity, are observed for signs of compression fractures of the vertebrae and pathological fractures of the long bones. If the patient complains of back or bone pain, this is brought to the attention of the physician. Extra care is also necessary to prevent falls and other injuries when the patient is confused or is allowed out of bed.

▶ Peptic ulcer has been associated with glucocorticoid therapy. Any complaints of epigastric burning or pain, or the passing of tarry stools is brought to the physician's attention immediately.

▶ The physician is always informed if signs of electrolyte imbalance or glucocorticoid drug effects are noted.

▶ If the patient is receiving alternate-day therapy, the drug must be given *before 9 AM.*

▶ *At no time must a glucocorticoid be discontinued suddenly.* When administration of a glucocorticoid extends beyond 5 days and the drug is to be discontinued, *the dosage is tapered* over several days. In some instances, it may be necessary to taper the dose over 7 to 10 or more days. Abrupt discontinuation of a glucocorticoid usually results in acute adrenal insufficiency, which, if not recognized in time, can result in death.

▶ The dose of a glucocorticoid must never be omitted. If the patient cannot take the drug orally because of nausea or vomiting, the physician is contacted immediately because the drug needs to be ordered given by the parenteral route. Patients who are receiving nothing by mouth for any reason must have the glucocorticoid given by the parenteral route.

ANXIETY. Depending on the situation, patients may experience anxiety because of the symptoms of their disorder, their diagnosis, or the required treatment regimen. The nurse may relieve some of the anxiety in these patients by assuring them that their symptoms will most likely be relieved. A thorough teaching plan may also help relieve anxiety due to prolonged therapy or alternate day therapy.

NONCOMPLIANCE AND KNOWLEDGE DEFICIT. To prevent noncompliance, it is most important that the patient and family receive thorough instructions and warnings about the drug regimen.

Short-Term Glucocorticoid Therapy

▶ Take exactly as directed in the prescription container. Do not increase, decrease, or omit a dose unless advised to do so by the physician.

▶ Follow the instructions for tapering the dose because they are extremely important.

▶ If the problem does not improve, contact the physician.

Alternate-Day Glucocorticoid Therapy

▶ Take this drug *before 9 AM once every other day.* Use a calendar or some other method to identify the days of each week the drug is taken.

▶ Do not stop taking the drug unless advised to do so by the physician.

▶ If the problem becomes worse, especially on the days the drug is not taken, contact the physician.

Note: Most of the teaching points given below may also apply to alternate-day therapy, especially when higher doses are used and therapy extends over many months.

Long-Term or High-Dose Glucocorticoid Therapy

▶ Do not omit this drug or increase or decrease the dosage except on the advice of the physician.

▶ Inform other physicians, dentists, and all medical personnel of therapy with this drug. Wear a Medic-Alert tag or bracelet or other form of identification to alert medical personnel of long-term therapy with a glucocorticoid.

▶ Do not take any nonprescription drug unless its use has been approved by the physician.

▶ Whenever possible, avoid exposure to infections. Contact the physician if minor cuts or abrasions fail to heal, persistent joint swelling or tenderness is noted, or fever, sore throat, upper respiratory infection, or other signs of infection occur.

▶ If the drug cannot be taken orally for any reason or if diarrhea occurs, contact the physician immediately. If unable to contact the physician before the next dose is due, go to the nearest hospital emergency department (preferably where the original treatment was started or where the physician is on the hospital staff) because the drug has to be given by injection.

▶ Weigh self weekly. If significant weight gain or swelling of the extremities is noted, contact the physician.

▶ If dietary recommendations are made by the physician, these are an important part of therapy and must be followed.

▶ Follow the physician's recommendations regarding periodic eye examinations and laboratory tests.

EVALUATION

▶ Anxiety is reduced

▶ Verbalizes an understanding of dosage regimen

▶ Verbalizes importance of complying with the prescribed treatment regimen and importance of continued follow-up care

▶ Patient and family demonstrate understanding of drug regimen

▶ Demonstrates understanding of importance in not suddenly discontinuing therapy (long-term or high-dose therapy)

28

Male and Female Hormones

On completion of this chapter the student will:

▶ *Discuss the medical uses of male and female hormones*

▶ *List and discuss the major adverse reactions associated with the administration male or female hormones*

▶ *Use the nursing process when administering male or female hormones*

▶ *Discuss the nursing implications associated with the administration of male and female hormones*

Male hormones—testosterone and its derivatives—are called **androgens.** Androgen secretion is under the influence of the anterior pituitary gland. The female hormones are **estrogen** and **progesterone,** and like the androgens, their production is under the influence of the anterior pituitary gland. Small amounts of male and female hormones are also produced by the adrenal cortex (see chap 26).

▶ THE MALE HORMONES

▷ Actions of the Male Hormones

Androgens

The male hormone testosterone and its derivatives actuate the reproductive potential in the adolescent male. From puberty onward, androgens continue to aid in the development and maintenance of secondary sex characteristics: facial hair, deep voice, body hair, body fat distribution, and muscle development. Testosterone also affects the accessory sex organs (penis, testes, vas deferens, prostate) at the time of puberty. Under the influence of testosterone, the accessory sex organs grow in size. The androgens also promote tissue-building processes (anabolism) and reverse tissue-depleting processes (catabolism). Examples of oral androgens are fluoxymesterone (Halotestin), methyltestosterone (Oreton), and testosterone.

Anabolic Steroids

The anabolic steroids are synthetic drugs chemically related to the androgens. Like the androgens, they promote tissue-building processes. Given in

209

normal doses, they have a minimal affect on the accessory sex organs and secondary sex characteristics. Examples of anabolic steroids are given in Summary Drug Table 28-1.

▷ Uses of the Male Hormones

Androgens

In the male, androgen therapy may be given as replacement therapy for testosterone deficiency. Deficiency states in the male, such as hypogonadism (failure of the testes to develop), selected cases of delayed puberty, and the development of testosterone deficiency after puberty may be treated with androgens.

In the female, androgen therapy may be used as part of the treatment for inoperable metastatic breast carcinoma in patients who are 1 to 5 years *past* menopause. Many breast carcinomas are "hormone-dependent" tumors, that is, their growth and spread are influenced by the female hormone estrogen. Administration of an androgen to these patients counteracts the effect of estrogen on these tumors. Androgens may also be administered to premenopausal women with metastatic breast carcinoma that is believed to be hormone-dependent and whose tumor growth and spread have been slowed after an oophorectomy (removal of the ovaries). Androgen therapy may also be used to reduce postpartum breast pain and engorgement.

The uses of the androgens are also given in Summary Drug Table 28-1.

Anabolic Steroids

Anabolic steroids may be used to promote weight gain in those who are underweight because of a recent illness or other factors that may contribute to catabolism. They are also used in the management of osteoporosis occurring past menopause and in reversing the profound catabolism that often occurs with the use of high doses of corticosteroids, in the control of metastatic breast cancer, and in the treatment of certain types of anemia.

The use of anabolic steroids to promote an increase in muscle mass and strength has become a serious problem. Anabolic steroids are *not* intended for this use. Unfortunately, there have been deaths in young, healthy individuals directly attributed to the use of these drugs.

The specific uses of the various anabolic steroids are listed in Summary Drug Table 28-1.

▷ Adverse Reactions Associated with the Administration of Male Hormones

Androgens

In the male, administration of an androgen may result in breast enlargement (gynecomastia), testicular atrophy, inhibition of testicular function, impotence, enlargement of the penis, nausea, jaundice, headache, anxiety, male pattern baldness, acne, and depression. Fluid and electrolyte imbalances, which include sodium, water, chloride, potassium, calcium, and phosphate retention, may also be seen.

In the female receiving an androgen preparation for breast carcinoma, the most common adverse reactions are amenorrhea and other menstrual irregularities, and virilization. Virilization in the female produces facial hair, a deepening of the voice, and enlargement of the clitoris. Male pattern baldness and acne may also be seen.

Adverse reactions are minimal when an androgen is given to the postpartum female because the drug is only given for 3 to 5 days.

Anabolic Steroids

Virilization in the female is the most common reaction associated with anabolic steroids, especially when higher doses are used. Acne occurs frequently in all age groups and both sexes. Nausea, vomiting, diarrhea, fluid and electrolyte imbalances (the same as for the androgens, discussed previously), testicular atrophy in the male, jaundice, anorexia, and muscle cramps may also be seen. Blood-filled cysts of the liver and sometimes the spleen, malignant and benign liver tumors, an increased risk of atherosclerosis, and mental changes are the most serious adverse reactions that may occur during prolonged use.

Many serious adverse drug reactions are being reported in healthy individuals using anabolic steroids. There is some indication that prolonged high-dose use has resulted in psychologic addiction and some individuals have required treatment in drug abuse centers. Severe mental changes such as uncontrolled rage ("roid rage"), severe depression, suicidal tendencies, inability to concentrate, and personality changes are not uncommon. In addition, the incidence of the severe adverse reactions cited earlier appears to be increased in those using anabolic steroids for this purpose.

SUMMARY DRUG TABLE 28–1
Male and Female Hormones

GENERIC NAME	TRADE NAME*	USES	ADVERSE REACTIONS	DOSE RANGES
ANDROGENS				
fluoxymesterone	Halotestin, *generic*	Males: hypogonadism, delayed puberty; females: inoperable breast cancer in those past menopause, postpartum breast pain and engorgement	Males: gynecomastia, virilization, testicular atrophy; females: virilization, amenorrhea, other menstrual irregularities	Males: 2.5–20 mg/d PO; females: postpartum 2.5–10 mg/d PO; malignancies: see Summary Drug Table 31-1
methyltestosterone	Android-10, *generic*	Same as fluoxymesterone	Same as fluoxymesterone	Males; 10–40 mg/d PO; females: postpartum 80 mg/d PO; malignancies: see Summary Drug Table 31-1
testosterone (aqueous suspension)	Andro 100, *generic*	Same as fluoxymesterone	Same as fluoxymesterone	Males: 10–50 mg IM; females: postpartum 25–50 mg/d IM; malignancies: see see Summary Drug Table 31-1
testosterone cypionate	Depo-Testosterone, *generic*	Males: hypogonadism, delayed puberty; females: inoperable breast cancer in those past menopause	Same as fluoxymesterone	Males: 50–400 mg IM; malignancies: see Summary Drug Table 31-1
ANABOLIC STEROIDS				
methandrostenolone	*Generic*	Senile and postmenopausal osteoporosis	Nausea, vomiting, diarrhea, virilization, fluid and electrolyte imbalance	2.5–5 mg/d PO
nandrolone phenpropionate	Durabolin, *generic*	Control of metastatic breast cancer	Same as methandrostenolone	50–100 mg/wk IM
oxymetholone	Anadrol	Anemias caused by deficient red cell production, aplastic anemia	Same as methandrostenolone	1–5 mg/kg/d PO
ESTROGENS				
chlorotrianisene	TACE	Postpartum breast engorgement, prostatic carcinoma, menopausal symptoms, female hypogonadism	See Table 28-1	Postpartum: 12 mg PO qid or 50 mg PO q6h; menopause, hypogonadism: 12–25 mg/d PO; malignancies: see Summary Drug Table 31-1
conjugated estrogens	Premarin, *generic*	Oral: menopausal symptoms, osteoporosis, mammary and prostatic carcinoma, postpartum breast engorgement, female hypogonadism; parenteral: abnormal uterine bleeding	See Table 28-1	Menopause: 0.3–1.25 mg/d PO; hypogonadism: 2.5–7.5 mg/d PO; osteoporosis: 0.625 mg/d PO; uterine bleeding: 25 mg IM, IV; malignancies: see Summary Drug Table 31-1
estradiol	Estrace	Menopausal symptoms, female hypogonadism, ovarian failure, breast and prostatic cancer	See Table 28-1	Menopause, hypogonadism: 1–2 mg/d PO; malignancies: see Summary Drug Table 31-1
estradiol transdermal system	Estraderm	Menopausal symptoms, female hypogonadism, ovarian failure	See Table 28-1	Apply system twice a week, 3 wk on and 1 wk off

(continued)

SUMMARY DRUG TABLE 28—1
(continued)

GENERIC NAME	TRADE NAME*	USES	ADVERSE REACTIONS	DOSE RANGES
ethinyl estradiol	Estinyl	Same as estradiol	See Table 28-1	Menopause: 0.02–1.5 mg/d PO; hypogonadism: 0.05 mg PO 1–3 times/d; malignancies: see Summary Drug Table 31-1
PROGESTINS				
hydroxypro-gesterone caproate in oil	Delalutin, *generic*	Amenorrhea, abnormal uterine bleeding	See Table 28-1	375 mg IM
medroxypro-gesterone acetate	Provera	Same as hydroxyproges-terone	See Table 28-1	5–10 mg/d PO
norethindrone	Norlutin	Amenorrhea, abnormal uterine bleeding, endometriosis	See Table 28-1	Amenorrhea, uterine bleeding: 5–20 mg/d PO; endometriosis: 10–30 mg/d PO
progesterone	*Generic*	Same as hyroxyproges-terone	See Table 28-1	5–10 mg/d IM

* The term generic *indicates that the drug is available in a generic form.*

▶ NURSING PROCESS
THE PATIENT RECEIVING AN ANDROGEN OR ANABOLIC STEROID

ASSESSMENT

Assessment of the patient receiving an androgen or anabolic steroid depends on the drug, the patient, and the reason for administration.

Androgens

In most instances, androgens are administered to the male on an outpatient basis. Before and during therapy, the physician may order electrolyte studies because use of these drugs can result in fluid and electrolyte imbalances. The physician also discusses the anticipated results of therapy with the patient, or in the case of a child, the parent.

When these drugs are given to the female patient with inoperable breast carcinoma, the patient's present status (physical, emotional, and nutritional) is carefully evaluated and the findings are recorded in the patient's chart. Problem areas, such as pain, any limitation of motion, and the ability to participate in the activities of daily living, are carefully evaluated and

recorded. The vital signs and weight are also taken and recorded. Baseline laboratory tests may include a complete blood count (CBC), hepatic function tests, serum electrolytes, and serum and urinary calcium levels.

When given as short-term therapy to the female patient with postpartum breast pain and engorgement, a summary of the patient's symptoms is recorded in the patient's chart.

Anabolic Steroids

The patient's physical and nutritional status is evaluated and recorded before starting therapy with anabolic steroids. The weight, blood pressure, pulse, and respiratory rate are taken. Baseline laboratory studies may include a CBC, hepatic function tests, and serum electrolytes and cholesterol levels.

NURSING DIAGNOSIS

Depending on the drug, dose, and reason for administration, one or more of the following nursing diagnoses may apply to a person receiving an androgen or anabolic steroid:

▶ Anxiety related to diagnosis, adverse effects of drug therapy (female patient), other factors

▶ Knowledge deficit of medication regimen, adverse drug effects, treatment modalities

PLANNING AND IMPLEMENTATION

The major goals of the patient may include a reduction in anxiety and an understanding of and compliance to the prescribed treatment regimen.

The major goals of nursing management may include a reduction in the patient's anxiety, recognition of adverse drug effects, and the development and implementation of an effective teaching plan.

The following areas may be included in a nursing care plan for the patient with inoperable breast carcinoma:

▶ The patient is weighed daily or as ordered by the physician. If the patient is on complete bed rest, weights may be taken every 3 to 4 days (or as ordered) using a bed scale. The physician is notified the physician if there is a significant increase or decrease in the weight.

▶ The patient is observed for adverse drug reactions, especially signs of fluid and electrolyte imbalance, jaundice (which may indicate hepatotoxicity), and virilization.

▶ Vital signs are monitored every 4 to 8 hours.

▶ The lower extremities are checked daily for signs of edema.

▶ Based on original assessments, the patient's response to drug therapy is evaluated. Responses that may be seen include a decrease in pain, an increase in the appetite, and a feeling of well-being.

The patient with postpartum breast pain and engorgement is evaluated for drug response. If breast pain or engorgement is not relieved, the physician is informed.

The male receiving an androgen or anabolic steroid is most often seen on an outpatient basis and is questioned by the physician regarding the effectiveness of drug therapy.

When anabolic steroids are used for weight gain, the patient is weighted at intervals ranging from daily to weekly. A good dietary regimen is necessary to promote weight gain. The dietitian is consulted if the patient eats poorly.

ADMINISTRATION. Some androgens are available in buccal form. The patient requires instruction in the placement of the tablet: he or she must be warned not to swallow the tablet but to allow it to dissolve in the mouth. The patient is also reminded not to smoke or drink water until the tablet is dissolved.

ADVERSE REACTIONS. Patients receiving an androgen or anabolic steroid are observed for signs of adverse drug reactions. In the female, masculinization may

been seen with long-term administration but must be tolerated to obtain the desired effect of the drug.

ANXIETY. With long-term administration, the female patient may develop mild to moderate masculine changes (virilization), namely, facial hair, a deepening of the voice, and enlargement of the clitoris. Male pattern baldness, patchy hair loss, skin pigmentation, and acne may also be seen. Although these adverse effects are not life-threatening, they often are distressing and only add to the patient's discomfort and anxiety. These problems may be easy to identify but they are not always easy to solve. If hair loss occurs, the wearing of a wig may be suggested. Mild skin pigmentation may be covered with makeup but severe and widespread pigmented areas and acne are often difficult to conceal. Each patient is different, and the emotional responses to these outward changes may range from severe depression to a positive attitude and acceptance. The nurse must work with the patient as an individual, first identifying the problems, and then helping the patient, whenever possible, to deal with these changes.

KNOWLEDGE DEFICIT. The dosage regimen and possible adverse drug reactions are explained to the patient and family.

The following points may be included in patient and family teaching plan:

Androgens

▶ Oral tablets—Take with food or a snack to avoid gastrointestinal (GI) upset.

▶ Buccal tablets—Place the tablet between the cheek and molars and allow it to dissolve in the mouth. Do not smoke or drink water until the tablet is dissolved.

▶ Notify the physician if any of the following occur: nausea, vomiting, swelling of the legs, jaundice. Female patients should report any signs of virilization to the physician.

Anabolic Steroids

▶ Anabolic steroids may cause nausea and GI upset. Take this drug with food or meals.

▶ Keep all physician or clinic visits because close monitoring of therapy is essential.

▶ Female patient—Notify the physician if signs of virilization occur.

EVALUATION

▶ Anxiety is reduced

▶ Adverse reactions are identified and reported to the physician

▶ Verbalizes importance of complying with the prescribed treatment regimen

▶ Patient and family demonstrate understanding of drug regimen

▶ Verbalizes an understanding of treatment modalities and importance of continued follow-up care

▶ THE FEMALE HORMONES

The two endogenous (natural) female hormones are the **estrogens** and **progesterone**. The natural estrogens are estradiol, estrone, and estriol. The most potent of these three estrogens is estradiol. There are natural and synthetic progesterones, which are collectively called **progestins** (see Summary Drug Table 28-1). Examples of estrogens used as drugs include chlorotrianisene (Tace) and estradiol (Estrace). Examples of progestins used as drugs include medroxyprogesterone (Provera) and norethindrone (Norlutin).

▷ Actions of the Female Hormones

Estrogens

The estrogens are secreted by the ovarian follicle and in smaller amounts by the adrenal cortex. Estrogens are important in the development and maintenance of the female reproductive system and the primary and secondary sex characteristics. At puberty, they promote growth and development of the vagina, uterus, and Fallopian tubes, and enlargement of the breasts. They also affect the release of pituitary gonadotropins (see chap 27). Other actions of estrogen include fluid retention, protein anabolism, thinning of the cervical mucus, and the inhibition of ovulation. Estrogens contribute to the conservation of calcium and phosphorus, the growth of pubic and axillary hair, and pigmentation of the breast nipples and genitals. Estrogens also stimulate contraction of the fallopian tubes (which promotes movement of the ovum), modify the physical and chemical properties of the cervical mucus, and restore the endometrium after menstruation.

Progestins

Progesterone is secreted by the corpus luteum, placenta, and, in small amounts, by the adrenal cortex. Progesterone and its derivatives (ie, the progestins) transform the proliferative endometrium into a secretory endometrium. Progestins are necessary for the development of the placenta and inhibit the secretion of pituitary gonadotropins, which, in turn, prevents maturation of the ovarian follicle and ovulation. The synthetic progestins are usually preferred for medical use because of the decreased effectiveness of progesterone when administered orally.

▷ Uses of the Female Hormones

Estrogens

The estrogens are used in the treatment of postpartum breast engorgement, inoperable prostatic carcinoma, the symptoms of menopause, female hypogonadism, atrophic vaginitis, osteoporosis in females past menopause, and in selected cases of inoperable breast carcinoma. The estrogens, in combination with a progestin, are also used as oral contraceptives (Summary Drug Table 28-2). The uses of individual estrogens are given in Summary Drug Table 28-1. The use of estrogens in the treatment of carcinoma are discussed in chapter 31.

Progestins

The progestins are used in the treatment of amenorrhea, endometriosis, and functional uterine bleeding. Progestins are also used as oral contraceptives, either alone or in combination with an estrogen (see Summary Drug Table 28-2).

Oral Contraceptives

Estrogens and progestins or progestins only are used as oral contraceptives. There are three types of estrogen and progestin combination oral contraceptives: monophasic, biphasic, and triphasic. The monophasic oral contraceptives provide a fixed dose of estrogen and progestin. The biphasic and triphasic oral contraceptives deliver hormones similar to the levels naturally produced by the body.

▷ Adverse Reactions Associated with the Administration of the Female Hormones

The adverse reactions seen with the administration of female hormones are given in Table 28-1. When used as oral contraceptives, the adverse reactions associated with the estrogens and the progestins must be considered.

The warnings associated with the use of oral contraceptives include cigarette smoking, which in-

SUMMARY DRUG TABLE 28–2
Oral Contraceptives

TABLET CONTENT	TRADE NAME
COMBINATION PRODUCTS (ESTROGEN AND PROGESTIN)*	
MONOPHASIC ORAL CONTRACEPTIVES	
50 mcg mestranol, 1 mg norethindrone	Genora 1/50, Norethin 1/50 M, Ortho-Novum 1/50
50 mcg ethinyl estradiol, 1 mg norethindrone	Ovcon-50
50 mcg ethinyl estradiol, 1 mg norethindrone acetate	Norlestrin, 1/50, Norlestrin Fe 1/50
50 mcg ethinyl estradiol, 1 mg ethynodiol diacetate	Demulen 1/50
50 mcg ethinyl estradiol, 2.5 mg norethindrone diacetate	Norlestrin 21 2.5/50, Norlestrin Fe 2.5/50
50 mcg ethinyl estradiol, 0.5 mg norgestrel	Ovral
35 mcg ethinyl estradiol, 1 mg norethindrone	Genora 1/35. Norethin 1/35 E, Ortho-Novum 1/35
35 mcg ethinyl estradiol, 0.5 mg norethindrone	Brevicon, Genora 0.5/35, Modi-con
35 mcg ethinyl estradiol, 0.4 mg norethindrone	Ovcon-35
35 mcg ethinyl estradiol, 1 mg ethynodiol	Demulen 1/35
30 mcg ethinyl estradiol, 1.5 mg norethindrone	Loestrin 21 1.5/30, Loestrin Fe 1.5/30
30 mcg ethinyl estradiol, 0.3 mg norgestrel	Lo/Ovral
30 mcg ethinyl estradiol, 0.15 mg levonorgestrel	Levlen, Nordette
20 mcg ethinyl estradiol, 1 mg norethindrone acetate	Loestrin 21 1/20, Loestrin Fe 1/20
BIPHASIC ORAL CONTRACEPTIVES	
Phase one: 35 mcg ethinyl estradiol, 0.5 mg norethindrone; *phase two:* 35 mcg ethinyl estradiol, 1 mg norethindrone	Nelova 10/11, Ortho-Novum 10/11
TRIPHASIC ORAL CONTRACEPTIVES	
Phase one: 35 mcg ethinyl estradiol, 0.5 mg norethindrone; *phase two:* 35 mcg ethinyl estradiol, 1 mg norethindrone; *phase three:* 35 mcg ethinyl estradiol, 0.5 mg norethindrone	Tri-Norinyl
Phase one: 35 mcg ethinyl estradiol, 0.5 mg norethindrone; *phase two:* 35 mcg ethinyl estradiol, 0.75 mg norethindrone; *phase three:* 35 mcg ethinyl estradiol, 1 mg norethindrone	Ortho-Novum 7/7/7
Phase one: 30 mcg ethinyl estradiol, 0.05 mg levonorgestrel; *phase two:* 40 mcg ethinyl estradiol, 0.075 mg levonorgestrel; *phase three:* 30 mcg ethinyl estradiol, 0.125 mg levonorgestrel	Tri-Levlen, Triphasil
PROGESTIN ONLY	
0.35 mg norethindrone	Micronor, Nor-Q.D.
0.075 mg norgestrel	Ovrette

* Estrogens are listed first and progestins seconds.

creases the risk of cardiovascular side effects, such as venous and arterial thromboembolism, myocardial infarction, and thrombotic and hemorrhagic stroke. Also reported with oral contraceptive use are hepatic adenomas and tumors, visual disturbances, gallbladder disease, hypertension, and fetal abnormalities.

▶ NURSING PROCESS
THE PATIENT RECEIVING A FEMALE HORMONE

ASSESSMENT

Before the administration of an estrogen or progestin, a complete health history is obtained including a menstrual history (menarche, menstrual pattern, and any changes in the menstrual pattern including a menopause history, when applicable). In those prescribed an estrogen (including oral contraceptives), a history of thrombophlebitis or other vascular disorders, a smoking history, and a history of liver diseases are obtained. The blood pressure, pulse, and respiratory rate are also obtained. The physician usually performs a breast and pelvic examination as well as obtains a Papanicolaou (Pap) smear before starting therapy. Hepatic function tests may also be ordered.

If the male or female patient is being treated for a malignancy, a general evaluation of the patient's physical and mental status should be determined and entered in the patient's record. The physician may also order laboratory tests, such as serum electrolytes and liver function tests.

NURSING DIAGNOSIS

Depending on the patient and reason for administration, one or more of the following may apply to the patient receiving a female hormone:

▶ Anxiety related to diagnosis, other factors

▶ Noncompliance related to lack of knowledge, other factors

▶ Knowledge deficit of medication regimen, adverse drug effects

PLANNING AND IMPLEMENTATION

The major goals of the patient may include a reduction in anxiety and an understanding of and compliance to the prescribed treatment regimen.

The major goals of nursing management may include a reduction in the patient's anxiety, recognition of adverse drug effects, and the development and implementation of an effective teaching plan.

TABLE 28–1
Adverse Effects of Female Hormones

ESTROGENS

Increased risk of endometrial carcinoma, hepatic adenoma, elevated blood pressure, hypercalcemia (in those with breast cancer and bone metastases), photosensitivity, thromboembolic disease, decrease in glucose tolerance, breakthrough bleeding, changes in menstrual flow, dysmenorrhea, premenstrual-like syndrome, amenorrhea, increase in the size of uterine fibromyomas, breast tenderness, breast enlargement, nausea, vomiting, abdominal cramps, bloating, cholestatic jaundice, colitis, intolerance to contact lenses, headache, migraine, dizziness, mental depression, urticaria, pain at the injection site, changes in libido, increase or decrease in weight, edema

PROGESTINS

Breakthrough bleeding, spotting, change in the menstrual flow, amenorrhea, edema, increase or decrease in weight, cholestatic jaundice, allergic rash, acne, melasma, mental depression, breast changes (tenderness, secretion), alopecia, hirsutism, masculinization of the female fetus

NOTE

Administration of progesterone is rarely accompanied by adverse reactions.

OBSERVATIONS AND NURSING MANAGEMENT. Evaluation of drug therapy, as well as nursing management, is based on the reason for use of the female hormone.

THE OUTPATIENT. At the time of each office or clinic visit, the blood pressure, pulse, respiratory rate, and weight are obtained. The patient is also questioned regarding any adverse drug effects, as well as the result of drug therapy. For example, if the patient is receiving an estrogen for the symptoms of menopause, she is asked to compare her original symptoms with the symptoms she is currently experiencing, if any. A periodic (usually annual) physical examination is performed by the physician and may include a pelvic examination, breast examination, Pap smear, and laboratory tests. The patient with a prostatic or breast carcinoma usually requires more frequent evaluations of response to drug therapy.

THE HOSPITAL PATIENT. The following are included in a nursing care plan for the hospitalized patient receiving a female hormone:

▶ The vital signs are monitored daily or more often, depending on the patient's physical condition and the reason for drug use.

▶ Diabetic patient—The physician is notified if the urine is positive for glucose or ketone bodies because a change in the dosage of insulin or the oral hypoglycemic agent may be required.

▶ The patient is observed for adverse drug reactions, especially those related to the liver (the development of jaundice) or the cardiovascular system (thromboembolism).

▶ The patient is weighed weekly or as ordered by the physician. Any significant weight gain or loss is reported to the physician.

▶ Patients with breast carcinoma or prostatic carcinoma should observe for and evaluate signs indicating a response to therapy, for example, a relief of pain, an increase in appetite, a feeling of well-being. In prostatic carcinoma, the response to therapy may be rapid, but in breast carcinoma the response is usually slow.

▶ Postpartum breast engorgement—A breast binder may be ordered for 3 days. The breast binder is removed and reapplied every 4 hours or as needed and the patient's response to therapy is recorded.

ANXIETY. The female patient taking female hormones may have many concerns about therapy with these drugs. Some concerns may be based on inaccurate knowledge, for example, the woman who hears of incorrect facts about certain dangers associated with female hormones. Although there are dangers associated with long-term use of female hormones, many of these adverse reactions occur in a small number of patients. When the patient is closely followed by the physician, the dangers associated with long-term use are often minimized.

The patient should be given time to ask questions about her therapy. Information that is inaccurate should be clarified before therapy is started. Questions that cannot or should not be answered by a nurse are referred to the physician.

The male patient with inoperable prostatic carcinoma also may have concerns over taking a female hormone. The patient should be assured that the dosage is carefully regulated and that feminizing effects, if they occur, are usually minimal.

NONCOMPLIANCE AND KNOWLEDGE DEFICIT. The patient should have a thorough explanation of the dose regimen and adverse reactions that may be seen with the prescribed drug. Patients taking oral contraceptives should be warned that skipping a dose could result in pregnancy.

In most instances, the physician performs periodic examinations, for example, laboratory tests, pelvic examination, or a Pap smear. The patient is encouraged to keep all appointments for follow-up evaluation of therapy.

Estrogens and Progestins

▶ A patient package insert is available with the drug. Read the information carefully. If there are any questions about this information, discuss them with the physician.

▶ If GI upset occurs, take the drug with food.

▶ Notify the physician if any of the following occurs: pain in the legs or groin area, sharp chest pain or sudden shortness of breath, lumps in the breast, sudden severe headache, dizziness or fainting, vision or speech disturbances, weakness or numbness in the arms or legs, severe abdominal pain, depression, or yellowing of the skin or eyes.

▶ Female patient—If pregnancy is suspected or abnormal vaginal bleeding occurs, stop taking the drug and contact the physician immediately.

▶ Avoid exposure to sunlight or ultraviolet light because a severe skin reaction (similar to a severe sunburn) may occur. A sunscreen (sun protection factor [SPF] of 12 or above) should be worn on exposed skin surfaces when exposure to the sun is necessary.

▶ Diabetic patient—Check urine daily or more often. Contact the physician if the urine is positive for glucose or ketones because a change in diabetic medication (insulin, oral hypoglycemic agent) or diet may be necessary.

Oral Contraceptives

▶ A patient package insert is available with the drug. Read the information carefully. If there are any questions about this information, discuss them with the physician.

▶ To obtain a maximum effect, take this drug as prescribed and at intervals not exceeding once every 24 hours. An oral contraceptive is best taken with the evening meal or at bedtime. The effectiveness of this drug depends on following the prescribed dosage schedule. Failure to comply with the dosage schedule may result in a pregnancy.

▶ Use an additional method of birth control (as recommended by the physician) until after the first week in the initial cycle.

▶ If there are any questions regarding what to do should a dose be missed, discuss the procedure to be followed with the physician.

EVALUATION

▶ Anxiety is reduced

▶ Verbalizes an understanding of dosage regimen and importance of continued follow-up care

▶ Verbalizes importance of complying with the prescribed treatment regimen

29

Thyroid and Antithyroid Drugs

On completion of this chapter the student will:

▶ *Discuss the role of the thyroid gland in the regulation of physiologic processes*

▶ *Discuss the actions and uses of thyroid and antithyroid drugs*

▶ *List the signs and symptoms of iodism and iodine allergy*

▶ *List the general adverse reactions associated with the administration of thyroid and antithyroid drugs*

▶ *Use the nursing process when administering a thyroid or antithyroid drug*

▶ *Discuss the nursing implications to be considered when administering a thyroid or antithyroid drug*

The thyroid gland is located in the neck, in front of the trachea. This highly vascular gland manufactures and secretes two hormones: **thyroxine** (T_4) and **triiodothyronine** (T_3). Iodine is an essential element for the manufacture of both of these hormones.

The activity of the thyroid gland is regulated by the anterior pituitary gland hormone thyroid-stimulating hormone (TSH; see Fig. 27-1). When the level of circulating thyroid hormones decreases, the anterior pituitary secretes TSH, which then activates the cells of the thyroid to release stored thyroid hormones. This is another example of the feedback mechanism (see chap 27).

Two diseases are related to the hormone-producing activity of the thyroid gland: (1) **hypothyroidism,** which is a *decrease* in the amount of thyroid hormones manufactured and secreted, and (2) **hyperthyroidism,** which is an *increase* in the amount of thyroid hormones manufactured and secreted. The symptoms of hypothyroidism and hyperthyroidism are given in Table 29-1.

▶ THE THYROID HORMONES

▷ Actions of the Thyroid Hormones

The thyroid hormones have an influence on every organ and tissue of the body. These hormones are principally concerned with increasing the metabolic rate of tissues, which results in increases in the

TABLE 29–1
Signs and Symptoms of Thyroid Dysfunction

BODY SYSTEM OR FUNCTION	HYPOTHYROIDISM	HYPERTHYROIDISM
Metabolism	*Decreased* with anorexia, intolerance to cold, low body temperature, weight gain despite anorexia	*Increased* with increased appetite, intolerance to heat, elevated body temperature, weight loss despite increased appetite
Cardiovascular	Bradycardia, moderate hypotension	Tachycardia, moderate hypertension
Central nervous system	Lethargy, sleepiness	Nervousness, anxiety, insomnia, tremors
Skin, skin structures	Pale, cool, dry skin, face appears puffy, hair coarse, nails thick and hard	Flushed, warm, moist skin
Ovarian function	Heavy menses, may be unable to conceive, loss of fetus possible	Irregular or scant menses
Testicular function	Low sperm count	

heart and respiratory rate, body temperature, cardiac output, oxygen consumption, and the metabolism of fats, proteins, and carbohydrates. The exact mechanisms by which the thyroid hormones exert their influence on body organs and tissues is not well understood.

Thyroid hormones used in medicine include both the natural and synthetic hormones. The synthetic hormones are generally preferred because they are more uniform in potency than the natural hormones obtained from animals. Thyroid hormones are listed in Summary Drug Table 29-1.

▷ Uses of Thyroid Hormones

Thyroid hormones are used as replacement therapy when the patient is hypothyroid. By supplementing the decreased endogenous thyroid production and secretion with exogenous thyroid hormones, an attempt is made to create a *euthyroid* (normal thyroid) state.

Thyroid hormones may also be used with antithyroid drugs in the treatment of thyrotoxicosis.

▷ Adverse Reactions Associated with the Administration of Thyroid Hormones

The dose of thyroid hormones must be carefully adjusted according to the patient's hormone re-

quirements. At times, several upward or downward dosage adjustments must be made until the optimal therapeutic dosage is reached and the patient becomes euthyroid. During initial therapy, the most common adverse reactions seen are signs of overdose and hyperthyroidism (see Table 29-1). Adverse reactions other than symptoms of hyperthyroidism are rare.

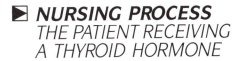 **NURSING PROCESS**
THE PATIENT RECEIVING A THYROID HORMONE

ASSESSMENT

After a diagnosis of hypothyroidism and before starting therapy, vital signs are taken and the patient is weighed. A history of the patient's signs and symptoms is obtained and a general physical assessment is performed to determine outward signs of hypothyroidism.

NURSING DIAGNOSIS

Depending on the individual and his or her symptoms, one or more of the following nursing diagnoses may apply to a person receiving a thyroid hormone:

▶ Anxiety related to diagnosis, symptoms of disorder

▶ Noncompliance related to indifference, lack of knowledge, other factors

▶ Knowledge deficit of medication regimen, adverse drug effects, treatment modalities

SUMMARY DRUG TABLE 29–2
Thyroid and Antithyroid Agents

GENERIC NAME	TRADE NAME*	USES	ADVERSE REACTIONS	DOSE RANGES
THYROID HORMONES				
levothyroxine sodium (T₄)	Levothroid, Synthroid, *generic*	Hypothyroidism, thyrotoxicosis	Symptoms of excessive dosage (hyperthyroidism); see Table 29-1	0.025–0.4 mg/d PO; 0.1–0.5 mg IV
liothyronine sodium (T₃)	Cytomel, *generic*	Same as levothyroxine	Same as levothyroxine	5–100 mcg/d PO
liotrix (T₃, T₄)	Euthroid, Thyrolar	Same as levothyroxine	Same as levothyroxine	15–30 mg/d PO and increased prn
thyroglobulin	Proloid	Same as levothyroxine	Same as levothyroxine	32–200 mg/d PO
thyroid desiccated	Armour Thyroid, *generic*	Same as levothyroxine	Same as levothyroxine	32–195 mg/d PO
ANTITHYROID PREPARATIONS				
methimazole	Tapazole	Hyperthyroidism, preparation for thyroidectomy	Agranulocytosis, headache, exfoliative dermatitis, granulocytopenia, thrombocytopenia, hepatitis, hypoprothrombinemia, jaundice, loss of hair, nausea, vomiting	5–60 mg/d PO, usually in divided doses at about 8-h intervals
propylthiouracil (PTU)	*Generic*	Same as methimazole	Same as methimazole	300–900 mg/d PO, usually in divided doses at about 8-h intervals
IODINE PRODUCTS				
strong iodine solution (Lugol's solution)	*Generic*	To prepare hyperthyroid patients for thyroid surgery	Rash, swelling of salivary glands, "iodism" (metallic taste, burning mouth and throat, sore teeth and gums, symptoms of a head cold, diarrhea, nausea), allergic reactions (fever, joint pains, swelling of parts of face and body)	2–6 drops PO tid for 10 d before surgery
sodium iodide	*Generic*	Thyrotoxicosis	Same as strong iodine solution	2 g/d IV
potassium iodide (parenteral)	*Generic*	Thyroid blocking in a radiation emergency	Same as strong iodine solution	Dosage determined by amount of radiation exposure; use and dosage directed by state or local public health authorities
potassium iodide (oral)	*Generic*	Same as potassium iodide, parenteral	Same as strong iodine solution	300–1500 mg tid PO

* The term generic *indicates that the drug is available in a generic form.*

PLANNING AND IMPLEMENTATION

The major goals of the patient may include a reduction in anxiety and an understanding of and compliance to the prescribed treatment regimen.

The major goals of nursing management may include a reduction in the patient's anxiety and the development and implementation of an effective teaching plan.

The full effects of thyroid hormone replacement therapy may not be apparent for several weeks or more but early effects may be apparent in as little as 48 hours. The vital signs are monitored daily or as ordered and the patient is observed for signs of hyperthyroidism, which is a sign of excessive drug dosage. If signs of hyperthyroidism are apparent, these are reported to the physician before the next dose is due because it may be necessary to decrease the daily dosage.

Signs of a therapeutic response include weight loss, mild diuresis, a sense of well-being, increased appetite, an increased pulse rate, an increase in mental activity, and decreased puffiness of the face, hands, and feet. If the dosage is inadequate, the patient will continue to experience signs of hypothyroidism.

Patients with diabetes mellitus are closely monitored during therapy, especially during the initial stages of dosage adjustment. The patient is observed for signs of hyperglycemia (see chap 20) and the physician is notified if this problem occurs.

ADMINISTRATION. Thyroid hormones are normally taken once a day, early in the morning and preferably before breakfast. An empty stomach increases the absorption of the oral preparation. Levothyroxine (Synthroid) can also be given intravenously (IV) and is prepared for administration immediately before use.

ANXIETY. Some patients may exhibit anxiety due to the symptoms of their disorder, as well as concern about relief of their symptoms. The patient should be reassured that although relief may not be immediate, symptoms should begin to decrease or even disappear in a few weeks.

NONCOMPLIANCE AND KNOWLEDGE DEFICIT. Thyroid hormones are usually given on an outpatient basis. The importance of taking the drug exactly as directed and not stopping the drug even though symptoms have improved should be emphasized.

The following information may be given to the patient and family when thyroid hormone replacement therapy is prescribed:

► Replacement therapy is for life (exception: transient hypothyroidism seen in those with thyroiditis).
► Do not increase, decrease, or skip a dose unless advised to do so by the physician.
► Take this drug in the morning, preferably before breakfast, unless advised by the physician to take it at a different time of day.
► Notify the physician if any of the following occur: headache, nervousness, palpitations, diarrhea, excessive sweating, heat intolerance, chest pain, increased pulse rate, or any unusual physical change or event.
► The dosage of this drug may require periodic adjustments; this is normal. Dosage changes are based on a response to therapy.
► Therapy needs to be evaluated at periodic intervals, which may vary from every 2 weeks during the beginning of therapy to every 6 to 12 months once symptoms are controlled.
► Weigh self weekly. Report any significant weight gain or loss to the physician.

EVALUATION

► Anxiety is reduced
► Verbalizes importance of complying with the prescribed treatment regimen
► Verbalizes an understanding of treatment modalities and importance of continued follow-up care
► Patient and family demonstrate understanding of drug regimen

► THE ANTITHYROID DRUGS

Hyperthyroidism may be treated with antithyroid drugs, surgical removal of some or almost all of the thyroid gland (subtotal thyroidectomy), or by the administration of radioactive iodine (^{131}I).

▷ Actions of the Antithyroid Drugs

Antithyroid drugs inhibit the manufacture of thyroid hormones. They do not affect existing thyroid hormones that are circulating in the blood or stored in the thyroid gland. They also do not interfere with exogenous thyroid hormones. Antithyroid drugs are listed in Summary Drug Table 29-1.

▷ Uses of the Antithyroid Drugs

Methimazole (Tapazole) and propylthiouracil (PTU) are used for the medical management of hyperthyroidism. Not all patients respond adequately to antithyroid drugs; therefore, a thyroidectomy may be necessary. Antithyroid drugs may also be administered before surgery in try to temporarily return the patient to a euthyroid state. When used for this reason, the vascularity of the thyroid gland is reduced and the tendency to bleed excessively during and immediately after surgery is decreased.

Strong iodine solution, also known as Lugol's solution, may be given orally with methimazole or PTU to prepare for thyroid surgery. Sodium iodide is given IV in the treatment of thyrotoxicosis, which is a state of severe hyperthyroidism and requires immediate treatment.

Potassium iodide (oral or parenteral) may be used in a radiation emergency to block the uptake of radiation by the thyroid gland. The drug is only available from state or local public health authorities. The dosage is determined by public health authorities and is based on the amount of radiation exposure.

Radioactive iodine (^{131}I) may be used for treatment of hyperthyroidism and selected cases of cancer of the thyroid. The drug is given orally either as a solution or in a gelatin capsule. Radioactive iodine has a half-life of 8.06 days.

▷ Adverse Reactions Associated with the Administration of Antithyroid Drugs

Methimazole and Propylthiouracil. The most serious adverse reaction associated with these drugs is agranulocytosis. Other major reactions include exfoliative dermatitis, granulocytopenia, thrombocytopenia, hypoprothrombinemia, and hepatitis. Minor reactions, such as nausea, vomiting, paresthesias, and skin rash may be also be seen.

Iodine Solutions.   Reactions that may be seen with strong iodine solution include symptoms of *iodism*, which are a metallic taste in the mouth, swelling and soreness of the parotid glands, burning of the mouth and throat, sore teeth and gums, symptoms of a head cold, and occasionally GI upset. Allergy to iodine may also be seen and can be serious. Symptoms of iodine allergy include swelling of parts of the face and body, fever, joint pains, and sometimes difficulty in breathing. The last problem requires immediate medical attention.

Reactions are seldom seen after the IV administration of sodium iodide; however, a marked allergic reaction to iodine may occur with swelling of the mouth, throat, and larynx, which can lead to severe respiratory difficulty and death. These symptoms may occur immediately or hours after sodium iodide is administered.

Radioactive Iodine (^{131}I).   Reactions after administration of radioactive iodine include sore throat, swelling in the neck, nausea, vomiting, cough, and pain on swallowing.

▶ NURSING PROCESS
THE PATIENT RECEIVING AN ANTITHYROID DRUG

ASSESSMENT

Before starting therapy with an antithyroid drug, a history of the symptoms of hyperthyroidism are obtained. The physical assessment includes vital signs, weight, and a notation regarding the outward symptoms of the hyperthyroidism (see Table 29-1). If the patient is prescribed an iodine solution, a careful allergy history, particularly to iodine or seafood (which contains iodine), is taken.

NURSING DIAGNOSIS

Depending on the individual, one or more of the following nursing diagnoses may apply to a person receiving an antithyroid drug:

▶ Anxiety related to symptoms of the disorder

▶ Noncompliance related to indifference, lack of knowledge, other factors

▶ Knowledge deficit of medication regimen, adverse drug effects, treatment modalities

PLANNING AND IMPLEMENTATION

The major goals of the patient may include a reduction in anxiety and an understanding of and compliance to the prescribed treatment regimen.

The major goals of nursing management may include a reduction in the patient's anxiety and the development and implementation of an effective teaching plan.

ADMINISTRATION. The patient with an enlarged thyroid gland may have difficulty swallowing the tablet. If this occurs, the problem is discussed with the physician.

Strong iodine solution is measured in drops, which are added to water or fruit juice. This drug has a strong, salty taste. The patient may experiment with various types of fruit juices to determine which one best disguises the taste of the drug.

Radioactive iodine is administered by the hospital's department of nuclear medicine.

ADVERSE DRUG REACTIONS. The patient is observed for adverse drug effects. During short-term therapy before surgery, adverse drug reactions are usually minimal. Long-term therapy is usually on an outpatient basis. The patient is questioned regarding a relief of symptoms, as well as signs or symptoms indicating an adverse reaction related to the blood cells such as fever, sore throat, easy bruising or bleeding, fever, cough, or any other signs of infection.

Once a euthyroid state is achieved, a thyroid hormone may be added to the therapeutic regimen to prevent or treat hypothyroidism, which may develop slowly during long-term antithyroid drug therapy or after administration of radioactive iodine.

When iodine solutions are administered, the patient is closely observed for symptoms of iodism and iodine allergy. If these occur, the drug is withheld and the physician is notified immediately. This is especially important if swelling around or in the mouth or difficulty in breathing occurs.

ANXIETY. The patient with hyperthyroidism may be concerned with the results of medical treatment and with the problem with taking the drug at regular intervals around the clock (usually every 8 hours). Whereas some patients may be awake early in the morning and retire late at night, others may experience difficulty in an every 8 hour dosage schedule. Another concern may be a tendency to forget the first dose early in the morning, thus, causing a problem with the two following doses.

If the patient expresses a concern about the dosage schedule, the nurse may be able to offer suggestions. For example, an 8 hour interval schedule may be suggested as 7 AM, 3 PM, and 11 PM. The nurse may also suggest pasting a notice on a bathroom mirror to remind the individual that the first dose is due immediately after rising. After a week or more of therapy, most patients remember to take their morning dose on time. If the first or last dose interferes with sleep, the nurse should suggest the patient discuss this with the physician.

NONCOMPLIANCE AND KNOWLEDGE DEFICIT. The dosage and times the drug is to be taken are reviewed with the patient and family. Additional teaching points include the following:

Methimazole and Propylthiouracil

▶ Take these drugs at regular intervals around the clock (eg, every 8 hours) unless directed otherwise by the physician.

▶ Do not take these drugs in larger doses or more frequently than as directed on the prescription container.

▶ Notify the physician promptly if any of the following occur: sore throat, fever, cough, easy bleeding or bruising, headache, or a general feeling of malaise.

▶ Record weight twice a week. Notify the physician if there is any sudden weight gain or loss. (*Note:* the physician may also want the patient to monitor pulse rate. If this is recommended, the patient needs instruction in the proper technique and a recommendation to record the pulse rate and bring the record to the physician's office or clinic).

▶ Avoid the use of nonprescription drugs unless the physician has approved the use of a specific drug.

Strong Iodine Solution

▶ Dilute the solution with water or fruit juice. Fruit juice often disguises the taste more than water does. Experiment with the types of fruit juice that best reduce the unpleasant taste of this drug.

▶ Discontinue the use of this drug and notify the physician if any of the following occur: skin rash, metallic taste in the mouth, swelling and soreness in front of the ears, sore teeth and gums, severe GI distress, or head-cold symptoms.

Radioactive Iodine

▶ Follow the directions of the department of nuclear medicine regarding precautions to be taken. (*Note:* In some instances, the dosage is small and no special precautions may be necessary).

▶ Thyroid hormone replacement therapy may be necessary.

▶ Follow-up evaluations of the thyroid gland and the effectiveness of treatment with this drug are necessary.

EVALUATION

▶ Anxiety is reduced

▶ Verbalizes an understanding of dosage regimen

▶ Verbalizes importance of complying with the prescribed treatment regimen

▶ Patient and family demonstrate understanding of drug regimen

30

Drugs Acting on the Uterus

On completion of this chapter the student will:

▶ *Discuss the actions and uses of drugs acting on the uterus*

▶ *List some of the major adverse reactions associated with the administration of drugs acting on the uterus*

▶ *Use the nursing process when administering an oxytocic drug, uterine relaxant, or abortifacient*

▶ *Discuss the nursing implications to be considered when administering an oxytocic drug, uterine relaxant, or abortifacient*

The three principal types of drugs used for their effect on the uterus are the **oxytocics,** the **uterine relaxants,** and the **abortifacients.** Drugs acting on the uterus are listed in Summary Drug Table 30-1.

▶ OXYTOCIC DRUGS

▷ Actions and Uses of Oxytocic Drugs

An oxytocic drug is one that stimulates the uterus. Included in this group of drugs are ergonovine (Ergotrate), methylergonovine (Methergine), and oxytocin (Pitocin).

Ergonovine and Methylergonovine. Ergonovine and methylergonovine both increase the strength, duration, and frequency of uterine contractions and decrease the incidence of uterine bleeding. They are given after the delivery of the placenta and are used to prevent postpartum and postabortal hemorrhage due to uterine atony (marked relaxation of the uterine muscle).

Oxytocin. Oxytocin is an endogenous hormone produced by the posterior pituitary gland (see chap 27). This hormone has uterine-stimulating properties, especially on the pregnant uterus. It also has antidiuretic and vasopressor effects. The exact role of oxytocin in normal labor and medically induced labor is not well understood.

Oxytocin is administered intravenously (IV) for starting or improving labor contractions to obtain an early vaginal delivery of the fetus. An early vaginal delivery may be used when there are fetal or

SUMMARY DRUG TABLE 30–1
Drugs Acting on the Uterus

GENERIC NAME	TRADE NAME*	USES	ADVERSE REACTIONS	DOSE RANGES
OXYTOCICS				
ergonovine maleate	Ergotrate, *generic*	Uterine atony	Nausea, vomiting, diarrhea, blood pressure elevation	0.2 mg IM, IV; 0.2–0.4 mg PO q6–12h
methyl-ergonovine maleate	Methergine	Routine management after delivery of the placenta, uterine atony and hemorrhage	Same as ergonovine maleate	0.2 mg IM, IV after delivery of the placenta; 0.2 mg PO tid, qid
oxytocin (parenteral)	Pitocin, Syntocinon, *generic*	Antepartum: to initiate or improve uterine contractions; postpartum: to produce uterine contractions in third stage of labor, control of postpartum bleeding and hemorrhage	Uterine rupture, fetal bradycardia, neonatal jaundice, anaphylactic reaction, nausea, vomiting, water intoxication, cardiac dysrhythmias	Induction of labor: 1–2 mU/min IV infusion; postpartum bleeding: IV infusion of 10–40 U in 1000 mL; 10 U IM
oxytocin, synthetic, nasal	Syntocinon	For initial milk let-down	Rare unless overdose occurs	1 spray in 1 or both nostrils
UTERINE RELAXANTS				
ritodrine hydrochloride	Yutopar	Preterm labor	Alterations in fetal and maternal heart rates and maternal blood pressure, palpitations, headache, nausea, vomiting	IV: 0.1 mg/min and increased depending on patient response; PO: 10–20 mg q2–6h
ABORTIFACIENTS				
carboprost tromethamine	Prostin/15 M	Termination of pregnancy	Nausea, vomiting, diarrhea, headache, paresthesia, perforated uterus or cervix	Initially: 250 mcg IM; subsequent doses of 250–500 mcg may be necessary
dinoprostone (prostaglandin E₂)	Prostin E2	Same as carboprost	Vomiting, diarrhea, nausea, headache, hypotension, chills	1 suppository high into vagina; may be repeated
sodium chloride 20%	*Generic*	Same as carboprost	Fever, flushing, fluid overload, pulmonary embolus, changes in the coagulation mechanism	Up to 250 mL by transabdominal intraamniotic instillation

* The term generic indicates that the drug is available in a generic form.

maternal problems, for example, a diabetic mother with a large fetus, Rh problems, premature rupture of the membranes, uterine inertia, and eclampsia or preeclampsia at or near term. Oxytocin may also be used in the management of inevitable or incomplete abortion.

Oxytocin may be given intramuscularly (IM) during the third stage of labor to produce uterine contractions and control postpartum bleeding and hemorrhage. It may also be used topically as a nasal spray to stimulate the milk ejection (milk letdown) reflex.

▷ Adverse Reactions Associated with Oxytocic Drugs

Ergonovine and Methylergonovine. The adverse reactions associated with ergonovine and methylergonovine include nausea, vomiting, diarrhea, elevated blood pressure, temporary chest pain, dizziness, and headache. Allergic reactions may also be seen.

Oxytocin. Administration of oxytocin may result in fetal bradycardia, uterine rupture, neonatal jaundice, nausea, vomiting, water intoxication (fluid overload, fluid volume excess), cardiac dysrhythmias, and anaphylactic reactions. When used as a nasal spray, adverse reactions are rare. Occasionally, abdominal cramping may be noted.

▶ NURSING PROCESS
THE PATIENT RECEIVING AN OXYTOCIC DRUG

ASSESSMENT

Before starting an IV infusion of oxytocin, an obstetric history (parity, gravidity, previous obstetric problems, type of labor, stillbirths, abortions, live birth infant abnormalities, and so forth) and a general health history are obtained.

When the patient is to receive ergonovine or methylergonovine, the blood pressure, pulse, and respiratory rate should be taken before administration of either of these drugs.

The fetal heart rate (FHR) and the mother's blood pressure, pulse, and respiratory rate are obtained immediately before starting an IV infusion of oxytocin for the induction of labor. In addition, the activity of the uterus (strength, duration, and frequency of contractions, if any) is recorded on a flow sheet.

NURSING DIAGNOSIS

Depending on the drug and reason for use, one or more of the following may apply to the patient receiving an oxytocic drug:

▶ Anxiety related to labor and delivery

▶ Fluid volume excess related to rapid administration of IV fluids containing oxytocin

▶ Knowledge deficit of treatment regimen

PLANNING AND IMPLEMENTATION

The major goals of the patient may include a reduction in anxiety, absence of a fluid volume excess (oxytocin administration), and an understanding of the treatment regimen.

The major goals of nursing management may include a reduction in the patient's anxiety, absence of a fluid volume excess (oxytocin administration), and a thorough explanation of the treatment regimen.

ERGONOVINE AND METHYLERGONOVINE. Ergonovine and methylergonovine are administered in the delivery room at the direction of the physician. Ergonovine is usually given during the third stage of labor after the placenta has been delivered. Methylergonovine is usu-

ally given at the time of the delivery of the anterior shoulder or after the delivery of the placenta. The mother's blood pressure, pulse, and respiratory rate are taken immediately before the drug is administered.

After injection of the drug, the blood pressure, pulse, and respiratory rate are monitored at the intervals ordered by the physician. After leaving the delivery room, the uterine fundus is palpated for firmness and position. Any excess bleeding is reported to the physician immediately.

Ergonovine and methylergonovine may also be given orally during the postpartum period to reduce the possibility of postpartum hemorrhage and prevent relaxation of the uterus. The vital signs are monitored every 4 hours. The patient may complain of abdominal cramping with the administration of these drugs. If cramping is moderately severe to severe, the physician is notified because it may be necessary to discontinue the medication.

OXYTOCIN. When oxytocin is prescribed, the physician orders the type and amount of IV fluid, the number of units of oxytocin added to the IV solution, and the initial IV infusion rate. Usually IV piggyback is used so that the infusion bottle containing oxytocin may be attached to the primary IV line, which is used to keep the vein open (KVO) when it is necessary to interrupt the infusion of oxytocin. An IV infusion pump is recommended for exact delivery of the IV solution containing oxytocin.

The physician establishes guidelines for the administration of the oxytocin solution and for increasing or decreasing the flow rate or discontinuing administration of oxytocin. Usually, the flow rate is increased every 15 minutes but this may vary according to the patient's response.

All patients receiving IV oxytocin must be under constant observation to identify complications. The patient's blood pressure, pulse, and respiratory rate and the FHR are monitored every 15 minutes or as ordered by the physician. Each uterine contraction is monitored and described on a flow sheet.

The physician is notified immediately if any of the following occurs:

▶ Any significant change in the FHR or rhythm

▶ Any marked change in the frequency, rate, or rhythm of uterine contractions: uterine contractions lasting more than 60 seconds or contractions occurring more frequently than every 2 to 3 minutes

▶ A marked increase or decrease in the patient's blood pressure or pulse or any significant change in the patient's general condition.

If any of the above are noted, the oxytocin infusion

is immediately discontinued and the primary IV line is run at KVO until the physician examines the patient.

Oxytocin may be given IM after delivery of the placenta. The blood pressure, pulse, and respiratory rate are obtained immediately before and every 5 to 10 minutes after the drug is administered. The fundus of the uterus is palpated for a response to the drug.

When administering oxytocin topically, the patient is placed in an upright position, and, with the squeeze bottle held upright, the prescribed number of sprays are delivered to one or both nostrils. The patient then waits 2 to 3 minutes before nursing the infant or pumping the breasts. If a breast pump is being used, the amount of milk pumped from the breasts is recorded. When the infant is being breastfed, the amount of milk produced during feeding is evaluated by the nurse and the patient.

The physician is notified if milk drips from the breast before or after nursing, if milk drips from the breast not being nursed, or if abdominal cramps occur during nursing, because the drug may need to be discontinued.

FLUID VOLUME EXCESS. When oxytocin is administered IV, there is a danger of a fluid volume excess because oxytocin has an antidiuretic effect. The intake and output are measured. In some instances, it may be necessary to measure the output hourly. The patient is also observed for signs of fluid overload (see chap 17). If these are apparent, the physician is notified *immediately* because it may be necessary to change the rate of infusion or discontinue the use of oxytocin.

ANXIETY AND KNOWLEDGE DEFICIT. When ergonovine or methylergonovine are administered in the delivery room, the purpose of the injection is briefly explained to the patient. If either of these drugs is given after delivery of the infant, the purpose of the drug, for example, to improve the tone of the uterus and help the uterus to return to its (near) normal size, is explained to the patient.

The patient receiving oxytocin to induce labor may have concern over the use of the drug to produce contractions. The purpose of the IV infusion and the results expected are explained to the patient. Since the patient receiving oxytocin must be closely supervised, spending time with the patient and offering encouragement and reassurance may help reduce anxiety.

EVALUATION

▶ Anxiety is reduced
▶ No evidence of a fluid volume excess (oxytocin administration)
▶ Patient demonstrates understanding of treatment

▶ UTERINE RELAXANTS

▷ Actions and Uses of Uterine Relaxants

Ritodrine (Yutopar) has an effect on beta-adrenergic receptors, principally those that innervate the uterus. Stimulation of these beta-adrenergic receptors inhibits uterine smooth muscle contractions. This drug is used in the management of preterm (or premature) labor. Ritodrine administration initially requires hospitalization. If treatment is successful, the patient may continue to take the drug orally at home.

▷ Adverse Reactions Associated with the Administration of Uterine Relaxants

Alterations in fetal and maternal heart rates and maternal blood pressure frequently occur when ritodrine is administered IV. Additional frequent adverse reactions associated with IV administration include nausea, vomiting, headache, palpitations, and erythema. Oral administration frequently produces a slight increase in the maternal heart rate. Palpitations, tremors, nausea, and vomiting also are seen in a small number of patients.

▶ NURSING PROCESS
THE PATIENT RECEIVING A UTERINE RELAXANT

ASSESSMENT

Before starting an IV infusion containing ritodrine, the patient's vital signs and the FHR are obtained.

NURSING DIAGNOSIS

▶ Anxiety related to preterm labor
▶ Knowledge deficit of treatment regimen

PLANNING AND IMPLEMENTATION

The major goals of the patient may include a reduction in anxiety and an understanding of the treatment of preterm labor.

The major goals of nursing management may include a reduction in the patient's anxiety and a thorough explanation of the treatment for preterm labor.

ADMINISTRATION. The IV solution is prepared by adding the prescribed dosage of ritodrine to 500 mL of the IV fluid ordered by the physician. A controlled infusion pump is recommended to control the rate of flow. A microdrip chamber is also recommended because it provides a convenient range of infusion rates. Ritodrine can be piggybacked to a primary line, with the primary line used to run the infusion at KVO should it be necessary to temporarily discontinue the ritodrine infusion. The patient is placed in a left lateral position, unless the physician orders a different position, after insertion of the IV line.

The following tasks are performed at 15- to 30-minute intervals:

▶ Blood pressure, pulse, and respiratory rate are obtained.

▶ FHR is obtained.

▶ The IV infusion rate is checked.

▶ The area around the IV needle insertion is examined for signs of extravasation.

▶ Uterine contractions (frequency, intensity, length) are monitored.

The physician is kept informed of the patient's response to the drug because a dosage change may be necessary. The physician establishes guidelines for the regulation of the IV infusion rate, as well as the blood pressure and pulse ranges that require stopping the IV infusion. The IV infusion is usually continued for at least 12 hours after uterine contractions have ceased.

Oral maintenance therapy is begun approximately 30 minutes before the IV infusion is discontinued. The patient may then be discharged from the hospital in 1 or more days and oral ritodrine therapy continued at home.

ANXIETY AND KNOWLEDGE DEFICIT. The patient in preterm labor may have many concerns about her pregnancy, as well as the effectiveness of drug therapy. The nurse can help the patient by offering emotional support and encouragement during the time the drug is being administered.

The treatment regimen is explained to the patient. The physician usually discusses the expected outcome of treatment with the patient.

The following instructions may be given to the patient taking oral ritodrine at home:

▶ Take the drug exactly as prescribed.

▶ Do not use any nonprescription drugs unless their use has been approved by the physician.

▶ Notify the physician immediately if any of the following occur: uterine contractions, nausea, vomiting, palpitations, or shortness of breath.

▶ Frequent examinations are necessary to monitor therapy.

EVALUATION

▶ Anxiety is reduced

▶ Demonstrates understanding of in-hospital treatment

▶ Demonstrates understanding of dosage regimen to be followed at home

▶ Verbalizes understanding of when to notify the physician if problems occur after discharge from the hospital

▶ ABORTIFACIENTS

Abortifacients are drugs that are used to abort or terminate a pregnancy. Administration of these drugs is one of several methods, such as a hysterotomy or dilation and curettage, that may be used to terminate a pregnancy. The method that is selected to terminate a pregnancy is individualized and is based on many factors, such as the health of the patient, the length of pregnancy, and the facilities available.

▷ Actions of the Abortifacients

Carboprost (Prostin/15 M) and dinoprostone (Prostin E2) are prostaglandins (fatty acid derivatives whose release is thought to increase the sensitivity of peripheral pain receptors), which stimulate the uterus to contract. By stimulating uterine contractions, the uterus is emptied of the products of pregnancy, that is, the fetus, the placenta, and the amniotic fluid. The manner in which each of these drugs stimulate the uterine muscle is not well understood.

Sodium chloride 20% is injected into the amniotic fluid and produces death of the fetus. The fetus is then expelled.

▷ Uses of the Abortifacients

Carboprost. Carboprost is given IM and is used to abort the fetus between the 13th and 20th weeks of pregnancy.

Dinoprostone. Dinoprostone is administered intravaginally and is used to abort the fetus between the 12th and 20th weeks of pregnancy.

Sodium Chloride 20%. Sodium chloride is administered transabdominally into the amniotic fluid. This procedure is performed by the physician. It is used to abort the fetus during the second trimester of pregnancy, preferably between the 16th and 22nd weeks of pregnancy.

▷ Adverse Reactions Associated with Administration of the Abortifacients

Carboprost. Adverse drug reactions to carboprost are usually temporary and disappear when therapy is completed. Adverse reactions include vomiting, diarrhea, nausea, headache, paresthesia, flushing, chills, and sweating. Rupture of the uterus has been reported.

Dinoprostone. After administration of dinoprostone, the most frequent adverse reactions seen are nausea, vomiting, hypotension, diarrhea, chills, and headache. Fever, joint inflammation and pain, and tightness in the chest may also be seen.

Sodium Chloride 20%. Accidental injection of the sodium chloride solution into the vascular system may occur when this drug is given. Additional adverse reactions include fever, flushing, fluid overload, pulmonary embolus, and changes in the blood coagulating mechanism.

▶ NURSING PROCESS
THE PATIENT RECEIVING AN ABORTIFACIENT

ASSESSMENT

Before the administration of an abortifacient, the patient's vital signs are taken. Some hospitals or clinics performing this procedure may also have additional assessments that are required before the procedure is begun.

NURSING DIAGNOSIS

▶ Anxiety related to procedure
▶ Knowledge deficit of abortion procedure

PLANNING AND IMPLEMENTATION

The major goals of the patient may include a reduction in anxiety and an understanding of the abortion procedure.

The major goals of nursing management may include a reduction in the patient's anxiety and a thorough and effective explanation of the abortion procedure.

ADMINISTRATION. When carboprost is to be used, the physician may order an antiemetic or an antidiarrheal agent before administration of carboprost. A tuberculin syringe is used to measure and administer this drug. Carboprost is given deep IM and injection sites are rotated if more than one injection is necessary.

Dinoprostone is administered as a vaginal suppository. The suppository is removed from the freezer and allowed to reach room temperature before insertion. The foil wrapper must be carefully removed from the suppository; contact with the fingers is avoided. The patient is placed in a supine position. Wearing a glove, the physician inserts the suppository high into the vagina. The patient should remain in the supine position for about 10 minutes after insertion of the suppository. The physician may allow ambulation after that time.

Sodium chloride is administered by the physician. About 250 mL is instilled into the amniotic sac by means of a transabdominal incision. The nurse is responsible for obtaining the necessary equipment for the procedure.

After administration of an abortifacient, the patient is observed for the onset of uterine contractions every 30 minutes to 1 hour. The time of the onset of labor, the length and intensity of each contraction, and the time interval between contractions are recorded on a flow sheet. The blood pressure, pulse, and respiratory rate are monitored every 1 to 4 hours or according to unit policy or the physician's orders.

The physician is notified if adverse drug reactions occur and is kept informed of the patient's response to the abortifacient. All tissue expelled is saved for examination either by the physician or by a laboratory. A vaginal examination may be performed by the physician after the fetus is passed.

ANXIETY. The procedure to be performed is thoroughly explained to the patient. The physician or the nurse should also explain some of the adverse reactions that may occur during and after the procedure.

Emotional support is needed before, during, and after the administration of an abortifacient. Many patients require reassurance and understanding; the amount depends on the individual.

KNOWLEDGE DEFICIT. The amount of time spent in a hospital or clinic after the administration of an abortifacient varies. In addition, the instructions given to the patient about the passage of the fetus and postabortion examination also vary. Some hospitals or clinics may allow the patient to leave the facility and return when uterine contractions begin. The postdischarge instructions given to the patient are usually established by the facility performing the procedure or by a physician. The nurse should advise the patient to follow the instructions given by the physician or facility.

EVALUATION

► Anxiety is reduced

► Verbalizes understanding of the abortion procedure

► Verbalizes understanding of the postprocedure directions given by the physician

31

Antineoplastic Drugs

On completion of this chapter the student will:

▶ *List the types of drugs used in the treatment of neoplastic diseases*

▶ *List the general adverse reactions associated with the administration of the antineoplastic drugs*

▶ *Use the nursing process when administering an antineoplastic drug*

▶ *Discuss the nursing implications to be considered when administering an antineoplastic drug*

Antineoplastic drugs are agents used in the treatment of malignant diseases. Although these drugs may not always effect a complete cure of the malignancy, they often slow the rate of tumor growth and delay metastasis. Use of these drugs is one of the tools in the treatment of cancer. The term *chemotherapy* is often used to refer to therapy with antineoplastic drugs.

The antineoplastic drugs covered in this chapter include the **alkylating agents, antibiotics, antimetabolites, hormones, mitotic inhibitors, and miscellaneous drugs.**

▷ Actions of Antineoplastic Drugs

Generally, most antineoplastic drugs affect cells that rapidly proliferate (divide and reproduce). Neoplasms, or cancerous tumors, usually consist of rapidly proliferating cells. The normal cells that line the oral cavity and gastrointestinal (GI) tract, and cells of the gonads, bone marrow, hair follicles, and lymph tissue are also rapidly dividing cells and are usually affected by these drugs. Thus, antineoplastic drugs may affect normal, as well as malignant, (neoplastic) cells.

Alkylating Agents.   Alkylating agents interfere with the process of cell division of malignant and normal cells. The malignant cells appear to be more susceptible to the effects of the alkylating agents. Examples of alkylating agents include mechlorethamine (Mustargen) and chlorambucil (Leukeran).

Antibiotics.   The antibiotics, unlike their antibiotic relatives, do not have antiinfective (against infection) ability. They appear to interfere with DNA and RNA synthesis, and therefore delay or inhibit cell division, including the reproducing ability of malignant cells. Examples of antineoplastic antibiotics include bleomycin (Blenoxane) and doxorubicin (Adriamycin).

Antimetabolites.   The antimetabolites interfere with various metabolic functions of cells, thereby disrupting normal cell functions. These drugs are most effective in the treatment of rapidly dividing neoplastic cells. Examples of the antimetabolites include methotrexate (Folex) and fluorouracil (Adrucil).

Hormones. The exact method of antineoplastic action of hormones is unclear. These drugs also appear to counteract the effect of male or female hormones in hormone-dependent tumors (see chap 28). Examples of hormones used as neoplastic agents include testolactone (Teslac), an androgen, polyestradiol (Estradurin), an estrogen, and megestrol (Megace), a progestin.

Gonadotropin-releasing hormone analogues, for example, leuprolide (Lupron), appear to act by inhibiting the anterior pituitary secretion of gonadotropins, thus suppressing the release of pituitary gonadotropins. These drugs primarily decrease serum testosterone levels and therefore are used in the treatment of advanced prostatic carcinomas.

Mitotic Inhibitors. Mitotic inhibitors interfere with or stop cell division. Examples of mitotic inhibitors include etoposide (VePesid) and vincristine (Oncovin).

Miscellaneous Antineoplastic Agents. The mechanism of action of this unrelated group of drugs is not entirely clear. Examples of miscellaneous antineoplastics include interferon Alpha-2a (Roferon-A) and hydroxyurea (Hydrea).

▷ Uses of Antineoplastic Drugs

Antineoplastic drugs may be given alone or in combination with other antineoplastic drugs. In many instances, a combination of these drugs produces better results than the use of a single antineoplastic agent.

Although many antineoplastic drugs share a similar activity (ie, they interfere in some way with cell division), their uses are not necessarily similar. The more common uses of specific antineoplastic drugs are given in Summary Drug Table 31-1.

▷ Adverse Reactions Associated with the Administration of Antineoplastic Drugs

Antineoplastic drugs often produce a wide variety of adverse reactions. Some of these reactions are dose dependent, that is, their occurrence is more common or their intensity is more severe when higher doses are used. Other adverse reactions occur primarily because of the effect the drug has on many cells of the body.

Some adverse reactions are desirable, for example, the depressing effect of certain antineoplastic drugs on the bone marrow because this adverse drug reaction is essential in the treatment of the leukemias. Other adverse reactions are not desirable, for example, severe vomiting or diarrhea.

Antineoplastic drugs are potentially toxic and their administration is often associated with many serious adverse reactions. At times, it is necessary to allow some of these adverse effects to occur because the only alternative is to stop treatment of the malignancy. What can be done is to develop a treatment plan that will prevent, lessen, or treat, most or all of the symptoms of a specific adverse reaction. An example of prevention is the giving of an antiemetic before administration of an antineoplastic drug known to cause severe nausea and vomiting. An example of treatment of the symptoms of an adverse reaction is the administration of an antiemetic, as well as intravenous (IV) fluids and electrolytes when severe vomiting occurs.

Adverse reactions seen with the administration of these drugs may range from very mild to life-threatening. Some of these reactions, such as the loss of hair (alopecia), may have little effect on the physical status of the patient but may definitely have a serious effect on the patient's mental health. Because nursing is concerned with the whole patient, some of these physically altering reactions can have a profound effect on the patient and must be considered when planning nursing management.

Some of the adverse reactions seen with antineoplastic agents are listed in Summary Drug Table 31-1. Appropriate references should be consulted when administering these drugs because there are a variety of uses, dose ranges, and, in some instances, many adverse reactions.

► NURSING PROCESS
THE PATIENT RECEIVING AN ANTINEOPLASTIC DRUG

ASSESSMENT

The extent of assessment depends on the type of malignancy and the patient's general physical condition.

The initial assessment of the patient scheduled for chemotherapy may include the following:

▶ The type and location of the neoplastic lesion (as stated on the patient's chart)

SUMMARY DRUG TABLE 31–1
Antineoplastic Drugs

GENERIC NAME	TRADE NAME*	USES	ADVERSE REACTIONS	DOSE RANGES†
ALKYLATING AGENTS				
busulfan	Myleran	Chronic myelogenous leukemia	Leukopenia, anemia, cataracts, hyperpigmentation of skin, thrombocytopenia	1–8 mg/d PO
carboplatin	Paraplatin	Ovarian carcinoma	Bone marrow suppression, pain, nausea, vomiting, diarrhea, electrolyte changes	360 mg/m² IV; smaller doses may be used when there is renal insufficiency or hematologic changes
carmustine	BiCNU	Brain tumors, multiple myeloma, Hodgkin's disease	Thrombocytopenia, burning at injection site, nausea, vomiting, azotemia, leukopenia	100–200 mg/m² IV
chlorambucil	Leukeran	Chronic lymphocytic leukemia, malignant lymphomas, Hodgkin's disease	Bone marrow depression, hyperuricemia, nausea, vomiting, diarrhea, hepatotoxicity	0.03–0.2 mg/kg/d PO
cisplatin	Platinol	Metastatic testicular and ovarian tumors, advanced bladder cancer	Nephrotoxicity, ototoxicity, marked nausea and vomiting, leukopenia, thrombocytopenia, hyperuricemia	Testicular tumors: 20 mg/m² IV; ovarian tumors: 50 mg/m² IV; bladder cancer: 50–70 mg/m² IV
cyclophosphamide	Cytoxan, Neosar	Malignant lymphomas, Hodgkin's disease, multiple myeloma, leukemia, carcinoma of the ovary and breast, neuroblastoma, retinoblastoma	Leukopenia, thrombocytopenia, anemia, anorexia, nausea, vomiting, diarrhea, cystitis, alopecia	Initial dose: 40–50 mg/kg IV; maintenance doses: 1–5 mg/kg/d PO; 3–15 mg/kg IV
ifosfamide	Ifex	Testicular cancer	Hemorrhagic cystitis, mental confusion, coma, alopecia, nausea, vomiting	1.2 g/m²/d IV
lomustine	CeeNu	Brain tumors, Hodgkin's disease	Nausea, vomiting, thrombocytopenia, leukopenia, alopecia, anemia	100–130 mg/m² PO
mechlorethamine hydrochloride	Mustargen	Hodgkin's disease, lymphosarcoma, bronchogenic carcinoma, leukemia	Nausea, vomiting, jaundice, alopecia, lymphocytopenia, granulocytopenia, thrombocytopenia, skin rash, diarrhea	0.4 mg/kg IV as a total dose for a course of therapy which may be given as a single or divided dose
melphalan	Alkeran	Multiple myeloma, carcinoma of the ovary	Nausea, vomiting, bone marrow depression, skin rash, alopecia	6–10 mg/d PO; dosage may also be based on weight
pipobroman	Vercyte	Polycythemia vera, chronic granulocytic leukemia	Nausea, vomiting, abdominal cramping, diarrhea, rash	1–3 mg/kg/d PO
streptozocin	Zanosar	Carcinoma of the pancreas	Renal toxicity, severe nausea and vomiting, diarrhea	500–1000 mg/m² IV depending on dosage intervals
thiotepa (tri-ethylenethiophosphoramide)	*Generic*	Carcinoma of the breast, ovary, Hodgkin's, lymphosarcomas, intracavity effusions due to localized metastatic diseases	Nausea, vomiting, pain at injection site, bone marrow depression	0.3–0.4 mg/kg IV; dosage is higher for intracavity or intratumor administration
uracil mustard	*Generic*	Chronic lymphocytic or myelogenous leukemia, non-Hodgkin's lymphomas	Bone marrow depression, nausea, vomiting, diarrhea	Adults: 0.15 mg/kg PO as a single weekly dose

(continued)

SUMMARY DRUG TABLE 31–1
(continued)

GENERIC NAME	TRADE NAME*	USES	ADVERSE REACTIONS	DOSE RANGES
ANTIBIOTICS				
bleomycin sulfate	Blenoxane	Carcinoma of the head and neck, lymphomas, testicular carcinoma	Pneumonitis, pulmonary fibrosis, erythema, rash, fever, chills, vomiting	0.25–0.5 U/kg IV, IM, SC
dactinomycin	Cosmegen	Wilms' tumor, choriocarcinoma, Ewing's sarcoma, testicular carcinoma	Anorexia, alopecia, bone marrow depression, nausea, vomiting	Up to 15 mcg/kg/d IV; may also be given by isolation perfusion at 0.035–0.05 mg/kg
daunorubicin hydrochloride	Cerubidine	Leukemia	Bone marrow depression, alopecia, acute nausea and vomiting, fever, chills	25–45 mg/m²/d IV
doxorubicin hydrochloride	Adriamycin	Acute leukemias, neuroblastoma, soft tissue and bone sarcomas, carcinomas of the breast, ovary, bladder, lymphomas, Wilms' tumor	Alopecia, acute nausea and vomiting, mucositis, chills, bone marrow depression, fever	30–75 mg/m² IV
mitomycin	Mutamycin	Adenocarcinoma of the stomach, pancreas	Bone marrow depression, anorexia, nausea, vomiting, headache, blurred vision, fever	20 mg/m² IV
mitoxantrone hydrochloride	Novantrone	Leukemia	CHF, GI bleeding, jaundice, nausea, vomiting, diarrhea, infections, dyspnea, headache, conjunctivitis, stomatitis	12 mg/m²/d IV infusion
plicamycin (mithramycin)	Mithracin	Malignant tumors of the testes, hypercalcemia and hypercalciuria associated with neoplasms	Hemorrhagic syndrome (epistaxis, hematemesis, widespread hemorrhage in the GI tract, generalized advanced bleeding), vomiting, diarrhea, anorexia, nausea, stomatitis	Testicular tumors: 25–30 mcg/kg/d IV; hypercalcemia, hypercalciuria: 25 mcg/kg/d IV for 3–4 d
ANTIMETABOLITES				
cytarabine	Cytosar-U	Acute myelocytic or lymphocytic leukemia	Bone marrow depression, nausea, vomiting, diarrhea, anorexia	100–200 mg/m²/d IV, SC
floxuridine	FUDR	GI adenocarcinoma metastatic to the liver	Diarrhea, anorexia, nausea, vomiting, alopecia, bone marrow depression	0.1–0.6 mg/kg/d by arterial infusion
fluorouracil (5-FU)	Adrucil, *generic*	Carcinoma of the breast, stomach, pancreas, colon	Same as floxuridine	3–12 mg/kg/d IV
mercaptopurine (6-mercaptopurine, 6-MP)	Purinethol	Acute lymphatic leukemia, acute or chronic myelogenous leukemia	Bone marrow depression, hyperuricemia, hepatotoxicity	1.5–2.5 mg/kg/d PO
methotrexate (MTX)	Folex, *generic*	Lymphosarcoma, severe psoriasis, cancer of the head, neck, breast, lung	Ulcerative stomatitis, nausea, rash, pruritus, renal failure, bone marrow depression, fatigue, fever, chills	Antineoplastic dosages vary widely depending on type of tumor; psoriasis: 10–50 mg/wk IV, IM, PO or up to 6.5 mg/d PO
thioguanine	*Generic*	Acute leukemias, chronic myelogenous leukemia	Bone marrow depression, hepatic toxicity, nausea, vomiting, stomatitis, hyperuricemia	2–3 mg/kg/d PO

(continued)

SUMMARY DRUG TABLE 31–1
(continued)

GENERIC NAME	TRADE NAME*	USES	ADVERSE REACTIONS	DOSE RANGES
HORMONES				
ANDROGENS				
fluoxy-mesterone	Halotestin, *generic*	Inoperable breast carcinoma	Virilization, amenorrhea, menstrual irregularities	10–40 mg/d PO in divided doses
methyltestos-terone	Android-10, *generic*	Breast carcinoma	Same as fluoxymesterone	200 mg/d PO
testolactone	Teslac	Breast cancer in post-menopausal women or pre-menopausal women when ovarian function has been terminated	Glossitis, anorexia, pares-thesia, hypertension, nau-sea, vomiting	250 mg PO qid
testosterone (aqueous suspension)	Andro 100, *generic*	Breast carcinoma	Same as fluoxymesterone	50–100 mg IM 3 times/wk
testosterone cypionate	Depo-Testos-terone, *generic*	Breast carcinoma	Same as fluoxymesterone	200–400 mg IM every 2–4 wk
ANTIANDROGEN				
flutamide	Eulexin	Metastatic prostate car-cinoma	Hot flashes, loss of libido, diarrhea, nausea, vomit-ing, impotence	250 mg PO tid at 8-h inter-vals
ANABOLIC STEROIDS				
nandrolone phenpropionate	Androlone, *generic*	Control of metastatic breast carcinoma	Nausea, vomiting, diarrhea, virilization, fluid and elec-trolyte imbalance	50–100 mg/wk IM
ESTROGENS				
chlorotrianisene	TACE	Prostatic carcinoma	Females: see Table 28-1; males: testicular atrophy, impotence, feminization of the genitalia, plus the ad-verse reactions in Table 28-1 except those per-taining to the female re-productive system	12–25 mg/d PO
conjugated estrogens, oral	Premarin, *generic*	Breast and prostatic car-cinoma	Same as chlorotrianisene	Breast carcinoma: 10 mg PO tid; prostatic carcinoma: 1.25–2.5 mg PO tid
diethylstil-bestrol (DES)	*Generic*	Breast and prostatic car-cinoma	Same as chlorotrianisene	Breast carcinoma: up to 15 mg/d PO; prostatic car-cinoma: 1–3 mg/d PO
diethylstil-bestrol diphos-phate	Stilphostrol	Inoperable prostatic car-cinoma	Same as chlorotrianisene	50–200 mg or more PO tid; drug may also be given IV
estradiol	Estrace	Breast and prostatic car-cinoma	Same as chlorotrianisene	Breast carcinoma: 10 mg PO tid; prostatic carcinoma: 1–2 mg PO tid
estramustine phosphate so-dium (estradiol and nonnitrogn mustard)	EMCYT	Metastatic or progressive prostatic carcinoma	Nausea, diarrhea, anorexia, fluid retention, increased risk of thrombosis, leukopenia, rash, throm-bopenia	14 mg/kg/d PO in 3–4 di-vided doses
ethinyl estradiol	Estinyl	Breast and prostatic car-cinoma	Same as chlorotrianisene	Breast carcinoma: 1 mg PO tid; prostatic carcinoma: 0.15–2 mg/d PO

(continued)

SUMMARY DRUG TABLE 31–1
(continued)

GENERIC NAME	TRADE NAME*	USES	ADVERSE REACTIONS	DOSE RANGES
polyestradiol phosphate	Estradurin	Prostatic carcinoma	Same as chlorotrianisene	40 mg IM
ANTIESTROGEN				
tamoxifen citrate	Nolvadex	Breast carcinoma in menopausal women	Hypercalcemia, ophthalmic changes, hot flashes, nausea, vomiting	10–20 mg PO bid
PROGESTINS				
medroxyprogesterone acetate	Depo-Provera	Endometrial or renal carcinoma	Breast tenderness, pruritus, thromboembolitic phenomena	400–1000 mg/wk IM
megestrol acetate	Megace	Advanced carcinoma of the breast, endometrium	Carpel tunnel syndrome, alopecia, deep vein thrombosis	Breast carcinoma: 40 mg PO qid; endometrial carcinoma: 40–320 mg/d PO in divided doses
GONADOTROPIN-RELEASING HORMONE ANALOGUE				
leuprolide acetate	Lupron	Advanced prostatic carcinoma	Edema, headache, dizziness, bone pain, nausea, vomiting, anorexia, ECG changes, hypertension	1 mg/d SC in divided doses
goserelin acetate	Zoladex	Same as leuprolide	Hot flashes, sexual dysfunction, lethargy, edema	3.6 mg SC every 28 d
MITOTIC INHIBITORS				
etoposide	VePesid	Testicular tumors, small cell lung cancer	Nausea, vomiting, anorexia, granulocytopenia, alopecia	Testicular cancer: 50–100 mg/m² IV; lung cancer: 35 mg/m² IV, oral dose is twice the IV dose
vinblastine sulfate (VLB)	Velban, *generic*	Hodgkin's disease, lymphoma, testicular carcinoma, Kaposi's sarcoma	Leukopenia, nausea, vomiting, paresthesias, malaise, weakness, mental depression, headache	3.7–18.5 mg/m²/wk IV
vincristine sulfate (VCR)	Oncovin, *generic*	Acute leukemia, lymphosarcoma, neuroblastoma, Wilms' tumor, Hodgkin's disease	Ataxia, headache, oral ulceration, vomiting, weight loss, fever, diarrhea	1.4 mg/m²/wk IV
MISCELLANEOUS ANTINEOPLASTIC DRUGS				
asparaginase	Elspar	Leukemia	Hypersensitivity reactions (rash, urticaria, arthralgia, respiratory distress, acute anaphylaxis), depression, somnolence, fatigue, coma, anorexia, nausea, vomiting	200–1000 IU/kg/d IV; 6000 IU/m²/d IM
dacarbazine	DTIC-Dome	Melanoma, Hodgkin's disease	Anorexia, nausea, vomiting	Melanoma: 2–4.5 mg/kg IV or 250 mg/m² IV; Hodgkin's: 150–375 mg/m² IV
hydroxyurea	Hydrea	Melanoma, leukemia, carcinoma of the ovary	Bone marrow depression, stomatitis, anorexia, nausea, vomiting, diarrhea, headache	20–80 mg/kg PO

(continued)

SUMMARY DRUG TABLE 31–1
(continued)

GENERIC NAME	TRADE NAME*	USES	ADVERSE REACTIONS	DOSE RANGES
MISCELLANEOUS ANTINEOPLASTIC DRUGS				
interferon alpha-2a	Roferon-A	AIDS-related Kaposi's sarcoma, hairy-cell leukemia	Fever, fatigue, myalgia, headache, chills, anorexia, nausea, diarrhea, vomiting, dizziness, cough, dyspnea, abdominal pain	Leukemia: 3 million IU per dose SC, IM; Kaposi's sarcoma: 36 million IU SC, IM per dose
interferon alpha-2b	Intron A	Same as interferon alpha-2a	Similar to interferon alpha-2a	Leukemia: 2 million IU/m^2 per dose SC, IM; Kaposi's sarcoma: 30 million IU/m^2 per dose IM, SC
mitotane	Lysodren	Adrenocortical carcinoma	Anorexia, nausea, vomiting, diarrhea, skin rash	2–10 g/d PO in divided doses
procarbazine hydrochloride	Matulane	Hodgkin's disease	Leukopenia, anemia, thrombocytopenia, nausea, vomiting, anorexia	1–6 mg/kg PO

* The term generic *indicates that the drug is available in a generic form.*
† *Dosages for some patients may vary from the dose ranges given here because dosages often depend on the stage of the tumor, the use of other antineoplastic drugs, and other factors. The frequency of administration may also be variable.*

▶ The stage of the disease; for example, early, metastatic, terminal

▶ The patient's general physical condition

▶ The patient's emotional response to his or her disease

▶ The anxiety or fears the patient may have regarding chemotherapy treatments

▶ Previous or concurrent treatments (if any), such as surgery, radiation therapy, other antineoplastic drugs

▶ Other current nonmalignant disease or disorder, for example, congestive heart failure or peptic ulcer, that may or may not be related to the malignant disease

▶ The patient's knowledge or understanding of the proposed chemotherapy regimen

▶ Other factors such as the patient's age, financial problems that may be associated with a long-term illness, family cooperation and interest in the patient, the adequacy of health insurance coverage (which may be of great concern to the patient), and so on

Immediately before administration of the first dose of an antineoplastic drug, the vital signs are taken. The patient is also weighed because the dose of some antineoplastic drugs is based on the patient's weight in kilograms or pounds. The dosages of some antineoplastic drugs also may be based on body surface measurements and are stated as a specific amount of drug per square meter (m^2) of body surface. Additional physical assessments may be necessary for certain antineoplastic agents.

A few antineoplastic agents require treatment measures before administration of the antineoplastic drug. An example of preadministration treatment is hydration of the patient with 1 to 2 liters of IV fluid infused before administration of cisplatin (Platinol), or administration of an antiemetic before the administration of mechlorethamine. These measures are ordered by the physician and, in some instances, may vary slightly from the manufacturer's recommendations.

When an antineoplastic drug has a depressing effect on the bone marrow, laboratory tests, such as a complete blood count (CBC), are ordered to determine the effect of the previous drug dosage. Before administration of the first dose of the drug, pretreatment laboratory tests provide baseline data for future reference. All laboratory tests are to be recorded on the patient's chart and the physician is to be notified of their results before the administration of successive doses of an antineoplastic agent. If these tests indicate a severe depressant effect on the bone marrow or other test abnormalities, the physician may reduce the next drug dose or temporarily stop chemotherapy to allow the affected body systems to recover.

NURSING DIAGNOSIS

The nursing diagnoses for the patient with a malignancy is usually extensive and should be based on many factors such as the patient's physical and emotional condition, the adverse reactions resulting from antineoplastic drug therapy, and the stage of the disease. The two diagnoses listed below apply only to the drug or drugs being administered and do not cover other possible areas that also may be added, for example, a high risk for a fluid volume deficit due to prolonged vomiting secondary to an adverse drug reaction, altered oral mucous membranes due to an adverse drug reaction, or anticipatory grieving.

▶ Anxiety related to diagnosis, necessary treatment measures, the occurrence of adverse reactions, other factors
▶ Knowledge deficit of treatment regimen, adverse reactions, dosage regimen

PLANNING AND IMPLEMENTATION

The major goals of the patient may include a reduction in anxiety and an understanding of the prescribed treatment modalities.

The major goals of nursing management may include a reduction in the patient's anxiety and the development and implementation of an effective teaching plan.

Management of the patient receiving an antineoplastic drug varies and often depends on factors such as the drug or combination of drugs given, the dosage of the drugs, the patient's physical response to therapy, the response of the tumor to chemotherapy, and the type and severity of adverse reactions.

In some hospitals, policies have been established to provide nursing personnel with specific guidelines for the assessment and management of patients receiving a single or combination chemotherapeutic drug regimen. If guidelines are not provided, the nurse should first review the drugs being given. Appropriate references should be consulted to obtain information regarding the preparation and administration of a particular drug, the average dose ranges, all the known adverse reactions, and the warnings and precautions given by the manufacturer.

ANXIETY. Patients and family members are usually devastated by the diagnosis of a malignancy. The emotional impact of the disease may be forgotten or put aside by members of the medical team as they plan and institute therapy to control the disease. Patients undergoing chemotherapy require a great deal of emotional support from all members of the medical team. Kindness and gentleness in giving care and an understanding of the strain placed on the patient and the family may help reduce some of the fear and anxiety experienced during treatment.

PREPARING AN ANTINEOPLASTIC DRUG FOR ADMINISTRATION. Although some of these drugs are given orally, others are given by the parenteral route. It is *most important* to follow the manufacturer's or physician's directions regarding the type of solution to be used for dilution or administration. For example, when carmustine (BiCNU) is prepared for administration, the manufacturer warns that only the diluent supplied with the drug is to be used for the first step in diluting the drug.

When preparing an antineoplastic drug for parenteral administration, the nurse must wear disposable plastic gloves. It has been shown that some of these drugs can be absorbed through the skin of the individual preparing these drugs. Because antineoplastic agents are highly toxic and can have an effect on many organs and systems of the body, the nurse must use measures to prevent absorption of the drug through the skin. Precautions are also taken to prevent accidental spilling or spraying of the drug into the eyes or onto unprotected areas of the skin. The hands must be thoroughly washed before and after preparing and administering an antineoplastic agent. This is especially important when the drug is given by the parenteral route.

Special directions for administration, stated by either the physician or manufacturer, are also important. For example, cisplatin cannot be prepared or administered with needles or IV administration sets containing aluminum because aluminum reacts with cisplatin, causing a precipitate formation and loss of potency.

ADMINISTRATION OF AN ANTINEOPLASTIC DRUG. Some antineoplastic agents have specific recommended administration techniques. For example, an infusion pump is recommended for the administration of cisplatin; lomustine (CeeNu) is given orally on an empty stomach; and plicamycin (Mithracin) is administered by slow IV infusion over 4 to 6 hours. If administration guidelines are not provided by the physician or the hospital, it is the nurse's responsibility to check with the appropriate authorities (physician, pharmacist) regarding the administration of a specific antineoplastic agent.

The package insert supplied with the drug should be read thoroughly before the drug is prepared and administered. The manufacturer's recommendations may include information such as storage of the drug, reconstitution procedures, stability of the drug after reconstitution, the rate of administration, the technique of administration, and so on.

POSTADMINISTRATION MANAGEMENT. After the administration of an antineoplastic agent, the planning of nursing management is based on the following:

▶ The patient's general condition

- The patient's individual response to the drug
- Adverse reactions that may occur
- Guidelines established by the physician or hospital
- Results of periodic laboratory tests

THE PATIENT'S GENERAL CONDITION. The patient who is acutely ill with many physical problems requires different nursing management than one who is ambulating and able to participate in the activities of daily living. Once the patient's general condition is assessed and his or her needs identified, a nursing care plan is developed to meet those needs. Patients receiving chemotherapy can be at different stages of their disease; therefore, nursing management of each patient must be individualized and not necessarily based on the type of drug administered.

THE PATIENT'S INDIVIDUAL RESPONSE TO THE DRUG. Not all patients respond in the same manner to a specific antineoplastic drug. For example, an antineoplastic agent may cause vomiting but the amount of fluid and electrolytes lost through vomiting may vary from patient to patient. One patient may require additional sips of water once nausea and vomiting has subsided, whereas another may require IV fluid and electrolyte replacement. Nursing management is not only geared to what may or what did happen, but is also based on the effects produced by a particular adverse reaction. In the example of the patient who is vomiting, it is important to accurately measure all fluid intake and all output from the GI and urinary tracts, as well as to observe the patient for signs of dehydration and electrolyte imbalances. These measurements and observations aid the physician in determining if fluid replacement is necessary.

ADVERSE DRUG REACTIONS. Knowing what adverse reactions may occur allows the nurse to prepare for any event that will happen. For example, a hemorrhagic syndrome may be seen with the administration of plicamycin. Knowing this, the nurse incorporates the assessments for hemorrhage in the nursing care plan. Another example is the development of hyperuricemia (elevated blood uric acid levels), which may be seen with drugs such as melphalan (Alkeran) or mercaptopurine (Purinethol). When this adverse reaction is known to occur, the nursing care plan must include intake and output measurements, as well as encourage a fluid intake of at least 2000 mL of oral fluid per day.

In some instances, the patient may need to be told what will happen. For example, if hair loss is associated with the antineoplastic drug being given, the patient must be told that hair loss may possibly occur. Depending on the patient, plans may need to be made in advance for the purchase of a wig or cap to disguise the hair loss until the hair grows back. Although this may

seem to be a minor problem when compared to the serious reactions that may be seen during chemotherapy, the loss of hair *is* a personal problem for most patients and requires as much nursing consideration as a serious or life-threatening situation.

GUIDELINES ESTABLISHED BY THE PHYSICIAN OR HOSPITAL. During chemotherapy, the physician may write orders for certain nursing procedures such as measuring intake and output, monitoring the vital signs at specific intervals, increasing the fluid intake to a certain amount, and so on. Even when orders are written, the nurse may increase the frequency of certain assessments, such as monitoring vital signs, if the patient's condition changes.

Some hospitals have written guidelines for nursing management when the patient is receiving a specific antineoplastic agent. These guidelines are incorporated into the nursing care plan with nursing observations and assessments geared to the individual patient. The nurse adds assessments to the nursing care plan when there has been a change in the patient's condition.

RESULTS OF PERIODIC LABORATORY TESTS. There are different types of laboratory tests that may be used to monitor the patient's response to therapy. Some of these tests, for example, a CBC, may be used to determine the response of the bone marrow to an antineoplastic agent. Other tests, for example, liver function tests, may be used to detect liver toxicity, which may be an adverse reaction that can be seen with the administration of some of these drugs. All recent laboratory tests are reviewed at the time they are reported. All significant changes or abnormal results are reported to the physician immediately because it may be necessary to treat the abnormal situation, temporarily stop chemotherapy, or change the dosage regimen.

Abnormal laboratory tests may also require a change in the nursing care plan. For example, a significant drop in the platelet count may result in bleeding episodes and will require measures, such as prolonged pressure on injection sites, to prevent bleeding or bruising episodes.

IMPORTANT POINTS TO REMEMBER. Antineoplastic drugs are potentially toxic agents that can cause a variety of effects during and after their administration. The following general areas should be considered when an antineoplastic drug is administered:

- Great care and accuracy are important in preparing and administering these drugs.
- Disposable plastic gloves are worn when preparing any of these drugs for parenteral administration.
- The patient is closely observed before, during, and after the administration of an antineoplastic drug.

▶ Nursing assessment, nursing diagnoses, and nursing care plans should be continually updated to meet the changing needs of the patient.

▶ The physician must be notified of all changes in the patient's general condition, the appearance of adverse reactions, and changes in laboratory test results.

▶ The patient and his or her family require physical *and* emotional support during treatment.

KNOWLEDGE DEFICIT. When the patient is hospitalized, all treatments and possible adverse effects should be explained to the patient before the initiation of therapy. The physician usually discusses the proposed treatment and possible adverse drug reactions with the patient and family members. The nurse can briefly review the physician's explanations immediately before parenteral administration of a drug.

Some of these drugs are taken orally at home. The areas included in a patient and family teaching plan for this type of treatment regimen is based on the drug prescribed, the physician's explanation of the chemotherapy regimen, the physician's instructions for taking the drug, and the needs of the individual patient. Some hospitals or physicians give printed instructions to the patient. These instructions are reviewed after they have been read by the patient, then time is allowed for the patient or family member to ask questions. The patient has a right to know the dangers associated with these drugs and what adverse reactions may occur.

Some patients are given antineoplastic drugs in a physician's office or outpatient clinic. Before the institution of therapy, the treatment regimen is thoroughly explained to the patient and family. In some instances, a medication to prevent nausea may be prescribed to be taken before administration of the drugs in the physician's office or clinic. To obtain the best possible effects, the patient must understand that the drug must be taken at the time specified by the physician.

The following points may be included in a patient and family teaching plan when oral therapy is prescribed:

▶ Take the drug only as directed on the prescription container. Follow specific directions, such as "take on an empty stomach" or "take at the same time each day"; they are extremely important.

▶ *Never* increase, decrease, or omit a dose unless advised to do so by the physician.

▶ If *any* problems (adverse reactions) occur, no matter how minor, contact the physician immediately.

▶ *All* recommendations given by the physician, such as increasing the fluid intake or eating or avoiding certain foods are important. The effectiveness or action of the drug could be altered if these directions are ignored. Other recommendations, such as checking the mouth for sores, rinsing the mouth thoroughly after eating or drinking, or drinking extra fluids are given to identify or minimize some of the effects these drugs have on the body. It is important that these recommendations be followed.

▶ Keep all appointments for chemotherapy. These drugs must be given at certain intervals to be effective.

▶ Do not take *any* nonprescription drug unless the use of a specific drug has been approved by the physician.

▶ Avoid drinking alcoholic beverages unless the physician approves of their use.

▶ Always inform other physicians, dentists, and other medical personnel of therapy with this drug.

▶ Keep all appointments for the laboratory tests ordered by the physician. If unable to keep a laboratory appointment, notify the physician immediately.

EVALUATION

▶ Anxiety is reduced

▶ Verbalizes understanding of dosage regimen

▶ Verbalizes an understanding of treatment modalities and importance of continued follow-up care

▶ Adverse reactions are identified and reported to the physician

▶ Verbalizes importance of complying with the prescribed treatment regimen

32

Anticonvulsant Drugs

On completion of this chapter the student will:

▶ *Describe the general drug action of anticonvulsant drugs*

▶ *List some of the adverse reactions associated with the administration of anticonvulsant drugs*

▶ *Use the nursing process when administering an anticonvulsant drug*

▶ *Discuss the nursing implications to be considered when administering an anticonvulsant drug*

The terms *convulsion* and *seizure* are often used interchangeably and basically have the same meaning. A seizure may be defined as a periodic attack of disturbed cerebral function. A seizure may also be described as an abnormal disturbance in the electrical activity in one or more areas of the brain. Examples of seizure (or convulsive) disorders include grand mal, petit mal, and focal seizures. Each different type of seizure disorder is characterized by a specific pattern of events, as well as a different pattern of motor or sensory manifestations. Examples of the manifestations of some seizure disorders include alternate contraction and relaxation of muscles, a loss of consciousness, and abnormal behavior.

Seizure disorders are generally classified as idiopathic or acquired. Idiopathic seizures have no known cause; acquired seizure disorders have a known cause. The causes of acquired seizures include high fever, electrolyte imbalances, uremia, hypoglycemia, hypoxia, brain tumors, and some drug withdrawal reactions. Once the cause is removed (if it can be removed), the seizures theoretically cease.

Epilepsy may be defined as a permanent, recurrent seizure disorder. Examples of the known causes of epilepsy include brain injury at birth, head injuries, and inborn errors of metabolism. In some patients, the cause of epilepsy is never determined.

Drugs used for the management of convulsive disorders are called *anticonvulsants*. Most anticonvulsants have specific uses, that is, they are of value only in the treatment of certain types of seizure disorders.

The types of anticonvulsants included in this chapter are the **barbiturates,** the **benzodiazepines,** the **hydantoins,** the **oxazolidinediones,** the **succinimides,** and **miscellaneous anticonvulsant preparations.**

▷ Actions of the Anticonvulsant Drugs

Generally, the anticonvulsants reduce the excitability of the neurons (nerve cells) of the brain. When neuron excitability is decreased, the seizures are theoretically reduced in intensity and frequency of occurrence or, in some instances, are virtually eliminated. For some patients, only partial control of the seizure disorder may be obtained with anticonvulsant drug therapy.

▷ Uses of the Anticonvulsant Drugs

The more common types of seizures responding to a specific anticonvulsant drug are given in Summary Drug Table 32-1. In some cases, the patient does not respond well to one drug, and another drug or a combination of anticonvulsant drugs must be tried. Dosage increases and decreases are often necessary during the initial period of treatment. Dosage adjustment may also be necessary during times of stress, severe illness, or when other drugs are being taken for treatment of conditions other than a seizure disorder. There also may be undetermined circumstances that require a dosage adjustment or change in the anticonvulsant drug.

▷ Adverse Reactions Associated with Administration of Anticonvulsant Drugs

The Barbiturates

The most common adverse reaction associated with mephobarbital (Mebaral) and phenobarbital is sedation, which can range from mild sleepiness or drowsiness to somnolence. These drugs may also cause nausea, vomiting, constipation, bradycardia, hypoventilation, skin rash, headache, fever, and diarrhea. Agitation, rather than sedation, may occur in some patients. Some of these adverse effects may be reduced or eliminated as therapy continues. Occasionally, a slight dosage reduction, without reducing the ability of the drug to control the seizures, will reduce or eliminate some of these adverse reactions.

The Benzodiazepines

As with the barbiturates, the most common adverse reaction seen with the use of clonazapam (Klonopin), clorazepate (Tranxene), and diazepam (Valium) is sedation in varying degrees. Additional adverse effects may include anorexia, constipation, or diarrhea. Some adverse reactions are dose-dependent, whereas others may diminish in intensity or cause few problems after several weeks of therapy.

The Hydantoins

Many adverse reactions are associated with the use of ethotoin (Peganone), mephenytoin (Mesantoin), and phenytoin (Dilantin). The adverse reactions most often seen are related to the central nervous system and include nystagmus, ataxia, slurred speech, and mental confusion. Other adverse reactions that may be seen include various types of skin rashes, nausea, vomiting, gingival hyperplasia (overgrowth of gum tissue), hematologic changes, and hepatotoxicity.

The Oxazolidinediones

Paramethadione (Paradione) and trimethadione (Tridione) administration may result in hematologic changes such as pancytopenia, leukopenia, aplastic anemia, and thrombocytopenia. Also reported are various types of skin rashes, diplopia, vomiting, changes in blood pressure, and fatal nephrosis.

The Succinimides

Gastrointestinal symptoms occur frequently with the administration of ethosuximide (Zarontin), methsuximide (Celontin Kapseals), and phensuximide (Milontin Kapseals). Mental confusion and other personality changes, pruritus, urticaria, urinary frequency, weight loss, and hematologic changes may also be seen.

Miscellaneous Anticonvulsant Drugs

The adverse reactions seen with the various miscellaneous anticonvulsants are given in Summary Drug Table 31-1.

▶ NURSING PROCESS
THE PATIENT RECEIVING AN ANTICONVULSANT DRUG

ASSESSMENT

Seizures that occur in the outpatient are almost always seen first by family members or friends rather than by a member of the medical profession. It is the abnormal behavior pattern or the convulsive movements that causes the patient to visit the physician's office or a neurologic clinic. Therefore, a thorough patient history

SUMMARY DRUG TABLE 32–1
Anticonvulsants

GENERIC NAME	TRADE NAME*	USES	ADVERSE REACTIONS	DOSE RANGES
BARBITURATES				
mephobarbital	Mebaral	Tonic-clonic (grand mal) epilepsy, absence seizures (petit mal)	Somnolence, agitation, nausea, vomiting, constipation, bradycardia, headache, fever, diarrhea, hypoventilation, rash, drowsiness	Adults: 400–600 mg/d PO; children: 16–64 mg/d PO
phenobarbital	*Generic*	Status epilepticus, generalized tonic-clonic and cortical focal seizures	Same as mephobarbital	Adults: 50–100 mg PO bid, tid; children: 15–50 mg PO bid, tid
phenobarbital sodium	*Generic*	Symptomatic control of acute convulsions	Same as mephobarbital	Adults: 120–800 mg IV, IM per dose with a maximum of 1–2 g/24 h; children: 6–20 mg/kg IV with a maximum of 40 mg/kg/24 h
BENZODIAZEPINES				
clonazepam	Klonopin	Absence seizures; variant, akinetic, and myoclonic seizures	Drowsiness, depression, lethargy, apathy, diarrhea, constipation, dry mouth, bradycardia, tachycardia, fatigue, visual disturbances, urticaria, anorexia, rash, pruritus	Adults: 1.5–20 mg/d PO; children: 0.05–0.2 mg/kg/d PO in divided doses
clorazepate dipotassium	Tranxene, *generic*	Partial seizures	Same as clonazepam	Adults: up to 90 mg/d PO in divided doses; children: up to 60 mg/d PO in divided doses
diazepam	Valium, *generic*	Adjunct in treatment of convulsive disorders	Same as clonazepam	Adults: 2–10 mg PO bid to qid; children: 1–2.5 mg PO tid, qid
HYDANTOINS				
ethotoin	Peganone	Tonic-clonic, psychomotor seizures	Nystagmus, ataxia, mental confusion, thrombocytopenia, leukopenia, agranulocytosis, pancytopenia, granulocytopenia, slurred speech, nausea, vomiting, rash, gingival hyperplasia, hepatotoxicity	Adults: initial—1 g/d or less PO in 4–6 divided doses; maintenance—2–3 g/d PO; children: initial—up to 750 mg/d PO in 4–6 divided doses; maintenance—500 mg–3 g/d PO in divided doses
mephenytoin	Mesantoin	Tonic-clonic, jacksonian, psychomotor, focal seizures	Same as ethotoin	Adults: 200–800 mg/d PO; children: 100–400 mg/d PO
phenytoin	Dilantin	Tonic-clonic, psychomotor seizures	Same as ethotoin	Adults: 100–600 mg/d PO in divided doses; children: 4–8 mg/kg/d PO in divided doses
phenytoin sodium, extended	Dilantin Kapseals, *generic*	Same as phenytoin	Same as ethotoin	300 mg PO taken once a day
phenytoin sodium, parenteral	Dilantin, *generic*	Status epilepticus of grand mal type, prevention and treatment of seizures during neurosurgery	Same as ethotoin	Status epilepticus: 150–250 mg IV; neurosurgery: 100–200 mg IM q4h

(continued)

SUMMARY DRUG TABLE 32–1
(continued)

GENERIC NAME	TRADE NAME*	USES	ADVERSE REACTIONS	DOSE RANGES
OXAZOLIDINEDIONES				
paramethadione	Paradione	Absence seizures	Aplastic anemia, nephrosis, rash, diplopia, vomiting, hematologic changes, changes in blood pressure	Adults: 900 mg–2.4 g/d PO in 3–4 divided doses; children: 300–900 mg/d PO in 3–4 divided doses
trimethadione	Tridione	Same as paramethadione	Same as paramethadione	Same as paramethadione
SUCCINIMIDES				
ethosuximide	Zarontin	Absence seizures	Nausea, vomiting, gastric cramps, anorexia, confusion, pruritus, urinary frequency, weight loss, hematologic changes, urticaria	Adults: 500 mg/d PO; children: up to 20 mg/kg/d PO
methsuximide	Celontin Kapseals	Same as ethosuximide	Same as ethosuximide	300 mg–1.2 g/d PO
phensuximide	Milontin	Same as ethosuximide	Same as ethosuximide	1–3 g/d PO in divided doses
MISCELLANEOUS PREPARATIONS				
acetazolamide	Diamox, *generic*	Absence, unlocalized seizures	Paresthesias, fever, rash, crystalluria, acidotic state, anorexia, nausea, vomiting	8–30 mg/kg/d PO in divided doses
carbamazepine	Tegretol, *generic*	Partial seizures, tonic-clonic seizures, mixed seizure patterns	Dizziness, drowsiness, nausea, vomiting, aplastic anemia, and other blood cell abnormalities	200–1600 mg/d PO in divided doses
magnesium sulfate	*Generic*	Prevention and control of seizures in preeclampsia or eclampsia and convulsions associated with epilepsy and other disorders	High magnesium blood levels with flushing, sweating, depressed reflexes, hypotension, cardiac and CNS depression	1–5 g of 25–50% solution IM; 1–4 g of 10–20% solution IV; 4 g in 250 mL of 5% dextrose by IV infusion
phenacemide	Phenurone	Severe epilepsy	GI disturbances, headache, drowsiness, dizziness, insomnia, weight loss	Adults: 2–3 g/d PO in divided doses; starting dose may be lower; children: 1/2 the adult dose
primidone	Mysoline, *generic*	Psychomotor, focal, tonic-clonic seizures	Ataxia, vertigo, nausea, anorexia, vomiting	Adults: 100–250 mg PO 1–4 times/d; children: 50–250 mg PO 1–3 times/d
valproic acid	Depakene, *generic*	Simple and complex absence seizures, multiple seizure types	Nausea, vomiting, sedative effects, rash, indigestion	15–60 mg/kg/d PO in single or divided doses

* The term generic *indicates that the drug is available in a generic form.*

is necessary to identify the type of seizure disorder. Information obtained from those who have observed the seizure should include the following:

▶ A description of the seizures (the motor or psychic activity occurring during the seizure)

▶ The frequency of the seizures (approximate number per day)

▶ The average length of the seizure

▶ A description of an aura, if any has occurred

▶ A description of the degree of impairment of consciousness

▶ What, if anything, appears to bring on the seizure

Additional patient information should include a family history of seizures (if any) and recent drug therapy (all drugs being presently used). Depending on the type of seizure disorder, other information may also be needed; for example, a history of a head injury or a through medical history.

Vital signs are taken at the time of the initial assessment to provide baseline data. The physician may order many laboratory and diagnostic tests, such as an electroencephalogram (EEG), computed tomographic (CT) scan, complete blood count (CBC), and hepatic and renal function tests to confirm the diagnosis and identify a possible cause of the seizure disorder, as well as provide a baseline during therapy with anticonvulsant drugs.

NURSING DIAGNOSIS

Depending on the patient and type of seizure disorder, one or more of the following nursing diagnoses may apply to a person receiving an anticonvulsant drug:

▶ Anxiety related to diagnosis, lifetime medication, other factors

▶ High risk for injury related to seizure disorder, adverse drug reactions (drowsiness, ataxia)

▶ Altered oral mucous membranes related to adverse drug reactions (hydantoins)

▶ Noncompliance related to indifference, lack of knowledge, other factors

▶ Knowledge deficit of medication regimen, adverse drug effects

PLANNING AND IMPLEMENTATION

The major goals of the patient may include a reduction in anxiety, absence of injury, normal oral mucous membranes, and an understanding of and compliance to the prescribed treatment regimen.

The major goals of nursing management may include a reduction in the patient's anxiety, prevention of injury, effective oral care, and the development and implementation of an effective teaching plan.

The dosage of the anticonvulsant may require frequent adjustments during the initial treatment period. Dosage adjustments are based on the patient's response to therapy (eg, the control of the seizures), as well as the occurrence of adverse reactions. It may also be necessary to add a second anticonvulsant to the therapeutic regimen or change from one anticonvulsant to another depending on the patient's response to therapy.

When a hospitalized patient is receiving an anticonvulsant, the most important observations made by the nurse are related to the patient's seizures, as well as response to drug therapy. Each seizure must be carefully documented with regard to the time of occurrence, the length of the seizure, and the psychic or motor activity occurring before, during, and after the seizure. Most seizures occur without warning and the nurse may not see the patient until the seizure begins or after the seizure is over. Any observations made during and after the seizure the seizure are important and may aid in the diagnosis of the type of seizure, as well as assist the physician in evaluating the effectiveness of drug therapy.

The vital signs are monitored daily or as ordered. The patient is observed for adverse drug reactions, which are reported to the physician.

It is *most important* that patients receive their anticonvulsant drug and that there is no accidental or intentional (except by order of the physician) omission of a dose. An abrupt interruption in therapy may result in a recurrence of the seizures. In some instances, abrupt withdrawal of an anticonvulsant can result in status epilepticus, which is a state of continuous seizures that can become life-threatening. Continuity of anticonvulsant administration can be aided by making a notation on the Kardex, as well as by informing all health team members of the importance of the medication.

ADMINISTRATION. To prevent gastric upset, oral anticonvulsant drugs may be given with food or soon after eating. Oral suspensions must be shaken well before measuring. Caution is used when giving an oral preparation if the patient appears drowsy because aspiration of the tablet, capsule, or liquid may occur. The swallowing ability of the patient can be tested by offering *small* sips of water before giving the drug. The drug should be withheld and the physician notified as soon as possible if the patient has difficulty in swallowing because a different route of administration may be necessary.

ANXIETY. The patient and family members are often distressed when epilepsy is first diagnosed. In addition, the development of a seizure disorder due to a known cause, for example, uremia, also is distressing to the patient and family.

Patients and their family need time to adjust to the diagnosis, as well as the opportunity to discuss treatment, expected results of treatment, and long-term management (epilepsy).

ALTERED ORAL MUCOUS MEMBRANES. Long-term administration of the hydantoins can cause gingivitis and gingival hyperplasia (overgrowth of gum tissue). Patients in a hospital or long-term clinical setting and receiving one of these drugs require periodic inspection of their teeth and gums. Any changes in the gums or teeth are reported to the physician. These patients also should receive oral care after each meal.

HIGH RISK FOR INJURY. Drowsiness is common, especially early in therapy. The patient should be assisted with all ambulatory activities. Precautions are taken to prevent falls and other injuries until seizures are controlled by medication. Injury may also occur when the patient has a seizure.

NONCOMPLIANCE AND KNOWLEDGE DEFICIT. If the patient is diagnosed as having epilepsy, the patient and family may need understanding and assistance in adjusting to the diagnosis.

Family members will require instruction in the care of the patient before, during, and after a seizure. The importance of restricting some activities until the seizures are controlled by medication is explained. What activities require restriction often depend on the age, sex, and occupation of the patient. For example, the mother with a seizure disorder and a newborn infant is advised to have help when caring for her child. Another example is the carpenter would be warned about climbing ladders or using power tools. For some patients, the restriction of activities may create a problem with employment, management of the home environment, caring for children, and so on. If a problem is recognized, the patient may need referral to a social service worker, discharge planning coordinator, or public health nurse.

The adverse drug reactions associated with the prescribed anticonvulsant should be reviewed with the patient and family members. The patient and family members are instructed to contact the physician before the next dose of the drug is due, if any adverse reactions occur. If adverse reactions occur, the drug must not be stopped until the patient or a family member discusses this problem with the physician.

Some patients, once their seizures are under control (eg, stop occurring or occur less frequently), may have a tendency to abruptly stop their medication or begin to occasionally omit a dose. It is most important that the patient and the family understand that the medication must *never* be abruptly discontinued or doses be omitted. If the patient experiences drowsiness during initial therapy, a family member should be responsible for administration of the medication.

The following points may be included in a patient and family teaching plan:

▶ Do *not* omit, increase, or decrease the prescribed dose.

▶ Never abruptly discontinue this drug except when recommended by the physician.

▶ If the physician finds it necessary to stop the drug, another drug usually is prescribed and should be started immediately, for example, at the time the next dose of the previous drug was due.

▶ This drug may cause drowsiness or dizziness. Observe caution when performing hazardous tasks.

▶ Avoid the use of alcohol unless use has been approved by the physician.

▶ Carry identification, such as Medic-Alert, indicating medication use and the type of seizure disorder.

▶ Do *not* use *any* nonprescription drug unless use of a specific drug has been approved by the physician.

▶ Inform the dentist and other physicians of use of this drug.

▶ Brush and floss the teeth after each meal and make periodic dental appointments for oral examination and care. (Note: this should be emphasized when the hydantoins are prescribed.)

▶ Keep a record of all seizures (date, time, length), as well as any minor problems (such as drowsiness, dizziness, lethargy, and so on) and bring this information to each clinic or office visit.

▶ Contact the local branches of agencies such as the Epilepsy Foundation of America for information and assistance with problems such as legal matters, insurance, driver's license, low cost prescription services, and job training or retraining.

EVALUATION

▶ Anxiety is reduced

▶ No evidence of injury

▶ Oral mucous membranes appear normal

▶ Verbalizes importance of complying with the prescribed treatment regimen

▶ Verbalizes an understanding of treatment modalities and importance of continued follow-up care

▶ Patient and family demonstrate understanding of drug regimen

33

Antiparkinsonism Drugs

On completion of this chapter the student will:

▶ *Define the terms* Parkinson's disease *and* parkinsonism

▶ *List the major adverse reactions associated with the administration of antiparkinsonism drugs*

▶ *Use the nursing process when administering an antiparkinsonism drug*

▶ *Discuss the nursing implications to be considered when administering an antiparkinsonism drug*

Parkinson's disease, also called paralysis agitans, is thought to be due to a deficiency of dopamine and an excess of acetylcholine within the central nervous system (CNS). This disease is characterized by fine tremors, and rigidity of some muscle groups and weakness of others. As the disease progresses, speech becomes slurred. There is a masklike and emotionless expression of the face and the patient may have difficulty chewing and swallowing. The patient may have a shuffling and unsteady gait and the upper part of the body is bent forward.

Parkinsonism is a term that refers to the symptoms of Parkinson's disease, as well as the Parkinson-like symptoms that may be seen with the use of certain drugs, head injuries, encephalitis, and so on.

▷ Actions of Antiparkinsonism Drugs

Levodopa (Larodopa). The symptoms of parkinsonism are due to a depletion of dopamine in the CNS. Dopamine, when given orally, does not cross the blood–brain barrier, and therefore is ineffective. Levodopa, the metabolic precursor of dopamine, does cross the blood–brain barrier and is then converted to dopamine.

Carbidopa (Lodosyn). Carbidopa is used with levodopa and has no effect when given alone. Administration of carbidopa with levodopa makes more levodopa available to cross the blood–brain barrier, thus reducing the dosage of levodopa.

Drugs with Anticholinergic Activity. Drugs with anticholinergic activity inhibit acetylcholine (which is produced in excess in Parkinson's disease) in the CNS. Drugs with anticholinergic activity are generally less effective than levodopa. Examples of drugs with anticholinergic activity include procyclidine (Kemadrin) and trihexyphenidyl (Artane).

Amantadine (Symmetrel) and Selegiline (Eldepryl). The mechanism of action of these drugs in the treatment of parkinsonism is not fully understood.

▷ Uses of Antiparkinsonism Drugs

As the term indicates, antiparkinsonism drugs are used in the treatment of parkinsonism. As with some other types of drugs, it may be necessary to change from one antiparkinsonism drug to another or to increase or decrease the dosage until maximum response is obtained (Summary Drug Table 33-1). Carbidopa is always given with levodopa, either as one medication or as two separate drugs. When it is necessary to titrate the dose of carbidopa, both carbidopa and levodopa may be given *at the same time* but as separate drugs. Selegiline is given to those being treated with carbidopa and levodopa but who have had a decreased response to therapy with these two drugs. Amantadine is also used as an antiviral agent (see chap 26).

▷ Adverse Reactions Associated with the Administration of Antiparkinsonism Drugs

Levodopa. The most serious and frequent adverse reactions seen with levodopa include choreiform and dystonic movements. Less frequent, but serious, reactions include mental changes such as depression, psychotic episodes, paranoia, and suicidal tendencies. Frequent and less serious adverse reactions include anorexia, nausea, vomiting, abdominal pain, dry mouth, difficulty in swallowing, increased hand tremor, headache, and dizziness.

Carbidopa. In recommended doses, carbidopa has no drug activity unless it is given with levodopa. The only adverse reactions seen with this drug are those seen with levodopa.

Drugs with Anticholinergic Activity. Frequently seen adverse reactions to drugs with anticholinergic activity include dry mouth, blurred vision, dizziness, mild nausea, and nervousness. These may become less pronounced as therapy progresses. Other adverse reactions that may be seen include skin rash, urticaria, urinary retention, dysuria, tachycardia, muscle weakness, disorientation, and confusion. If any of these reactions are severe, the drug may be discontinued for several days and restarted at a lower dosage or a different antiparkinsonism agent may be prescribed.

Amantadine. The most frequent serious adverse reactions to amantadine are depression, congestive heart failure, orthostatic hypotension, psychosis, urinary retention, convulsions, leukopenia, and neutropenia. Less serious reactions include hallucinations, confusion, anxiety, anorexia, nausea, and constipation. This drug may be given alone or in combination with an antiparkinsonism agent with anticholinergic activity.

Selegiline. Nausea, hallucinations, confusion, depression, loss of balance, and dizziness may be seen with the use of this drug.

▶ NURSING PROCESS
THE PATIENT RECEIVING AN ANTIPARKINSONISM DRUG

ASSESSMENT

Because of memory impairment and alterations in thinking in some patients with parkinsonism, a history obtained from the patient may be unreliable. When necessary, the history should be obtained from a family member or relative and should include information regarding the symptoms of the disorder, the length of time the symptoms have been present, the ability of the patient to carry on activities of daily living, and the patient's present mental condition (eg, impairment in memory, signs of depression or withdrawal, and so on).

Physical assessment should include an evaluation of the patient's neurologic status, which should be performed before starting drug therapy to provide a baseline for future evaluations of drug therapy. The neurologic evaluation includes looking for the following:

▶ Tremors of the hands or head while the patient is at rest

▶ A masklike facial expression

▶ Changes (from the normal) in walking

▶ The type of speech pattern (halting, monotone)

SUMMARY DRUG TABLE 33–1
Antiparkinsonism Agents

GENERIC NAME	TRADE NAME*	USES	ADVERSE REACTIONS	DOSE RANGES
DRUGS WITH ANTICHOLINERGIC ACTIVITY				
benztropine mesylate	Cogentin, *generic*	All forms of parkinsonism	Skin rash, urticaria, dry mouth, blurred vision, urinary retention, dysuria, muscle weakness, disorientation, confusion, tachycardia	0.5–8 mg/d PO, IM in single or divided doses; 1–2 mg IV
biperiden	Akineton	Same as benztropine mesylate	Same as benztropine mesylate	2 mg PO 1–4 times/d; 2 mg IM, IV
diphenhydramine	Benadryl, *generic*	Parkinsonism, drug-induced extrapyramidal reactions	Same as benztropine mesylate	25–50 mg PO 3–4 times/d; 10–100 mg IM, IV
ethopropazine hydrochloride	Parsidol	Same as diphenhydramine	Same as benztropine mesylate	50–600 mg/d PO in single or divided doses
procyclidine	Kemadrin	Same as diphenhydramine	Same as benztropine mesylate	2.5–5 mg PO tid
trihexyphenidyl hydrochloride	Artane, *generic*	Same as benztropine mesylate	Same as benztropine mesylate	1–15 mg/d PO in divided doses
OTHER AGENTS				
amantadine hydrochloride	Symmetrel, *generic*	All forms of parkinsonism; influenza A respiratory tract illness	Depression, congestive heart failure, orthostatic hypotension, psychosis, urinary retention, confusion, nausea	Parkinsonism: 100–400 mg/d PO in divided doses; influenza: see Summary Drug Table 26-1
carbidopa	Lodosyn	Given with levodopa for all forms of parkinsonism	None; adverse reactions when used with levodopa are due to levodopa	Maximum daily dose: 200 mg PO; used as a single agent when individualized titrations of carbidopa and levodopa are necessary
carbidopa and levodopa	Sinemet 10/100, Sinemet 25/100, Sinemet 25/250	Same as benztropine mesylate	Due to levodopa (see below)	1 tablet 3–4 times/d PO
levodopa	Dopar, Larodopa, *generic*	Same as benztropine mesylate	Choreiform or dystonic movements, anorexia, nausea, vomiting, abdominal pain, dysphagia, dry mouth, mental changes, headache, dizziness, increased hand tremor	0.5–8 g/d PO in divided doses
pergolide mesylate	Permax	Adjunctive treatment to carbidopa and levodopa therapy	Nausea, dyskinesia, dizziness, hallucinations, somnolence, rhinitis, peripheral edema, constipation	Up to 5 mg/d PO in divided doses
selegiline hydrochloride	Eldepryl	Parkinson patients being treated with carbidopa and levodopa who have a decreased response to these drugs	Nausea, hallucinations, confusion, depression, loss of balance, dizziness	10 mg/d PO in divided doses; dose may be reduced if response is adequate

* The term generic *indicates that the drug is available in a generic form.*

▶ Postural deformities

▶ Muscular rigidity

▶ Drooling, difficulty in chewing or swallowing

▶ Changes in thought processes

▶ Ability of the patient to carry out any or all of the activities of daily living (bathing, ambulating, dressing, and so on)

NURSING DIAGNOSIS

Depending on the degree of severity and the individual, one or more of the following nursing diagnoses may apply to the patient receiving an antiparkinsonism drug:

▶ Anxiety related to diagnosis, therapeutic regimen, other factors

▶ High risk for injury related to parkinsonism, adverse drug reactions (dizziness, light-headedness, loss of balance)

▶ Noncompliance related to failure of drug therapy, lack of knowledge, inability to assume responsibility for the prescribed drug therapy, other factors

▶ Knowledge deficit of medication regimen, adverse drug reactions

PLANNING AND IMPLEMENTATION

The major goals of the patient may include a reduction in anxiety, absence of injury, and an understanding of and compliance to the prescribed treatment regimen.

The major goals of nursing management may include a reduction in the patient's anxiety, an absence of injury, recognition of adverse drug reactions, and the development and implementation of an effective teaching plan.

The patient's response to drug therapy is evaluated by neurologic observations, which are compared to the data obtained during the initial physical assessment. Although drug response may occur slowly in some patients, these observations aid the physician in adjusting the dosage of the drug upward or downward to obtain the desired therapeutic results.

When these drugs are used to treat the parkinsonism that may occur with the administration of some of the psychotherapeutic drugs (see chap 34), antiparkinsonism drugs may exacerbate mental symptoms and precipitate a psychosis. The patient's behavior is observed at frequent intervals and if sudden behavioral changes are noted, the next dose of the drug is withheld and the physician is immediately notified.

Patients receiving levodopa or carbidopa *and* levodopa, are observed for the occurrence of choreiform and dystonic movements, such as facial grimacing, protruding tongue, exaggerated chewing motions and head movements, and jerking movements of the arms and legs. If these occur, the next dose of the drug is withheld and the physician is notified because it may be necessary to reduce the dosage of levodopa or discontinue the drug.

The diabetic patient receiving levodopa may require an adjustment in the dosage of insulin or oral hypoglycemic agent. These patients are closely observed for signs of hypoglycemia or hyperglycemia (see chap 20) and the urine is tested for glucose and ketones four times a day.

ANXIETY. The patient with early signs of Parkinson's disease may exhibit anxiety over the diagnosis, as well as the ability of medication to control symptoms. Patients should be allowed time to discuss the prescribed medication regimen and ask questions about their drug therapy. Patients should be assured that the physician will closely monitor their drug therapy and that it may be several weeks or more before a relief of symptoms may occur.

ADVERSE DRUG REACTIONS. The patient is observed daily for the development of adverse reactions. All adverse reactions are reported to the physician because a dosage adjustment or change to a different antiparkinsonism drug may be necessary with the occurrence of the more serious adverse reactions. Some adverse reactions, although not serious, may be uncomfortable. An example of a less serious but uncomfortable adverse reaction is dryness of the mouth, which may be relieved by offering frequent sips of water, ice chips, or hard candy (if allowed).

Some patients with parkinsonism communicate poorly and do not tell the physician or nurse that problems are occurring. The patient with parkinsonism must be observed for outward changes that may indicate one or more adverse reactions. For example, a sudden change in the facial expression or changes in posture may indicate abdominal pain or discomfort, which may be due to urinary retention, paralytic ileus, or constipation. Sudden changes in behavior may indicate hallucinations, depression, or other psychotic episodes. Visual difficulties (eg, adverse reactions of blurred vision, diplopia, and so on) may be evidenced by the patient's sudden refusal to read or watch television or by bumping into objects when ambulating. Any sudden changes in the patient's behavior or activity are carefully evaluated and then reported to the physician.

HIGH RISK FOR INJURY. The patient with parkinsonism may have difficulty in ambulating. Adverse reactions such as dizziness, muscle weakness, and ataxia may further increase difficulty with ambulatory activities. The patient should be assisted in getting out of the bed or a chair, walking, and other self-care activities; these individuals are especially prone to falls and other accidents due to their disease process and possible adverse drug reactions.

NONCOMPLIANCE AND KNOWLEDGE DEFICIT. The nurse must evaluate the patient's ability to understand his or her therapeutic drug regimen. Patients are also evaluated for their ability to care for themselves in the home environment, as well as to comply with the prescribed drug therapy. If it is determined that the patient will require any type of assistance, a referral to the discharge planning coordinator or social service worker may be necessary.

If the patient requires supervision or help with daily activities and his or her medication regimen, the family is encouraged to create a home environment that is least likely to result in accidents or falls. Changes such as removing throw rugs, installing a handrail next to the toilet, and moving obstacles that can result in tripping or falling can be made at little or no expense to the family.

The following points may be included in a patient and family teaching plan:

▶ Take this drug as prescribed. Do not increase, decrease, or omit a dose or stop taking the drug unless advised to do so by the physician.

▶ If dizziness, drowsiness, or blurred vision occurs, avoid driving or performing other tasks that require alertness.

▶ Avoid the use of alcohol unless use has been approved by the physician.

▶ Relieve dry mouth by hard candy (unless the patient is a diabetic) or frequent sips of water.

▶ Consult a dentist if dryness of the mouth interferes with wearing, inserting, or removing dentures or causes other dental problems.

▶ Notify the physician if any of these problems occur: severe dry mouth, inability to chew or swallow food, inability to urinate, feelings of depression, severe dizziness or drowsiness, rapid heartbeat, abdominal pain, and unusual (new) movements of the head, eyes, arms, legs, feet, mouth, or tongue.

▶ Keep all physician or clinic appointments because close monitoring of therapy is necessary.

▶ Diabetics taking levodopa: perform urine testing as recommended by the physician. Notify the physician if the urine is positive for glucose or ketones because it may be necessary to change the insulin or oral hypoglycemic drug dosage. If signs of hypoglycemia occur, notify the physician immediately.

EVALUATION

▶ Anxiety is reduced

▶ No evidence of injury

▶ Adverse reactions are identified and reported to the physician

▶ Verbalizes an understanding of treatment modalities, adverse reactions, and importance of continued follow-up care

▶ Patient and family demonstrate understanding of drug regimen

34

Psychotherapeutic Drugs

On completion of this chapter the student will:

► *Name the types of psychotherapeutic drugs*

► *List the general adverse reactions associated with the administration of the psychotherapeutic drugs*

► *Use the nursing process when administering a psychotherapeutic drug*

► *Discuss the nursing implications to be considered when administering a psychotherapeutic drug*

By definition, a **psychotherapeutic drug** is one that is used to treat disorders of the mind. A drug that affects the mind is called a **psychotropic** drug. Narcotics, sedatives and hypnotics, alcohol, hallucinogens, and psychotherapeutic drugs are examples of psychotropic agents.

The types of psychotherapeutic drugs used in the treatment of mental illness are the **antianxiety** drugs (tranquilizers), the **antidepressant** drugs, and the **antipsychotic** drugs. Examples of types of antipsychotic drugs are given in Summary Drug Table 34-1.

▷ Actions of Psychotherapeutic Drugs

Antianxiety Drugs

Antianxiety drugs act on subcortical (beneath the cortex) areas of the brain. Their exact mechanism of action is not fully understood but it is believed that their effect on areas such as the limbic system and the reticular formation results in a reduction of anxiety. Examples of antianxiety drugs include ox-

SUMMARY DRUG TABLE 34–1
Psychotherapeutic Drugs

GENERIC NAME	TRADE NAME*	USES	ADVERSE REACTIONS	DOSE RANGES
ANTIANXIETY DRUGS				
alprazolam	Xanax	Anxiety disorders, symptoms of anxiety	Sedation, sleepiness, lethargy, constipation, pruritus, diarrhea, apathy, incontinence, depression, urticaria, fever, hiccups, visual disturbances, nausea, vomiting	0.25–0.5 mg PO tid increased to 4 mg/d if required
buspirone hydrochloride	BuSpar	Same as alprazolam	Dizziness, drowsiness, nervousness, headache, fatigue, nausea, dry mouth	Up to 60 mg/d PO in divided doses
chlordiazepoxide	Librium, *generic*	Same as alprazolam; acute alcohol withdrawal, preoperative anxiety	Same as alprazolam	Anxiety: 5–25 mg PO tid, qid; alcohol withdrawal: 50–100 mg PO, IM, IV; preoperative anxiety: 5–10 mg PO on days before surgery, 50–100 mg IM 1 h before surgery
clorazepate dipotassium	Tranxene	Same as alprazolam; acute alcohol withdrawal, partial seizures	Same as alprazolam	Anxiety: 15–60 mg/d PO in divided doses; alcohol withdrawal: 15–90 mg/d PO in divided doses; anticonvulsant: see Summary Drug Table 32-1
diazepam	Valium, *generic*	Same as alprazolam; acute alcohol withdrawal, skeletal muscle spasm, preoperative anxiety, convulsive disorders	Same as alprazolam	Anxiety: 2–10 mg PO 2–4 times/d; acute alcohol withdrawal: 5–10 mg PO tid, qid; muscle relaxant: see Summary Drug Table 42-1; anticonvulsant: see Summary Drug Table 32-1
halazepam	Paxipam	Same as alprazolam	Same as alprazolam	20–40 mg PO tid, qid
hydroxyzine	Atarax, Vistaril, *generic*	Same as alprazolam; pruritus, preoperative and postoperative sedation, nausea and vomiting, psychiatric and emotional emergencies, prepartum and postpartum adjunctive therapy	Dry mouth, drowsiness, hypersensitivity reactions	Anxiety: 50–100 mg PO qid; pruritus: 25 mg PO tid, qid; preoperative and postoperative: 25–100 mg IM; psychiatric emergencies: 100 mg IM; nausea, vomiting: 25–100 mg IM; prepartum and postpartum: 25–100 mg PO
lorazepam	Ativan, *generic*	Anxiety disorders, preanesthetic sedation	Same as alprazolam	Anxiety: 1–10 mg/d PO in divided doses; preoperative sedation: up to 4 mg IM or 2 mg IV
meprobamate	Equanil, Miltown, *generic*	Same as alprazolam	Drowsiness, ataxia, nausea, vomiting, diarrhea, palpitations, tachycardia, rash, slurred speech, dizziness	1200–2400 mg/d PO in divided doses
oxazepam	Serax, *generic*	Same as alprazolam	Same as alprazolam	10–30 mg PO tid, qid
ANTIDEPRESSANTS				
amitriptyline hydrochloride	Elavil, Endep, *generic*	Depression	Sedation, confusion, nasal congestion, rash, numbness, blurred vision, hypertension,	Up to 300 mg/d PO in divided doses; 20–30 mg IM qid

(continued)

SUMMARY DRUG TABLE 34–1
(continued)

GENERIC NAME	TRADE NAME*	USES	ADVERSE REACTIONS	DOSE RANGES
			orthostatic hypotension, dry mouth, nausea, vomiting, pruritus	
amoxapine	Asendin, *generic*	Same as amitriptyline	Same as amitriptyline	Up to 300 mg/d PO in divided doses
bupropion hydrochloride	Wellbutrin	Same as amitriptyline	Agitation, dry mouth, insomnia, headache, nausea, vomiting, constipation, tremor, weight loss, anorexia, seizures (with doses exceeding 450 mg/d)	200–450 mg/d PO in divided doses
clomipramine hydrochloride	Anafranil	Obsessions and compulsions in those with obsessive-compulsive disorders (OCD)	Same as amitriptyline	25–250 mg/d PO
desipramine hydrochloride	Norpramin, *generic*	Same as amitriptyline	Same as amitriptyline	Up to 300 mg/d PO in single dose or divided doses
doxepin hydrochloride	Adapin, Sinequan, *generic*	Anxiety or depression, emotional symptoms accompanying organic disease	Same as amitriptyline	25–300 mg/d PO in single or divided doses
fluoxetine hydrochloride	Prozac	Same as amitriptyline	Anxiety, nervousness, insomnia, drowsiness, fatigue, asthenia, tremor, sweating, dizziness, lightheadedness, anorexia, nausea, diarrhea, headache	20 mg/d PO in the morning or 40–80 mg/d PO in divided doses
imipramine hydrochloride or pamoate	Tofranil, *generic*	Same as amitriptyline	Same as amitriptyline	75–200 mg/d PO in divided doses; up to 100 mg/d IM in divided doses
maprotiline hydrochloride	Ludiomil, *generic*	Depressive neurosis, manic-depressive illness, anxiety associated with depression	Same as amitriptyline	25–300 mg/d PO in single dose or divided doses
nortriptyline hydrochloride	Aventyl	Same as amitriptyline	Same as amitriptyline	25 mg PO tid, qid
trimipramine maleate	Surmontil	Same as amitriptyline	Same as amitriptyline	Up to 200 mg/d PO in divided doses
trazodone hydrochloride	Desyrel, *generic*	Same as amitriptyline	Skin conditions, tinnitus, anger, hostility, anemia, hypertension, blurred vision, abdominal/gastric disorder, hypotension, dry mouth, nausea, vomiting, diarrhea	150–600 mg/d PO in divided doses
MAOI ANTIDEPRESSANTS				
isocarboxazid	Marplan	Same as amitriptyline	Orthostatic hypotension, dizziness, vertigo, nausea, constipation, dry mouth, diarrhea, headache	10–30 mg/d PO in single or divided doses
phenelzine	Nardil	Same as amitriptyline	Same as isocarboxazid	Up to 60 mg/d PO in divided doses
tranylcypromine	Parnate	Same as amitriptyline	Same as isocarboxazid	Up to 60 mg/d PO in divided doses

(continued)

SUMMARY DRUG TABLE 34–1

(continued)

GENERIC NAME	TRADE NAME*	USES	ADVERSE REACTIONS	DOSE RANGES
ANTIPSYCHOTIC DRUGS				
chlorpromazine hydrochloride	Promapar, Thorazine, *generic*	Psychotic disorders, nausea, vomiting, intractable hiccups	Hypotension, postural hypotension, tardive dyskinesia, photophobia, urticaria, nasal congestion, dry mouth, pseudoparkinsonism, behavioral changes, headache, photosensitivity	Psychiatric disorders: up to 500 mg/d PO in divided doses, 25–400 mg IM; nausea and vomiting: 10–25 mg PO, 25 mg IM, 50–100 mg rectal; hiccups: 25–50 mg PO, IM
chlorprothixene	Taractan	Psychotic disorders	Same as chlorpromazine	Up to 600 mg/d PO in divided doses; 12–25 mg IM tid, qid
clozapine	Clozaril	Severely ill schizophrenic patients not responding to other therapies	Drowsiness, sedation, seizures, dizziness, syncope, tachycardia, hypotension, nausea, vomiting	Up to 900 mg/d PO in divided doses
fluphenazine hydrochloride	Permitil, Prolixin	Same as chlorprothixene	Same as chlorpromazine	0.5–10 mg/d PO in divided doses; 2.5–10 mg/d IM in divided doses
haloperidol	Haldol	Psychotic disorders, Tourette's disorder	Same as chlorpromazine	0.5–5 mg PO bid, tid with dosages up to 100 mg/d in divided doses; 2–5 mg IM
lithium	Eskalith, Lithane, *generic*	Manic episodes of manic-depressive illness	See Table 34-1	Based on lithium serum levels; average dose range is 900–1800 mg/d PO in divided doses
loxapine	Loxitane	Same as chlorprothixene	Same as chlorpromazine	20–100 mg/d PO in divided doses; 12.5–50 mg IM
molindone hydrochloride	Moban	Same as chlorprothixene	Same as chlorpromazine	15–100 mg/d PO in divided doses
perphenazine	Trilafon, *generic*	Psychotic disorders, nausea and vomiting	Same as chlorpromazine	Psychotic disorders: 4–16 mg PO bid to qid, 5–10 mg IM; nausea, vomiting: see Summary Drug Table 37-1
pimozide	Orap	Tourette's disorder	Parkinson-like symptoms, motor restlessness, dystonia, oculogyric crisis, tardive dyskinesia, dry mouth, diarrhea, headache, drowsiness, rash	Initial dose: 1–2 mg/d PO; maintenance doses: up to 10 mg/d PO
prochlorperazine	Compazine, Chlorazine, *generic*	Same as perphenazine	Same as chlorpromazine	Psychotic disorders: up to 100 mg/d PO, 10–20 mg IM; nausea, vomiting: see Summary Drug Table 37-1
promazine hydrochloride	Sparine, *generic*	Same as chlorprothixene	Same as chlorpromazine	10–200 mg PO, IM q4–6h
thioridazine hydrochloride	Mellaril, *generic*	Psychotic disorders and agitation, depressed mood, tension, fears, sleep disturbances, anxiety in the elderly	Same as chlorpromazine	Psychotic disorders: up to 800 mg/d PO in divided doses; elderly: 20–200 mg/d PO in divided doses
trifluoperazine hydrochloride	Stelazine, *generic*	Same as chlorprothixene	Same as chlorpromazine	1–5 mg PO bid and up to 20 mg/d PO in divided doses; up to 6 mg/d IM in divided doses

* The term *generic* indicates that the drug is available in a generic form.

azepam (Serax), chlordiazepoxide (Librium), diazepam (Valium), and buspirone (BuSpar).

Antidepressant Drugs

There are three types of antidepressants: the tricyclic antidepressants, the monoamine oxidase inhibitors, and a group of miscellaneous, unrelated drugs.

The tricyclic antidepressants, for example, amitriptyline (Elavil) and doxepin (Sinequan) block the reuptake of the endogenous neurohormones, norepinephrine (see chap 6) and serotonin, which then results in stimulation of the central nervous system.

Drugs classified as monoamine oxidase inhibitors (MAOIs) inhibit the activity of monoamine oxidase—a complex enzyme system that is responsible for breaking down amines. This results in an increase in endogenous epinephrine, norepinephrine, and serotonin in the nervous system. An increase in these neurohormones results in central nervous system stimulation.

The mechanism of action of most of the miscellaneous antidepressants is not clearly understood. Examples of this group of drugs include fluoxetine (Prozac) and bupropion (Wellbutrin).

Antipsychotic Drugs

The exact mechanism of action of antipsychotic drugs is not well understood. The effects of these drugs include an alteration or inhibition of the release of the neurohormone dopamine and an increase in the firing of nerve cells in certain areas of the brain. These effects may be responsible for the ability of these drugs to suppress the symptoms of certain psychotic disorders. Examples of antipsychotic drugs include chlorpromazine (Thorazine), thioridazine (Mellaril), haloperidol (Haldol), and lithium.

▷ Uses of Psychotherapeutic Drugs

Antianxiety Drugs

Antianxiety drugs are used in the short-term treatment of the symptoms of anxiety. Anxiety may be seen in many types of situations ranging from the anxiety that may accompany one's employment to the acute anxiety that may be seen during withdrawal from alcohol. Long-term use of these drugs is usually not recommended because prolonged therapy can result in drug dependence and serious withdrawal symptoms.

A few of these drugs may have additional uses. For example, clorazepate (Tranxene) and diazepam are also used as anticonvulsants (see chap 32).

Antidepressant Drugs

Antidepressant drugs are used in the management of various types of depression or depression accompanied by anxiety. The uses of individual antidepressants are given in Summary Drug Table 34-1.

Antipsychotic Drugs

Antipsychotic drugs are used in the management of various psychotic disorders. Some of these drugs have specific uses, such as the use of lithium in the management of manic-depressive illness. More specific uses of these drugs are given in Summary Drug Table 34-1.

▷ Adverse Reactions Associated with the Administration of Psychotherapeutic Drugs

Antianxiety Drugs

Drowsiness and sedation are common adverse reactions seen during initial therapy with antianxiety drugs. Depending on the severity of anxiety or other circumstances, it may be desirable to allow some degree of sedation to occur during early therapy. Other adverse reactions include constipation, diarrhea, dry mouth, nausea, vomiting, visual disturbances, and incontinence. Some adverse reactions may only be seen when higher dosages are used.

Long-term use of antianxiety drugs may result in physical drug dependence. These drugs must never be discontinued abruptly because withdrawal symptoms, which can be extremely severe, may occur.

Antidepressant Drugs

Sedation and dry mouth are the most common adverse reactions seen with the antidepressants. Orthostatic hypotension, hypertension, mental confusion, disorientation, rash, nausea, vomiting, visual disturbances, and nasal congestion may also be seen.

Orthostatic hypotension is a common adverse reaction seen with the administration of the MAOIs. Other common adverse reactions include dizziness, vertigo, nausea, constipation, dry mouth, diarrhea, headache, and overactivity. One serious adverse reaction associated with the use of the MAOIs is hypertensive crisis (extremely high blood pressure), which may occur when foods containing tyramine are eaten. Examples of foods containing tyramine are aged cheeses, beef or chicken livers, some meats, meat tenderizer, some sausages, imported beers and ales, red wine, figs, bananas, raisins, soy sauce, and avocados.

One of the earliest symptoms of hypertensive crisis is headache (usually occipital), followed by other symptoms such as a stiff or sore neck, nausea, vomiting, sweating, fever, chest pain, dilated pupils, and bradycardia or tachycardia. If a hypertensive crisis occurs, immediate medical intervention is necessary to reduce the blood pressure. Strokes (cerebrovascular accidents) and death have been reported.

Trazodone administration may result in hypertension or hypotension, hostility, tinnitus, anemia, visual disturbances, dry mouth, nausea, and vomiting.

Antipsychotic Drugs

Administration of these drugs may result in a wide variety of adverse reactions.

The adverse reactions seen with the use of some of these drugs may include hypotension, postural hypotension, tardive dyskinesia, dry mouth, nasal congestion, photophobia, urticaria, Parkinson-like symptoms, photosensitivity, behavior changes, and headache. Some of these adverse reactions, for example, tardive dyskinesia and Parkinson-like symptoms (see chap 33), are usually seen only at higher dosages.

Tardive dyskinesia is characterized by rhythmic, involuntary movements of the tongue, face, mouth, or jaw, and sometimes the extremities. The tongue may protrude and there may be chewing movements, puckering of the mouth, and facial grimacing. When these symptoms occur, the drug must be discontinued. Depending on the severity of the condition being treated, the physician may slowly taper the drug dose because abrupt discontinuation may result in a return of the psychotic symptoms.

When higher doses of some of these drugs are used, the physician may prescribe an antiparkinsonism drug to reduce the possibility of the occurrence of Parkinson-like symptoms.

Behavioral changes may also occur with the use of the antipsychotics. These changes include a catatonic-like state, an increase in the intensity of the psychotic symptoms, lethargy, hyperactivity, paranoid reactions, agitation, and confusion. A decrease in dosage may eliminate some of these symptoms but it also may be necessary to try another drug.

Adverse reactions are seldom seen with lithium administration, but toxic reactions may be seen when certain lithium blood levels are reached (Table 34-1). Because some of these toxic reactions are potentially serious, lithium blood levels are usually drawn during therapy and the dosage of lithium adjusted according to the results.

▶ NURSING PROCESS
THE PATIENT RECEIVING A PSYCHOTHERAPEUTIC DRUG

ASSESSMENT

A patient receiving a psychotherapeutic drug may be treated in the hospital or in an outpatient setting.

Before starting therapy for the hospitalized patient, a complete psychiatric and medical history is obtained. In the case of mild depression or anxiety, patients may (but sometimes may not) give a reliable history of their illness. When a severe psychosis is present, the psychiatric history must be obtained from a family member or friend. During the time the history is taken, the patient is observed for what appear to be deviations from normal behavior patterns. Examples of deviations are poor eye contact, failure to answer questions completely, inappropriate answers to questions, a monotone speech pattern, and inappropriate laughter, sadness, or crying.

Physical assessments should include the blood pressure on both arms and in a sitting position, pulse, respiratory rate, and weight.

TABLE 34-1
Signs of Lithium Toxicity

SERUM LEVEL	SIGNS OF TOXICITY
<1.5 mEq/L	Nausea, vomiting, diarrhea, thirst, polyuria, lethargy, slurred speech, muscle weakness, hand tremor
1.5–2 mEq/L	Persistent GI upset, coarse hand tremor, mental confusion, hyperexcitabiilty of muscles, ECG changes, drowsiness, incoordination
2–2.5 mEq/L	Ataxia, giddiness, large output of dilute urine, serious ECG changes, fasciculations, tinnitus, blurred vision, clonic movements, seizures, stupor, severe hypertension, coma
>2.5 mEq/L	A complex picture involving many organ systems may be seen

The hospitalized patient may ultimately be discharged from the psychiatric setting. There are also patients, such as those with mild anxiety or depression, who do not require inpatient care. These patients are usually seen as periodic intervals in the physician's office or in a psychiatric outpatient setting.

The initial assessments of the outpatient are basically the same as those for the hospitalized patient. A complete medical history and a history of the symptoms of the mental disorder are obtained from the patient, a family member, or the patient's hospital records. During the initial interview, the nurse should observe the patient for what appear to be deviations from a normal behavior pattern. The initial physical assessment should also include vital signs and weight.

NURSING DIAGNOSIS

Depending on the drug, dose, and reason for administration, one or more of the following nursing diagnoses may apply to a person receiving an psychotherapeutic drug. Additional nursing diagnoses pertaining to the patient's mental and physical status may need to be added.

- ▶ Noncompliance related to indifference, lack of knowledge, other factors
- ▶ High risk for injury related to an adverse drug reaction (eg, drowsiness or ataxia)
- ▶ Knowledge deficit of medication regimen, adverse drug effects, treatment modalities

PLANNING AND IMPLEMENTATION

The major goals of the patient may include an absence of injury and a knowledge of and compliance to the prescribed treatment regimen.

The major goals of nursing management may include an absence of injury, recognition of adverse drug reactions, and the development and implementation of an effective teaching plan.

Many psychotherapeutic agents are administered for a long time. The exception is the antianxiety agents which are not recommended for long-term use. The nurse plays an important role in the administration of these drugs in both the psychiatric and nonpsychiatric setting for several reasons: (1) the patient's response to drug therapy on an inpatient basis requires around-the-clock assessments because frequent dosage adjustments may be necessary during therapy; and (2) accurate assessments for the appearance of adverse drug effects assume a greater importance when the patient may not be able to verbalize physical changes to the physician or nurse.

HOSPITALIZED PATIENTS. A nursing care plan must be developed to meet the patient's individual needs. The vital signs are monitored at least daily. In some instances, such as when hypotensive episodes occur, it may be necessary to monitor the vital signs every 4 hours. Any significant change in the vital signs is reported to the physician.

Patients receiving lithium must increase their oral fluid intake to about 3000 mL/d. The patient must have fluids readily available and be offered extra fluids throughout waking hours. If there is any question regarding the oral fluid intake, the intake and output are measured.

Patients receiving MAOIs require strict dietary control because foods containing tyramine must not be eaten. Family members and visitors should be asked not to bring food to the patient and should be told why this is important. The patient may also require close observation when eating in a community setting so that he or she does not take or accept food from other patients. If the patient complains of a headache (especially an occipital headache), hypertensive crisis may be occurring. The blood pressure is taken and if elevated, the physician is notified immediately. The blood pressure is then monitored at 30-minute intervals. Any further appearance of the symptoms of hypertensive crisis requires notifying the physician again and closely observing the patient.

Behavioral records should be written at periodic intervals, with their frequency depending on hospital or unit guidelines. An accurate description of the patient's behavior aids the physician in planning therapy, and, thus, becomes an important part of nursing management. Patients responding poorly to drug therapy may require dosage changes, a change to another psychotherapeutic drug, or the addition of other therapies to the treatment regimen.

DRUG ADMINISTRATION. When given parenterally, these drugs are given intramuscularly in a large muscle mass such as the gluteus muscle. The patient should remain lying down (when possible) for about 30 minutes after the drug is given.

Oral administration requires great care because some patients may have difficulty swallowing (due to a dry mouth or other causes), or be so withdrawn that they fail to swallow an oral medication. Other patients may refuse to take their medication. *At no time* should any patient be force-fed an oral medication. If the patient refuses his or her medication, the physician is contacted regarding this problem because parenteral administration of the drug may be necessary.

After administration of an oral medication, the patient's oral cavity is inspected to be sure the medication has been swallowed. If the patient resists having his or her oral cavity checked, this is reported to the physician.

HIGH RISK FOR INJURY. The patient experiencing extreme sedation requires total assistance with activities of daily living including eating, dressing, and ambulation. On the other hand, extremely hyperactive patients must be protected from injuring themselves or others.

ADVERSE DRUG REACTIONS. During initial therapy or whenever the dosage is increased or decreased, the patient is closely observed for adverse drug reactions and *any* behavioral changes. Any change in behavior or the appearance of adverse reactions is reported to the physician because a further increase or decrease in dosage may be necessary or the drug may need to be discontinued.

Some adverse reactions, such as dry mouth, episodes of postural hypotension, and drowsiness, may need to be tolerated because drug therapy must continue. Nursing interventions to relieve some of these reactions may include offering the patient frequent sips of water, assisting the patient out of the bed or chair, and supervising all ambulatory activities.

THE OUTPATIENT. At the time of each physician's office or clinic visit, the patient is observed for his or her response to therapy. In some instances, the patient or a family member may be questioned about the response to therapy. The type of questions asked depends on the patient and the diagnosis and may include questions such as "How are you feeling?", "Do you seem to be less nervous?", or "Would you like to tell me how everything is going?" Many times questions may need to be rephrased or the conversation directed toward other subjects until these patients feel comfortable and are able to discuss their therapy.

The patient or a family member must also be asked about adverse drug reactions or any other problems that are occurring during therapy. These reactions or problems are then brought to the attention of the physician. A general summary of the patient's outward behavior and any complaints or problems are entered in the patient's record and compared to previous notations and observations.

NONCOMPLIANCE AND KNOWLEDGE DEFICIT. Noncompliance is a problem with some patients once they are discharged to the home setting. Outpatients or hospitalized patients ready for discharge require an evaluation of their ability to be responsible for taking their medications at home. The administration of psychotherapeutic drugs becomes a family responsibility if the outpatient appears to be unable to manage his or her own drug therapy.

Any adverse reactions that may occur with a specific psychotherapeutic drug are explained and the patient or family member is encouraged to contact the physician immediately if a serious drug reaction occurs.

The following points may be included in a teaching plan for the patient or family member:

▶ Take the drug exactly as directed. Do *not* increase, decrease, or omit a dose or discontinue this drug unless directed to do so by the physician.

▶ Do not drive or perform other hazardous tasks if drowsiness occurs.

▶ Do not take *any* nonprescription drug unless use of a specific drug has been approved by the physician.

▶ Inform physicians, dentists, and other medical personnel of therapy with this drug.

▶ Do not drink alcoholic beverages unless approval is obtained from the physician.

▶ If dizziness occurs when changing position, rise slowly when getting out of bed or a chair. If dizziness is severe, always have help when changing positions.

▶ If dryness of the mouth occurs, it may be relieved by frequent sips of water, hard candy, or chewing gum (preferably sugarless).

▶ MAOIs—A list of foods containing tyramine must be given to the patient with emphasis on not eating *any* of the foods on the list.

▶ Lithium—Drink at least 10 large glasses of fluid each day and add extra salt to food. If any of the following occurs, do not take the next dose and notify the physician immediately: diarrhea, vomiting, tremors, drowsiness, lack of muscle coordination, muscle weakness.

▶ Keep all physician or clinic appointments because close monitoring of therapy is essential.

▶ Report any unusual changes or physical effects to the physician.

EVALUATION

▶ Verbalizes an understanding of treatment modalities and importance of continued follow-up care

▶ Verbalizes importance of complying with the prescribed treatment regimen

▶ Patient and family demonstrate understanding of drug regimen

▶ Adverse reactions are identified and reported to the physician

▶ No evidence of injury

35

Drugs Used for Allergic and Respiratory Disorders

On completion of this chapter the student will:

▶ *List the various types of drugs used for allergic and respiratory disorders*

▶ *Describe the uses and actions of drugs used for allergic and respiratory disorders*

▶ *List some of the adverse reactions associated with drugs used in the treatment of allergic and respiratory disorders*

▶ *Use the nursing process when administering a drug for an allergic or respiratory disorder*

▶ *Discuss the nursing implications to be considered when administering a drug for an allergic or respiratory disorder*

▶ ANTIHISTAMINES

Histamine is a substance present in various tissues of the body, such as the liver, lungs, intestines, and skin. The highest concentration of histamine is found in basophils (a type of white blood cell) and the mast cells that are found near capillaries. Histamine is produced in response to injury. Histamine acts on areas such as the vascular system and smooth muscle, producing dilatation of arterioles and an increased permeability of capillaries and venules. Dilatation of the arterioles results in localized redness. An increase in the permeability of small blood vessels produces an escape of fluid from these blood vessels into the surrounding tissues, which produces localized swelling. The release of histamine produces an inflammatory response.

Antihistamines are drugs used to counteract the effects of histamine on body organs and structures. Examples of antihistamines include diphenhydramine (Benadryl), terfenadine (Seldane), brompheniramine (Dimetane), and astemizole (Hismanal).

▷ Actions of the Antihistamines

Antihistamines block most, but not all, of the effects of histamine. They do this by competing for histamine at histamine receptor sites, thereby preventing histamine from entering these receptor sites and producing an effect on body tissues. Some antihistamines have additional effects such as an antipruritic effect, an antiemetic effect, and a sedative effect.

▷ Uses of the Antihistamines

The general uses of the antihistamines are the following:

▷ Relief of the symptoms of seasonal and perennial allergies
▷ Allergic and vasomotor rhinitis
▷ Allergic conjunctivitis
▷ Mild and uncomplicated angioneurotic edema and urticaria
▷ Relief of allergic reactions to drugs, blood, or plasma
▷ Relief of coughs due to colds or allergy
▷ Adjunctive therapy in anaphylactic shock
▷ Treatment of parkinsonism
▷ Relief of nausea and vomiting
▷ Relief of motion sickness
▷ Sedation
▷ As adjuncts to analgesics

Each antihistamine may be used for one or more of these reasons. The more specific uses of the various antihistamine preparations are given in Summary Drug Table 35-1.

▷ Adverse Reactions Associated with the Administration of the Antihistamines

Drowsiness and sedation are common adverse reactions seen with the use of many of the antihistamines. Some antihistamines appear to cause more drowsiness and sedation than others. Several newer preparations, for example, astemizole and terfenadine cause little, if any, drowsiness in most individuals.

Some antihistamines may cause dizziness, disturbed coordination, fatigue, hypotension, headache, and epigastric distress. Even though these drugs are sometimes used in the treatment of allergies, a drug allergy can occur with the use of an antihistamine. Symptoms that may indicate an allergy to these drugs include skin rash, urticaria, and anaphylactic shock. These drugs may also have anticholinergic (cholinergic blocking) effects, which may result in dryness of the mouth, nose, and throat and a thickening of bronchial secretions.

► NURSING PROCESS
THE PATIENT RECEIVING AN ANTIHISTAMINE

ASSESSMENT

Assessment of the patient receiving these drugs depends on the reason for use. Examples of assessments that may be performed include an assessment of the involved areas (eyes, nose, upper and lower respiratory tract) if the patient is receiving an antihistamine for the relief of symptoms of an allergy. If promethazine (Phenergan) is used with a narcotic to enhance the effects and reduce the dosage of the narcotic, the blood pressure, pulse, and respiratory rate are taken before the drug is given.

NURSING DIAGNOSIS

Depending on the reason for administration, one or more of the following nursing diagnoses may apply to a person receiving an antihistamine:

► Anxiety related to symptoms
► High risk for injury related to adverse drug reactions (drowsiness, dizziness, disturbed coordination)
► Knowledge deficit of medication regimen, adverse drug effects, treatment modalities

PLANNING AND IMPLEMENTATION

The major goals of the patient may include a reduction in anxiety, an absence of injury, and an understanding of compliance to the prescribed treatment regimen.

The major goals of nursing management may include a reduction in the patient's anxiety, protection from injury, and the development and implementation of an effective teaching plan.

The patient is observed for the expected effects of the antihistamine. If the antihistamine is given for a serious situation, such as a blood transfusion reaction or a severe drug allergy, the patient is assessed at

SUMMARY DRUG TABLE 35—1
Antihistamines

GENERIC NAME	TRADE NAME*	USES	ADVERSE REACTIONS	DOSE RANGES
astemizole	Hismanal	Allergic symptoms	Headache, increased appetite, weight gain, nausea, nervousness, dizziness, diarrhea	10 mg/d PO
bromphen-iramine maleate	Bromphen, Dimetane, *generic*	Allergic symptoms; allergic reactions to blood or plasma; adjunctive therapy in anaphylactic reactions	Drowsiness, sedation, dizziness, disturbed coordination, fatigue, hypotension, headache, epigastric distress, thickening of bronchial secretions	4 mg PO q4–6h; 8–12 mg PO of sustained-release form q12h; up to 40 mg/d IM, SC, IV in divided doses
chlorphen-iramine maleate	Chlor-Trimeton, *generic*	Same as brompheniramine	Same as brompheniramine	4 mg PO 3–6 times/d; sustained-release form: 8–12 mg PO q8–12h; 10–20 mg IM, SC, IV
clemastine fumarate	Tavist	Same as astemizole	Same as brompheniramine	1.34 mg PO bid to 2.68 mg PO tid
diphenhydra-mine hydro-chloride	Benadryl, Bendylate, *generic*	Same as brompheniramine; motion sickness, parkinsonism, control of coughs due to colds or allergy	Same as brompheniramine	25–50 mg PO tid, qid; 10–100 mg IM, IV
promethazine hydrochloride	Phenergan, Anergan, *generic*	Same as brompheniramine; motion sickness, nausea and vomiting associated with anesthesia and surgery, as an adjunct to analgesics, sedation and apprehension, preoperative and postoperative sedation	See Summary Drug Table 34-1, adverse reactions of chlorpromazine sedation	Allergy: 12.5–25 mg PO, 25 mg IM, IV; motion sickness, nausea, vomiting: 12.5–25 mg PO, IM, IV; 25–50 mg PO, IM, IV; preoperative: 25–50 mg IM or PO the night before surgery
terfenadine	Seldane	Same as astemizole	Alopecia, bronchospasm, visual disturbances, itching, urticaria, rash	60 mg PO bid

* *The term* generic *indicates that the drug is available in a generic form.*

frequent intervals until the symptoms appear relieved and for about 24 hours after the incident.

ADVERSE DRUG REACTIONS, HIGH RISK FOR INJURY. Dryness of the mouth, nose, and throat may occur. These symptoms may be relieved by frequent sips of water. If drowsiness is severe or if other problems such as dizziness or a disturbance in muscle coordination occur, the patient may require assistance with ambulatory activities. Adverse reactions are reported to the physician. In some instances, for example, drowsiness or sedation when given to relieve preoperative anxiety, these adverse reactions are expected and are allowed to occur.

KNOWLEDGE DEFICIT. The dosage regimen and possible adverse drug reactions are reviewed with the patient. The following points may be included in a patient teaching plan:

▶ Do not drive or perform other hazardous tasks if drowsiness occurs.

▶ Avoid the use of alcohol, as well as other drugs that cause sleepiness or drowsiness, while taking these drugs.

▶ These drugs may cause dryness of the mouth and throat. Frequent sips of water, hard candy, or chewing gum (preferably sugarless) may relieve this problem.

▶ Take this drug with food or meals because it may cause gastrointestinal (GI) upset.

▶ If the condition is not relieved, discuss this with the physician.

EVALUATION

► Anxiety is reduced
► No evidence of injury
► Adverse reactions are identified and reported to the physician
► Patient demonstrates understanding of drug regimen, adverse drug effects

► SYSTEMIC AND TOPICAL BRONCHODILATORS AND DECONGESTANTS

A **bronchodilator** is a drug used to relieve bronchospasm associated with respiratory disorders such as bronchial asthma, chronic bronchitis, and emphysema. A **decongestant** is a drug that reduces swelling of the nasal passages, which, in turn, opens clogged nasal passages and enhances drainage of the sinuses.

▷ Actions of Bronchodilators and Decongestants

Bronchodilators

There are two types of bronchodilators: the *sympathomimetics* and the *xanthine derivatives*. Examples of sympathomimetic bronchodilators include terbutaline (Bricanyl) and albuterol (Ventolin). Examples of the xanthine derivatives are theophylline and aminophylline. Additional bronchodilators are listed in Summary Drug Table 35-2.

The sympathomimetics have beta-adrenergic activity (see chap 6), and therefore dilate the bronchi. The xanthine derivatives, although a different class of drugs, also have bronchodilating activity by means of their direct relaxation of the smooth muscles of the bronchi.

When bronchospasm occurs, there is a decrease in the lumen (or inside diameter) of the bronchi, which decreases the amount of air taken into the lungs with each breath. A decrease in the amount of air taken into the lungs results in respiratory distress. Use of a bronchodilating drug dilates the bronchi and allows more air to enter the lungs, which, in turn, completely or partially relieves respiratory distress.

Decongestants

The nasal decongestants are sympathomimetic agents, which produce localized vasoconstriction of the small blood vessels of the nasal membranes. Vasoconstriction reduces swelling in the nasal passages (decongestive activity). Nasal decongestants may be applied topically and a few are available for oral use. Examples of nasal decongestants include phenylephrine (Neo-Synephrine) and oxymetazoline (Afrin), which are available as nasal sprays or drops and pseudoephedrine (Sudafed) which is taken orally. Additional nasal decongestants are listed in Summary Drug Table 35-3.

▷ Adverse Reactions Associated with the Administration of Bronchodilators and Decongestants

Bronchodilators

Administration of a sympathomimetic bronchodilator may result in restlessness, anxiety, increase in blood pressure, palpitations, cardiac dysrhythmias, and insomnia. Adverse reactions associated with administration of the xanthine derivatives include nausea, vomiting, restlessness, headache, palpitations, increased respirations, fever, hyperglycemia, and electrocardiographic (ECG) changes.

Decongestants

When used topically in prescribed doses, there are usually minimal systemic effects in most individuals. On occasion, nasal burning, stinging, and dryness may be seen. *Overuse* of the topical form of these drugs can cause "rebound" nasal congestion, that is, the congestion becomes worse with the use of the drug. Although congestion may be relieved for a *brief* time after the drug is used, it recurs within a short time, which then prompts the patient to use the drug at more frequent intervals. When the topical form is used frequently or if the liquid is swallowed, the same adverse reactions seen with the oral decongestants may occur.

Use of oral decongestants may result in tachycardia and other cardiac dysrhythmias, nervousness, restlessness, insomnia, blurred vision, nausea, and vomiting.

Nonprescription nasal decongestants should not be used by those with hypertension or heart disease unless use is approved by the physician.

SUMMARY DRUG TABLE 35–2
Systemic and Topical Bronchodilators

GENERIC NAME	TRADE NAME*	USES	ADVERSE REACTIONS	DOSE RANGES
SYMPATHOMIMETICS				
albuterol sulfate	Proventil, Ventolin	Bronchospasm	Restlessness, anxiety, fear, hypertension, palpitations, tachycardia, insomnia	2–4 mg PO tid, qid; 1–2 inhalations q4–6h
ephedrine sulfate	*Generic*	Allergic disorders such as bronchial asthma	Same as albuterol sulfate	25–50 mg PO, IM, SC, slow IV
epinephrine	Adrenalin, Sus-Phrine, *generic*	Bronchial asthma, bronchospasm, hypersensitivity reactions to drugs, sera, insect stings, or other allergens	Same as albuterol sulfate	1 : 1000 solution: 0.3–0.5 mL (0.3–0.5 mg) SC, IM; 1 : 200 suspension: 0.1–0.3 mL SC; also may be given by inhalation or nebulization
ethylnorepinephrine hydrochloride	Bronkephrine	Same as albuterol sulfate	Same as albuterol sulfate	0.3–1 mL SC, IM
isoproterenol hydrochloride	Isuprel	Bronchodilator in bronchopulmonary diseases, bronchospasm during anesthesia	Same as albuterol sulfate	10–20 mg sublingual; bronchospasm under anesthesia: 0.01–0.02 mg IV; may also be given by nebulization aerosol or metered-dose inhaler
metaproterenol hydrochloride	Alupent, Metaprel	Bronchial asthma, bronchospasm due to bronchitis, emphysema	Same as albuterol sulfate	20 mg PO tid, qid; 2–3 inhalations q3–4h
terbutaline sulfate	Brethine, Bricanyl, Brethaire	Same as metaproterenol hydrochloride	Same as albuterol sulfate	2.5–5 mg PO tid; 0.25 mg SC; 2 inhalations q4–6 h
XANTHINE DERIVATIVES				
aminophylline	Amoline, Truphylline, *generic*	Bronchial asthma, bronchospasm	Nausea, vomiting, restlessness, headache, palpitations, fever, increased respirations, hyperglycemia, ECG changes	100–200 mg PO; dosage may also be based on serum levels or body weight; IV infusion requires dilution and is given at a rate not exeeding 25 mg/min
dyphylline	Dilor, *generic*	Same as aminophylline	Same as aminophylline	Up to 15 mg/kg PO q6h; 250–500 mg IM
oxtriphylline	Choledyl, *generic*	Same as aminophylline	Same as aminophylline	200 mg PO qid
theophylline	Slo-Phyllin, Elixophyllin, *generic*	Same as aminophylline	Same as aminophylline	2–6 mg/kg PO; dosage may also be based on serum levels

* The term generic *indicates that the drug is available in a generic form.*

SUMMARY DRUG TABLE 35–3
Systemic and Topical Nasal Decongestants

GENERIC NAME	TRADE NAME*	USES	ADVERSE REACTIONS	DOSE RANGES
ephedrine	Efedron	Nasal congestion	Nasal burning, stinging, dryness, rebound nasal congestion	2–3 drops or small amount of jelly in each nostril q4–6h
epinephrine hydrochloride	Adrenalin Chloride	Same as ephedrine	Same as ephedrine	1–2 drops in each nostril q4–6h
naphazoline hydrochloride	Privine	Same as ephedrine	Same as ephedrine	2 drops in each nostril prn
oxymetazoline hydrochloride	Afrin, Dristan Long Lasting, *generic*	Same as ephedrine	Same as ephedrine	2–3 drops or sprays q12h
phenylephrine hydrochloride	Neo-Syn-ephrine, Al-conefrin	Same as ephedrine	Same as ephedrine	1–2 drops or sprays in each nostril
phenylpropanol-lamine hydro-chloride	Propagest, *generic*	Same as ephedrine	Anxiety, restlessness, anorexia, dysrhythmias, nervousness, nausea, vomiting, blurred vision	25 mg PO q4h; 50 mg PO q8h
pseudoephedrine hydrochloride	Sudafed, *generic*	Same as ephedrine	Same as phenyl-propanolamine	60 mg PO q4–6 h
tetrahydrozoline hydrochloride	Tyzine	Same as ephedrine	Same as phenyl-propanolamine	2–4 drops in each nostril
xylomethazoline hydrochloride	Otrivin, *generic*	Same as ephedrine	Same as ephedrine	2–3 drops or sprays in each nostril q8–10h

* The term generic *indicates that the drug is available in a generic form.*

▶ NURSING PROCESS
THE PATIENT RECEIVING A BRONCHODILATOR

ASSESSMENT

The blood pressure, pulse, and respiratory rate are taken before bronchodilator therapy is initiated. The lungs are auscultated and the sounds heard are described on the patient's chart. If the patient is raising sputum, a description of the sputum is also recorded. The patient's general physical condition is noted and recorded.

NURSING DIAGNOSIS

Depending on the severity of bronchospasm. one or more of the following nursing diagnoses may apply to the patient receiving a bronchodilator:

▶ Anxiety related to difficulty breathing
▶ Knowledge deficit of medication regimen, adverse drug effects

PLANNING AND IMPLEMENTATION

The major goals of the patient may include a reduction in anxiety and an understanding of and compliance to the prescribed treatment regimen.

The major goals of nursing management may include a reduction in the patient's anxiety and the development and implementation of an effective teaching plan.

ANXIETY. The patient having difficulty breathing is bound to have anxiety, the extent of which depends on the degree of respiratory difficulty. The nurse should reassure the patient that the medication being administered will most likely relieve his or her respiratory distress in a short time. Patients who are extremely apprehensive may require more frequent observation until their respirations are near normal.

ADMINISTRATION. Oral preparations may be given with food or milk if gastric upset occurs. If a nebulizer or aerosol inhaler is used for administration, the patient must be shown how to use this method of delivering the drug to the lungs.

Some of these drugs, for example, aminophylline,

may be given intravenously (IV), either direct IV or as an IV infusion. Some of the sympathomimetics are extremely potent drugs. Great care must be exercised in reading the physician's order when preparing these drugs for administration. Note that the dose of drugs such as epinephrine and ethylnorepinephrine (Bronkephrine) are measured in *tenths* of a milliliter. A tuberculin syringe should be used for measuring and administering these drugs by the parenteral route.

POSTADMINISTRATION OBSERVATIONS. After administration of the drug, the patient is observed for the effectiveness of drug therapy. Breathing should improve and the patient will appear less anxious. If relief does not occur, the physician is notified because a different drug or an increase in dosage may be necessary.

If the patient has acute bronchospasm, the blood pressure, pulse, respiratory rate, and response to the drug should be monitored every 15 to 30 minutes until the patient's condition stabilizes and respiratory distress is relieved. If a drug is given by IV infusion, the infusion rate is monitored every 15 minutes. These patients may be extremely restless and the IV infusion site must be checked at frequent intervals.

If aminophylline is given as a rectal suppository, the patient should be checked every 15 to 30 minutes to be sure the suppository has been retained. If the patient is unable to retain the suppository, the physician is contacted because another route of administration may be necessary.

ADVERSE DRUG REACTIONS. The patient should be observed for adverse drug reactions. The next dose is withheld and the physician is contacted if adverse reactions occur. Patients who have difficulty breathing and are receiving a sympathomimetic drug may experience extreme anxiety, nervousness, and restlessness, which may be due to their breathing difficulty, as well as the action of the sympathomimetic drug. In these patients, it may be difficult for the physician to determine if the patient is having an adverse drug reaction or if the problem is related to their respiratory disorder.

KNOWLEDGE DEFICIT. If an aerosol inhalator is to be used for administration of the bronchodilator, the patient requires a thorough explanation of its use. Each brand is slightly different. An instruction sheet describing how the unit is assembled, used, and cleaned is provided with these products and is carefully reviewed with the patient.

The following points may be included in a patient teaching plan:

▶ If symptoms become worse, do *not* increase the dose or frequency of use unless directed to do so by the physician.

▶ If GI upset occurs, take this drug with food or milk (oral form).

▶ Do not use nonprescription drugs (some may contain sympathomimetic drugs) unless use has been approved by the physician.

▶ Avoid smoking (when applicable). Smoking may make it difficult to adjust the dosage and may worsen breathing problems.

▶ These drugs may cause nervousness, insomnia, and restlessness (especially the sympathomimetics). Contact the physician if these symptoms become severe.

EVALUATION

▶ Anxiety is reduced

▶ Patient demonstrates understanding of drug regimen, use of nebulizer, or aerosol inhalator

▶ NURSING PROCESS
THE PATIENT USING A NASAL DECONGESTANT

ASSESSMENT

Decongestants are used only occasionally in the clinical setting. Since some of these products are available without a prescription, the use of these products may be discovered during a patient history for other medical disorders. A history of the use of these products should be obtained and include the product used and frequency of use.

NURSING DIAGNOSIS

▶ Knowledge deficit of medication regimen, adverse drug effects

PLANNING AND IMPLEMENTATION

The major goal of the patient may include an understanding of the use and adverse reactions associated with nasal decongestants.

The major goal of nursing management may include the development and implementation of an effective teaching plan.

The nurse should inform the physician if nasal congestion is not relieved.

KNOWLEDGE DEFICIT. The following points may be included in a patient teaching plan:

▶ Use this product as directed by the physician or on

the container label. Overuse of topical nasal decongestants can make the symptoms *worse*.

▶ Nasal burning and stinging may occur with the topical decongestants. If this becomes severe, discontinue use and discuss this problem with the physician, who may prescribe or recommend another drug.

EVALUATION

▶ Verbalizes understanding of use of a decongestant and adverse reactions associated with use

▶ ANTITUSSIVES

An **antitussive** is a drug used to relieve coughing. Many antitussive drugs are combined with other drugs, such as an antihistamine or expectorant, and sold as nonprescription cough medicines. Other antitussives, either alone or in combination with other drugs, are available by prescription only.

▷ Actions of the Antitussives

Antitussives that depress the cough center located in the medulla are called centrally acting agents. Codeine and dextromethorphan are examples of these types of antitussives. Other antitussives are peripherally acting agents and act by anesthetizing stretch receptors in the respiratory passages, thereby decreasing coughing. An example of this type of antitussive is benzonatate (Tessalon Perles). Other antitussives act locally, that is, they soothe irritated areas in the mouth and throat for a brief time. These syruplike agents are usually combined with other ingredients in a cough mixture preparation.

▷ Uses of the Antitussives

Antitussives are used for the relief of a nonproductive cough. When the cough is productive of sputum, it should be treated by a physician.

▷ Adverse Reactions Associated with the Administration of the Antitussives

Use of codeine may result in respiratory depression, euphoria, light-headedness, sedation, nausea, vomiting, and hypersensitivity reactions. When used as directed, the nonprescription cough medicines have few adverse reactions (Summary Drug Table 35-4).

One problem associated with the use of an antitussive is related to its drug action. Although not an adverse reaction, depression of the cough reflex can cause a pooling of secretions in the lungs. A pooling of secretions, which normally are removed by coughing, may result in a more serious problem such as pneumonia. Another problem associated with the use of these drugs is when the patient uses a nonprescription cough medicine for self-treatment of a chronic cough, which could be a symptom of a more serious problem such as lung cancer or emphysema.

▶ NURSING PROCESS
THE PATIENT RECEIVING AN ANTITUSSIVE DRUG

ASSESSMENT

A hospitalized patient may occasionally have an antitussive preparation prescribed, especially when a nonproductive cough causes discomfort, or may cause more serious problems such as raising pressure in the eye (increased intraocular pressure) following eye surgery and increased intracranial pressure in those with disorders of the central nervous system. Assessment should include documentation of the type of cough (productive, nonproductive).

NURSING DIAGNOSIS

Depending on the reason for administration, one or more of the following nursing diagnoses may apply to a person receiving an adrenergic drug:

▶ Anxiety related to need to cough frequently, pain or discomfort associated with coughing
▶ Knowledge deficit of medication regimen, adverse drug effects

PLANNING AND IMPLEMENTATION

The major goals of the patient may include a reduction in anxiety and an understanding of the prescribed treatment regimen.

The major goals of nursing management may include a reduction in the patient's anxiety and the development and implementation of an effective teaching plan.

ANXIETY. If the patient appears anxious over the need to cough at frequent intervals, the nurse should reas-

SUMMARY DRUG TABLE 35–4
Antitussives*

GENERIC NAME	TRADE NAME†	USES	ADVERSE REACTIONS	DOSE RANGES
NARCOTICS				
codeine sulfate	Generic	Nonproductive cough	Respiratory depression, euphoria, lightheadedness, sedation, nausea, vomiting	10–20 mg PO q4–6h
NONNARCOTICS				
benzonatate	Tessalon Perles	Same as codeine sulfate	Sedation, headache, dizziness, constipation, nausea, pruritus	100 mg PO tid
dextromethorphan hydrobromide	Mediquell, Sucrets Cough Control, Hold	Same as codeine sulfate	Rare	10–30 mg PO q4–8h
diphenhydramine hydrochloride	Benylin Cough, generic	Same as codeine sulfate	See Summary Drug Table 35-1	25 mg PO q4h

* Some cold preparations contain an antitussive, such as one of those listed above, as well as other ingredients, which may include one or more other agents such as an antihistamine, an expectorant, or a decongestant.
† The term generic indicates that the drug is available in a generic form.

sure the patient that the medication will most likely relieve this problem. If the cough is not relieved, the physician is notified.

KNOWLEDGE DEFICIT. The nurse should discourage the indiscriminate use of nonprescription cough medicines and advise the patient to read the label carefully, follow the dosage recommendations, and consult a physician if the cough persists for more than 10 days or if fever or chest pain occurs. If the patient is prescribed an antitussive, the following points may be included in a patient teaching plan:

► Do not exceed the recommended dose.
► If chills, fever, chest pain, or sputum production occurs, contact the physician as soon as possible.
► Oral capsules—Do not chew or break the capsules open; swallow them whole.
► If the cough is not relieved or becomes worse, contact the physician.

► MUCOLYTICS AND EXPECTORANTS

A **mucolytic** is a drug that loosens respiratory secretions. An **expectorant** is a drug that aids in raising thick, tenacious mucus from the respiratory passages.

▷ Actions of Mucolytics and Expectorants

Mucolytics. Mucolytic drugs appear to reduce the thickness (viscosity) of respiratory secretions by direct action on the mucus. The only mucolytic presently in use is acetylcysteine (Mucomyst).

Expectorants. Expectorants increase the production of respiratory secretions, which, in turn, appears to decrease the thickness of the mucus. An example of an expectorant is guaifenesin (Hytuss).

▷ Uses of Mucolytics and Expectorants

Mucolytics. Mucolytic agents may be used as part of the treatment of bronchopulmonary diseases such as emphysema. They are primarily given by nebulization.

Expectorants. Expectorants, which may be included in some prescription and nonprescription cough medicines, are used to help raise respiratory secretions.

▷ Adverse Reactions Associated with the Administration of Mucolytics and Expectorants

The more common adverse reactions associated with mucolytic and expectorant drugs are listed in Summary Drug Table 35-5.

▶ NURSING PROCESS
THE PATIENT RECEIVING A MUCOLYTIC OR AN EXPECTORANT

ASSESSMENT

The patient's degree of respiratory congestion is determined by auscultation of the lungs.

NURSING DIAGNOSIS

▶ Anxiety related to respiratory difficulty, inability to raise sputum

▶ Knowledge deficit of medication regimen, adverse drug effects, treatment modalities

PLANNING AND IMPLEMENTATION

The major goals of the patient may include a reduction in anxiety and an understanding of the medication regimen.

The major goal of nursing management may include a reduction in the patient's anxiety and the development and implementation of an effective teaching plan.

When the mucolytic acetylcystine is administered by nebulization, the nurse must explain the treatment to the patient. In some instances, it may be necessary to remain with the patient during the first few treatments, especially when the patient is elderly or exhibits anxiety. If this drug is ordered to be inserted into a tracheostomy, suction equipment is placed at the bedside to be immediately available for aspiration of secretions.

The patient is supplied with tissues and a paper bag for disposal of the tissues. These are placed within the patient's reach. Immediately before and after treatment, the lungs are auscultated. The findings of both assessments are recorded on the patient's chart. Between treatments, the patient's respiratory status should be evaluated and the findings are recorded on the patient's chart. These evaluations aid the physician in determining the effectiveness of therapy. If any prob-

SUMMARY DRUG TABLE 35–5
Mucolytics and Expectorants

GENERIC NAME	TRADE NAME*	USES	ADVERSE REACTIONS	DOSE RANGES
MUCOLYTICS				
acetylcysteine	Mucomyst	Mucus secretions in bronchopulmonary diseases (acute, chronic)	Bronchospasm, stomatitis, nausea, vomiting	Nebulization: 1–10 mL of 20% solution; 2–20 mL of 10% solution q2–6h; may also be instilled into tracheostomy
EXPECTORANTS				
guaifenesin	Hytuss, Nortussin, *generic*	Respiratory conditions with dry, nonproductive cough	Vomiting, nausea, gastric disturbances, drowsiness	100–400 mg PO q3–6h
potassium iodide (tablets, oral solution)	*Generic*	Chronic pulmonary diseases with tenacious mucus	Iodine sensitivity or iodism (sore mouth, metallic taste, increased salivation, nausea, vomiting, epigastric pain, parotid swelling, and pain)	Tablets: 300–1000 mg PO tid PC; oral solution: 0.3–0.6 mL 3–4 times/d
terpin hydrate (contains 42% alcohol)	*Generic*	Cough due to cold or minor bronchial irritations	Drowsiness, epigastric pain	85 mg (5 mL) PO q3–4h

* The term generic *indicates that the drug is available in a generic form.*

lem occurs during or after treatment, or if the patient is uncooperative, the problem is discussed with the physician.

When expectorants are given to those with chronic pulmonary disease, the effectiveness of drug therapy (ie, the patient's ability to raise sputum) is evaluated and recorded in the patient's chart.

ANXIETY. The patient should be reassured that the prescribed therapy will most likely help in raising secretions.

KNOWLEDGE DEFICIT. Acetylcysteine usually is administered in the hospital but may be prescribed for the patient being discharged and renting or buying respiratory therapy equipment may be recommended. The patient or a family member needs full instruction in the use and maintenance of the equipment, as well as the technique of administration of acetylcysteine.

When an expectorant is prescribed, the patient is instructed to take the drug as directed and to contact his or her physician if any unusual symptoms or other problems occur during use of the drug or if the drug appears to be ineffective.

EVALUATION

► Anxiety is reduced
► Patient and family demonstrate understanding of drug regimen, use of equipment to administer the drug (mucolytic)

36

Drugs Used in the Management of Gastrointestinal Disorders

On completion of this chapter the student will:

▶ *List the type of drugs prescribed or recommended for gastrointestinal disorders*

▶ *Discuss the actions and adverse reactions associated with gastrointestinal drugs*

▶ *Use the nursing process when administering a gastrointestinal drug*

▶ *Discuss the nursing implications to be considered when administering a gastrointestinal drug*

The gastrointestinal (GI) tract is subject to more diseases and disorders than any other system of the body. Some disorders, such as constipation, may be self-treated, although, in some instances, this practice can be dangerous. Other disorders, such as peptic ulcer, may require a variety of drugs in the medical management of this disease.

The drugs presented in this chapter include the antacids, anticholinergics, histamine H_2 antagonists, antidiarrheals, antiflatulents, digestive enzymes, emetics, gallstone-solubilizing agents, and laxatives. Some of the more common preparations

and their individual uses are listed in Summary Drug Table 36-1.

▷ Actions of the Drugs Used in the Management of GI Disorders

Antacids. Antacids neutralize or reduce the acidity of gastric contents. Examples of antacids include

271

(c̄ Magnesium = diarrhea)
(aluminum = constipation)

SUMMARY DRUG TABLE 36–1
Gastrointestinal Drugs

GENERIC NAME	TRADE NAME*	DOSE RANGES
ANTACIDS† Local / Systemic Ulcers Give last		
aluminum carbonate gel, basic	Basaljel	2 capsules or tablets; 10 mL of liquid suspension PO q2h
aluminum hydroxide gel	Alu-Cap, Amphojel, *generic*	500–1800 mg PO 3–6 times/d between meals and hs
aluminum phosphate gel	Phosphaljel	15–30 mL PO q2h between meals and hs
calcium carbonate	Dicarbosil, Tums, *generic*	0.5–1.5 g PO prn
dihydroxyaluminum sodium carbonate	Rolaids Antacid	1–2 tablets chewed prn
magaldrate	Riopan	480–1080 mg PO between meals and hs
magnesia (magnesium hydroxide)	*Generic*, (milk of magnesia)	5–10 mL PO or 650 mg–1.3 g PO qid
magnesium oxide	Maox, Mag-Ox 400, Uro-Mag	Capsules: 140 mg PO tid, qid; tablets: 400–840 mg/d PO
sodium bicarbonate → Systemic	Soda Mint, *generic*	0.3–2 g PO 1–4 times/d
ANTICHOLINERGICS		
See Summary Drug Table 9-1		
ANTIDIARRHEAL DRUGS		
camphorated tincture of opium (paregoric)	*Generic*	5–10 mL PO, 1–4 times/d
diphenoxin hydrochloride with atropine sulfate	Motofen	Initial dose: 2 tablets, then 1 tablet after each loose stool
diphenoxylate hydrochloride with atropine sulfate	Lomotil, *generic*	5 mg PO qid; once control is achieved, dosage may be decreased
loperamide hydrocholoride	Imodium	Initial dose: 4 mg PO then 2 mg after each un-formed stool
ANTIFLATULENTS		
charcoal	Charcocaps, *generic*	520–975 mg PO ac
simethicone	Silain, Mylicon, Gas-X	Capsules: 125 mg PO qid; tablets: 40–125 mg PO qid; drops: 40 mg PO qid
DIGESTIVE ENZYMES		
pancreatin	Pancreatin Enseals, *generic*	1–3 tablets PO with meals
pancrelipase	Cotazym, Pancrease, Viokase, *generic*	1–3 capsules, tablets before or with meals; powder: 0.7 g with meals
EMETICS		
apomorphine hydrochloride	*Generic*	2–10 mg SC
ipecac syrup	*Generic*	5–20 mL PO followed by 1/2–4 glasses of water (dosage and amount of water depend on age of individual)
HISTAMINE H₂ ANTAGONISTS		
cimetidine	Tagamet	300 mg PO qid and up to 2400 mg/d in divided doses; alternate dosage schedules include 400–800 mg PO hs, 400 mg PO bid; par-enteral: 300 mg IM, IV, intermittent IV infusion q6h or up to 2400 mg/d IM, IV, intermittent IV infusion in divided doses
famotidine	Pepcid	20 mg PO bid or 40 mg PO daily at hs; par-enteral: 20 mg IV, IV infusion q12h
nizatidine	Axid	150–300 mg PO sid hs
ranitidine	Zantac	150 mg PO bid or daily at hs; 50 mg IM, IV q6–8h; 50 mg diluted in 0.9% sodium chloride by IV infusion q6–8h

(continued)

Handwritten annotations:
- Local Acting Coat Stomach Ex ulcer
- Na Bicarbonate NaHCO₃ Systemic Antacid + Rebound = Metabolic RXN. alkalosis
- over neutralize — Metabolic alkalosis
- Makes more acid rebound effect
- Sch V Controlled drug
- monitor stools — report/record fl. elect imbalance
- ↑ Hyperactive Means = has gas RBS
- Give to people c̄ C Fibrosis replacing enz.
- Controlled
- Hist blocker Creates HCL (vagotomy) Makes HCL
- Ulcers Systemic used

* Know for pharm

*[handwritten top margin: Adrenergic – ediphine – ephrine – Sympathetic N System; atropine alone dilitates eye 3/4 1 eye mg; Cholinergic (Parasympathetic N System (atropine) ↓ gastric Motility; 2) Pre-op ↓ or to dry secretion (Pre-op & Dureal (relax anxiety) drivers (operations) easier to relax when giving anesthesia; 3) pupils would Be Constricted when given a narcotic; * all narcotic analgics are resp depressants fall VTS before giving Morphine – resp 12↑ daily ↓ notify MD; Demerol Narc. over powers atropine in OR eye contricts]*

SUMMARY DRUG TABLE 36–1
(continued)

GENERIC NAME	TRADE NAME*	USES	ADVERSE REACTIONS	DOSE RANGES
LAXATIVES‡				
BULK-FORMING LAXATIVES				
polycarbophil	FiberCon			1 g PO qid or prn
psyllium	Konsyl D, Metamucil			1 rounded tsp stirred into 1 glass of liquid 1–3 times/d
EMOLLIENT LAXATIVES				
mineral oil	Agoral Plain, *generic*			5–20 mL PO hs
FECAL SOFTENERS				
docusate calcium	Surfak, *generic*			240 mg/d PO
docusate potassium	Dialose, Kasof			100–300 mg/d PO
docusate sodium	Colase, Modane Soft, *generic*			50–500 mg/d
HYPEROSMOLAR AGENTS				
glycerin	*Generic*			1 rectal suppository
IRRITANT OR STIMULANT LAXATIVES				
bisacodyl	Dulcolax, Theralax, *generic*			10–15 mg PO
cascara sagrada	*Generic*			Tablets: 325 mg; aromatic fluid extract: 5 mL PO
castor oil	Alphamul, *generic*			15–60 mL PO
phenolphthalein	Ex-Lax, Correctol, Phenolax			60–194 mg PO
senna	Senokot, Senolax, Genna			Varies according to product used; consult package labeling
SALINE LAXATIVES				
citrate of magnesia	Citroma, *generic*			1 glass (about 240 mL)
magnesium hydroxide (milk of magnesia)	*Generic*			15–30 mL PO; concentrated form: 10–20 mL PO
sodium phosphate and sodium biphosphate	Phospho-Soda, *generic*			20–30 mL mixed with 1/2 glass of cold water
GALLSTONE-SOLUBILIZING AGENTS				
chenodiol	Chenix			13–16 mg/kg/d PO in 2 divided doses
ursodiol	Actigall			8–10 mg/kg/d PO in 2–3 divided doses

[handwritten annotations in table: "Bulk forming ↑ Fl. & Med gives stool form." beside psyllium; "Cathartics ↑ fl bulk in diet" beside fecal softeners; "OTC" beside glycerin, phenolphthalein, senna; "diarrhea" and "Bowel prep" in saline laxatives area]

* The term *generic* indicates that the drug is available in a generic form.
† Other antacids offer a combination of drugs and may contain one or more of the agents listed.
‡ Some laxatives offer a combination of drugs and may contain one or more of the agents listed.

aluminum hydroxide gel (Amphojel), magnesium hydroxide (Magnesia, Milk of Magnesia), and magaldrate (Riopan).

Anticholinergics. Anticholinergics (cholinergic blocking drugs) reduce gastric motility and decrease the amount of acid secreted by the stomach (see chap 9). Examples of anticholinergics used for GI disorders include clidinium (Quarzan) and glycopyrrolate (Robinul).

Histamine H₂ Antagonists. These drugs inhibit the action of histamine at histamine H₂ receptor cells of the stomach, which then reduces gastric acid secretion. Examples of histamine H₂ antagonists include cimetidine (Tagamet), ranitidine (Zantac), famotidine (Pepcid), and nizatidine (Axid).

Antidiarrheals. Antidiarrheals decrease intestinal peristalsis, which is usually increased when the patient has diarrhea. Examples of these drugs include difenoxin (Motofen), diphenoxylate (Lomotil), and loperamide (Imodium).

Antiflatulents. Simethicone (Mylicon) and charcoal are used as antiflatulents. Simethicone has a defoaming action that disperses and prevents the formation of mucus-surrounded gas pockets in the intestine. Charcoal is an absorbent which reduces the amount of intestinal gas.

1F tablet

Digestive Enzymes. The pancreatic enzymes pancreatin and pancrelipase are responsible for the breakdown of fats, starches, and proteins and are necessary for the breakdown and digestion of food.

Emetics. Apomorphine promotes vomiting by its direct action on the vomiting center (chemoreceptor trigger zone or CTZ) of the medulla. Ipecac causes vomiting because of its local irritating effect on the stomach, as well as by stimulation of the vomiting center in the medulla.

Gallstone-Solubilizing Agents. Chenodiol (Chenix) and ursodiol (Actigall) suppress the manufacture of cholesterol and cholic acid by the liver, which ultimately result in a decrease in the size of radiolucent gallstones.

Laxatives. There are various types of laxatives (see the following list and Summary Drug Table 36-1). The action of each laxative is somewhat different, yet produces the same result—the relief of constipation. *drink lots of fluids = laxatives*

▷ **Bulk-forming laxatives** are not digested by the body and therefore add bulk and water to the contents of the intestines. The added bulk in the intestines stimulates peristalsis, moves the products of digestion through the intestine, and encourages evacuation of the stool. Examples of bulk-forming laxatives are psyllium (Metamucil) and polycarbophil (FiberCon).

▷ **Emollient laxatives** lubricate the intestinal walls and soften the stool, thereby enhancing passage of fecal material. Mineral oil is an emollient laxative.

▷ **Fecal softeners** promote water retention in the fecal mass and soften the stool. One difference between emollient laxatives and fecal softeners is that the emollient laxatives do not promote the retention of water in the stool. Examples of fecal softeners include docusate sodium (Colace) and docusate calcium (Surfak).

▷ **Hyperosmolar agents** dehydrate local tissues, which causes irritation and increased peristalsis with consequent evacuation of the fecal mass. Glycerin is a hyperosmolar agent.

▷ **Irritant or stimulant laxatives** increase peristalsis by direct action on the intestine. An example of an irritant laxative is cascara sagrada.

▷ **Saline laxatives** attract or pull water into the intestine, thereby increasing pressure in the intestine followed by an increase in peristalsis. Magnesium hydroxide (Milk of Magnesia) is a saline laxative.

▷ Uses of Drugs Used in the Management of GI Disorders

Antacids. Antacids are used in the treatment of gastric distress, such as heartburn and acid indigestion, and in the medical treatment of peptic ulcer. Many antacid preparations contain more than one ingredient, for example, Maalox, which consists of aluminum hydroxide and magnesium hydroxide.

Anticholinergics. Some anticholinergic drugs (see Summary Drug Table 9-1) are used in the medical treatment of peptic ulcer. These drugs have been largely replaced by histamine H_2 antagonists, which appear to be more effective and have less adverse drug reactions.

Histamine H_2 Antagonists. These drugs are used for medical treatment of a gastric or duodenal ulcer, gastric hypersecretory conditions, and gastroesophageal reflux disease.

Antidiarrheals. Antidiarrheals are used in the treatment of diarrhea.

Antiflatulents. Antiflatulents are used to reduce gas formation in the intestines. Simethicone may also be included in some antacid combination products, for example, Mylanta.

Digestive Enzymes. These drugs are prescribed as replacement therapy for those with pancreatic enzyme insufficiency. Conditions or diseases that may cause a decrease in or absence of pancreatic digestive enzymes include cystic fibrosis, chronic pancreatitis, cancer of the pancreas, the malabsorption syndrome, surgical removal of all or part of the stomach, and surgical removal of all or part of the pancreas.

Emetics. Emetics are used to cause vomiting and thereby empty the stomach rapidly when an individual has accidentally or intentionally ingested a poison or drug overdose. Not all poison ingestions or drug overdoses are treated with emetics.

Gallstone-Solubilizing Agents. These drugs are used in the nonsurgical treatment of radiolucent gallstones. They are not effective for all types of gallstones.

Laxatives. A laxative may be ordered for the short-term relief or prevention of constipation, for prevention of straining at stool when this is contraindicated, before examination of the rectum, and in preparation for surgery and diagnostic tests, such as radiographic examination of the bowel.

▷ Adverse Reactions Associated with the Administration of Drugs Used in the Management of GI Disorders

Antacids. The magnesium-containing antacids may have a laxative effect and produce diarrhea. Aluminum-containing and calcium-containing products tend to produce constipation.

Anticholinergics. Dry mouth, blurred vision, urinary hesitancy, urinary retention, nausea, vomiting, palpitations, and headache are some of the adverse reactions that may be seen with the use of anticholinergic drugs. See also Summary Drug Table 9-1.

Histamine H₂ Antagonists. There is a low incidence of adverse reactions seen with the administration of these drugs. Mild and transient diarrhea, dizziness, and fatigue have been reported with the use of cimetidine. Famotidine administration may result in headache and dizziness.

Antidiarrheals. Diphenoxylate use may result in anorexia, nausea, vomiting, constipation, rash, dizziness, drowsiness, sedation, euphoria, and headache. This drug is a narcotic-related drug that has no analgesic activity but has sedative and euphoric effects and drug dependence potential. To discourage abuse, it is combined with atropine (an anticholinergic or cholinergic blocking drug), which causes dry mouth and other mild adverse effects. Loperamide is not a narcotic-related drug; minimal adverse reactions are associated with its use. Occasionally, abdominal discomfort, pain, and distention have been seen, but these symptoms are also seen with severe diarrhea and are difficult to distinguish from an adverse drug reaction.

Antiflatulents. No adverse reactions have been reported with the use of antiflatulents.

Digestive Enzymes. No adverse reactions have been reported with the use of digestive enzymes; however, high doses may cause nausea and diarrhea.

Emetics. Therapeutic doses of apomorphine may cause central nervous system (CNS) depression. There are no apparent adverse reactions to ipecac. Although not an adverse reaction, a danger associated with an emetic is the aspiration of vomitus.

Gallstone-Solubilizing Agents. Diarrhea, cramps, nausea, and vomiting are the more common adverse drug reactions. A reduction in the dose may reduce or eliminate these problems.

Laxatives. Laxative use can cause diarrhea and a loss of water and electrolytes. Laxatives may also cause abdominal pain or discomfort, nausea, vomiting, perianal irritation, and weakness. Prolonged use of a laxative can result in the "laxative habit" or a dependency on a laxative to have a bowel movement.

▶ NURSING PROCESS
THE PATIENT RECEIVING A DRUG FOR A GI DISORDER

ASSESSMENT

The patient's chart is reviewed for the medical diagnosis and reason for administration of the prescribed drug. The patient should be questioned regarding the type and intensity of symptoms (pain, discomfort, diarrhea, constipation, and so on) to provide a baseline for evaluation of the effectiveness of drug therapy.

If the antacid is left at the bedside for self-administration, the patient's understanding of the treatment regimen is evaluated.

Before an emetic is given, it is extremely important to know the chemicals that have been ingested, the time it or they were ingested, and what symptoms were noted before seeking medical treatment. This information will probably be obtained from a family member or friend, but the adult patient may also contribute to the history. The physician or nurse may also contact the local poison center to obtain information regarding treatment.

NURSING DIAGNOSIS

Depending on the patient's symptoms and reason for administration, one or more of the following nursing diagnoses may apply to a person receiving a GI drug:

- ▶ Anxiety related to diagnosis, symptoms, adverse drug reactions, other factors
- ▶ Noncompliance related to lack of knowledge, other factors
- ▶ Knowledge deficit of medication regimen

PLANNING AND IMPLEMENTATION

The major goals of the patient may include a reduction in anxiety and an understanding of and compliance to the prescribed treatment regimen.

The major goals of nursing management may include a reduction in the patient's anxiety and the development and implementation of an effective teaching plan.

ADMINISTRATION. Special considerations for the administration of certain GI preparations are listed in the following sections.

ANTACIDS. Liquid antacid preparations must be shaken thoroughly immediately before administration. If tablets are given, the patient is instructed to chew the tablets thoroughly before swallowing and then drink a full glass of water or milk. Liquid antacids are followed by a small amount of water or milk. Antacids may be ordered to be left at the patient's bedside for self-administration. An adequate supply of water and cups for measuring the dose are made available.

HISTAMINE H₂ ANTAGONISTS. Ranitidine may be given without regard to meals, but oral cimetidine is given immediately before or with meals. Nizatidine and famotidine are given at bedtime. In certain situations or disorders, cimetidine and ranitidine may also be given by intermittent intravenous (IV) infusion or direct IV injection.

ANTIDIARRHEALS. These drugs may be ordered to be given after each loose bowel movement. Each bowel movement is inspected before the nurse makes a decision to administer the drug.

DIGESTIVE ENZYMES. When digestive enzymes are given in capsule or enteric-coated tablet form, the patient is instructed not to bite or chew the capsule or tablet.

EMETICS. An emetic must *not* be given when a corrosive substance (such as lye) or a petroleum distillate (paint thinner, kerosene, and so on) has been ingested. In many cases of poisoning, it is preferable to insert a nasogastric tube to empty stomach contents. These drugs are used with great caution, if at all, when the substance ingested is unknown or in question.

Because treatment of poison ingestion is of an emergency nature, equipment for treatment is readied immediately. Along with the drug, an emesis basin, towels, specimen containers (for sending contents of the stomach to the laboratory for analysis), and a suction machine are placed near the patient. Vital signs are monitored and the physician or nurse performs a physical examination to determine what other damages or injuries, if any, may have occurred. An emetic is never given to a patient who is unconscious or semiconscious because aspiration of vomitus may occur.

Activated charcoal may be given before or after administration of apomorphine. Apomorphine is given by the subcutaneous route. Oral fluids are given immediately after administration of the drug to dilute the poison and encourage vomiting. The patient is positioned on his or her side before or immediately after the drug is given. When emesis occurs, the patient is suctioned as needed and observed closely for the possible aspiration of vomitus. Vital signs are monitored every 5 to 10 minutes until stable.

Ipecac is available without a prescription for use in the home. The instructions for use and the recommended dose are printed on the label.

LAXATIVES. Bulk-producing or fecal-softening laxatives are given with a *full* glass of water or juice. Administration of a bulk-producing laxative is followed by an additional full glass of water. Mineral oil is preferably given on an empty stomach in the evening. Laxatives in powder, flake, or granule form are mixed and stirred thoroughly immediately before administration. If the laxative has an unpleasant or salty taste, this is explained to the patient. Chilling some preparations, adding to juice, or pouring over cracked ice may help disguise the taste.

OBSERVATIONS AND NURSING MANAGEMENT. The patient receiving a GI drug is assessed for relief of symptoms (diarrhea, pain, constipation, and so on). If the drug fails to relieve symptoms, the physician is contacted.

Vital signs are monitored daily and more frequently if the patient has a bleeding peptic ulcer, severe diarrhea, or other condition that may warrant more frequent observation. The effectiveness of drug therapy should be evaluated by a daily comparison of symptoms with those experienced before starting therapy. In some instances, frequent evaluation of the patient's response to therapy may be necessary.

ANTACIDS. A record of bowel movements is kept because use of these drugs may cause constipation or diarrhea. If the patient expresses a dislike for the taste of the antacid or has difficulty chewing the tablet form, the physician is informed of this problem. A flavored antacid may be ordered if the taste is a problem, or a liquid form if there is a problem chewing a tablet.

ANTICHOLINERGICS. Urinary retention or hesitancy may be seen during therapy with these drugs. This can be avoided by instructing the patient to void before taking the drug. If urinary retention is suspected, the intake and output are monitored.

These drugs may cause drowsiness, dizziness, and blurred vision. Some patients may require assistance with ambulatory activities. If photophobia occurs, the room may be kept semidark. Cycloplegia and mydriasis may interfere with activities such as reading or watching television.

HISTAMINE H₂ ANTAGONISTS. When one of these drugs is given by the parenteral route, the rate of infusion is monitored at frequent intervals. Too rapid an infusion has been reported to occasionally result in cardiac dysrhythmias.

ANTIDIARRHEALS. The physician is notified if an elevation in temperature occurs or if severe abdominal pain or abdominal rigidity or distention occurs because this may indicate a complication of the disorder, such as infection or intestinal perforation. If diarrhea is severe, additional treatment measures, such as IV fluids and electrolyte replacement, may be necessary.

Drowsiness or dizziness may occur with these drugs. The patient may require assistance with ambulatory activities. If diarrhea is chronic, the patient is encouraged to drink extra fluids. In some instances, the physician may prescribe an oral electrolyte supplement to replace electrolytes lost by frequent loose stools.

DIGESTIVE ENZYMES. The patient is observed for nausea and diarrhea. If these occur, the physician is notified before the next dose is due because dosage may need to be reduced. The patient's tray is checked after each meal. If the diet is taken poorly or if certain foods are not eaten, this is brought to the attention of the physician. The patient is weighed weekly (or as ordered) and any significant or steady weight loss is brought to the attention of the physician.

The appearance of each stool is noted and recorded. Periodic stool examinations, as well as ongoing descriptions of the appearance of the stools, help the physician determine the effectiveness of therapy.

EMETICS. After the administration of an emetic, the patient is closely observed for signs of shock, respiratory depression, or other signs and symptoms that may be part of the clinical picture of the specific poison or drug that was accidentally or purposely taken by the patient.

LAXATIVES. The results of administration are recorded on the patient's chart. If excessive bowel movements or severe prolonged diarrhea occurs or if the laxative is ineffective, the physician is notified. If a laxative is ordered for constipation, a liberal fluid intake is encouraged to prevent a repeat of this problem.

ADVERSE DRUG REACTIONS. The patient should be observed for adverse drug reactions associated with the specific GI drug being administered. Adverse reactions are reported to the physician.

ANXIETY. Some patients may experience anxiety over circumstances such as their diagnosis, the symptoms of their disorder, or the adverse drug reactions that may be seen with the administration of some of these drugs. The patient should be allowed time to discuss his or her problems or to ask questions. Once problems that may be causing anxiety are identified, the nurse can often relieve anxiety by simple explanations. For example, a patient may be concerned over certain adverse reactions, such as a dry mouth (anticholinergics) or constipation (some antacids). The nurse can explain that these may need to be tolerated and that these adverse reactions may lessen over time. In addition, suggestions can be made to help relieve some adverse drug reactions, such as frequent sips of water to relieve a dry mouth or an increase in fluid intake to correct constipation.

NONCOMPLIANCE AND KNOWLEDGE DEFICIT. When a GI drug must be taken for a long time, there is a possibility that the patient may begin to skip doses or stop the drug. Patients are encouraged to take the prescribed drug as directed by the physician and not to stop taking the drug unless advised to do so by the physician.

The following information may be included in a patient and family teaching plan when a drug is prescribed or recommended for the treatment of a GI disorder:

Antacids

► Chew tablets thoroughly before swallowing and then drink a full glass of water.
► Adhere to the dosage schedule recommended by the physician. Do not increase the frequency of use or the dose if symptoms become worse. Instead, see the physician as soon as possible.
► Antacids impair the absorption of some drugs. Do not take other drugs within 1 to 2 hours before or after taking the antacid unless use of an antacid with a drug is recommended by the physician.
► If pain or discomfort remains the same or becomes worse, if the stools turn black, or if other symptoms occur, contact the physician as soon as possible.
► Antacids may change the color of the stool (white, white streaks); this is normal.

Anticholinergics

► If an aversion to light occurs (photophobia), wear sunglasses when outside, keep rooms dimly lit, and schedule outdoor activities (when necessary) before the first dose of the drug is taken, such as early in the morning.
► If a dry mouth occurs, take frequent sips of cool water during the day. Take several sips of water before taking oral medications and sip water frequently during meals.
► Constipation may be avoided by drinking plenty of fluids during the day.
► Drowsiness may occur with these drugs. Schedule tasks requiring alertness during times when drowsiness does not occur, such as early in the morning before the first dose of the drug is taken.

Histamine H₂ Antagonists

fx of ulcers

- ▶ Keep the physician informed of the results of therapy, that is, relief of pain or discomfort.
- ▶ Take as directed (eg, with meals, at bedtime) on the prescription container.
- ▶ Follow physician's recommendations regarding additional treatment, such as eliminating certain foods, avoiding the use of alcohol, using of additional drugs, such as an antacid, and so on.
- ▶ Cimetidine — If drowsiness occurs, avoid driving or performing other hazardous tasks.

Antidiarrheals

- ▶ Do not exceed the recommended dosage.
- ▶ The drug may cause drowsiness. Observe caution when driving or performing other hazardous tasks.
- ▶ Avoid the use of alcohol or other CNS depressants (tranquilizers, sleeping pills) and other non-prescription drugs unless use has been approved by the physician.
- ▶ Notify the physician if diarrhea persists or becomes more severe.

Antiflatulents

- ▶ If the problem of gas is not relieved, discuss this with the physician.

Digestive Enzymes

- ▶ Take as directed by the physician.
- ▶ Do not exceed the recommended dose.
- ▶ Do not chew tablets or capsules.
- ▶ Powder form may be sprinkled over small quantities of food. All the food sprinkled with the powder must be eaten.

Emetics (Ipecac Syrup)

- ▶ Read the directions on the label after the drug is purchased and be familiar with these instructions before an emergency occurs.
- ▶ In case of accidental or intentional poisoning, contact the nearest poison center *before* using or giving this drug. *Not all poisoning can be treated with this drug.*
- ▶ *Do not give this drug to semiconscious, unconscious, or convulsing individuals.*
- ▶ Vomiting should occur in 20 to 30 minutes. Seek medical attention immediately after contacting the poison center and giving this drug.

Gallstone-Solubilizing Agents

- ▶ Periodic laboratory tests (liver function studies) and ultrasound or radiologic examinations of the gallbladder may be scheduled by the physician.
- ▶ If diarrhea occurs, contact the physician.
- ▶ If symptoms of gallbladder disease (pain, nausea, vomiting) occur, contact the physician immediately.

Laxatives

Habit / dependant

- ▶ Avoid long-term use of these products unless use of the product has been recommended by the physician. Long-term use may result in the laxative habit, which is a dependence on a laxative to have a bowel movement. *loose stiller*
- ▶ Avoid long-term use of mineral oil. Daily use of this product may interfere with the absorption of some vitamins (vitamins A, D, E, K). *no Fat Sol Vit Stored*
- ▶ Read and follow the directions on the label.
- ▶ Do not use these products in the presence of abdominal pain, nausea, or vomiting.
- ▶ Notify the physician if constipation is not relieved or if rectal bleeding or other symptoms occur.
- ▶ Bulk-producing or fecal-softening laxatives — Drink a full glass of water or juice, followed by more glasses of fluid in the next few hours. *Metamucil*
- ▶ Mineral oil — Take on an empty stomach, preferably at bedtime.
- ▶ Bisacodyl (Dulcolax) — Do not chew the tablets and do not take within 1 hour of taking antacids or milk.
- ▶ To avoid constipation, drink plenty of fluids, exercise, and eat foods high in bulk or roughage.

EVALUATION

- ▶ Anxiety is reduced
- ▶ Adverse reactions are identified and reported to the physician
- ▶ Patient and family demonstrate understanding of drug regimen
- ▶ Verbalizes importance of complying with the prescribed treatment regimen
- ▶ Verbalizes an understanding of treatment modalities and importance of continued follow-up care

37

Antiemetic and Antivertigo Drugs

dizzy

On completion of this chapter the student will:

▶ *Define the terms* antiemetic *and* antivertigo

▶ *List the actions, uses, and adverse reactions associated with the administration of antiemetic and antivertigo drugs*

▶ *Use the nursing process when administering an antiemetic or antivertigo drug*

▶ *Discuss the nursing implications to be considered when administering an antiemetic or antivertigo drug*

Benadryl —

An **antiemetic** is a drug used to treat or prevent nausea or vomiting. An **antivertigo** drug is used to treat or prevent vertigo that may occur with motion sickness, Meniere's disease of the ear, and middle and inner ear surgery.

▷ Actions of Antiemetic and Antivertigo Drugs

Vomiting due to drugs, radiation, and metabolic disorders usually occurs because of stimulation of the chemoreceptor trigger zone (CTZ) of the medulla, which, in turn, stimulates the vomiting center in the brain. The vomiting center may also be directly stimulated by gastrointestinal irritation, motion sickness, vestibular neuritis (inflammation of the vestibular nerve), and so on.

These drugs appear to act primarily by inhibition of the CTZ or by depressing the sensitivity of the vestibular apparatus of the inner ear. Those that act on the vestibular apparatus of the inner ear are more effective for motion sickness and middle and inner ear surgeries, whereas those that act on the CTZ are more effective for vomiting due to stimulation of the CTZ.

Some of the more common preparations and their uses are listed in Summary Drug Table 37-1.

SUMMARY DRUG TABLE 37–1
Antiemetic and Antivertigo Drugs

[handwritten: + Dramamine OTC]

GENERIC NAME	TRADE NAME*	USES	ADVERSE REACTIONS	DOSE RANGES
buclizine hydrochloride	Bucladin-S Softabs	Nausea, vomiting, dizziness of motion sickness	Drowsiness, dry mouth, headache	50 mg PO bid
cyclizine	Marezine	Same as buclizine	Urticaria, rash, dry mouth, nose, and throat	50 mg PO
chlorpromazine hydrochloride	Thorazine, *generic*	Nausea, vomiting; see Summary Drug Table 34-1 for other uses	See Summary Drug Table 34-1	10–25 mg PO; 25–50 mg IM; 50–100 mg rectally
dimenhydrinate	Dimentabs, Marmine, *generic*	Same as buclizine	Drowsiness, confusion, nervousness, nausea, vomiting, blurred vision	50–100 mg PO, 50 mg IM, 50 mg in 10 mL of sodium chloride IV over 2 min
diphenhydramine hydrochloride	Benadryl, Bendylate, *generic*	Motion sickness; see Summary Drug Table 35-1 for other uses	See Summary Drug Table 35-1	25–50 mg PO tid, qid; 10–100 mg IV, IM
diphenidol	Vontrol	Vertigo and associated nausea and vomiting as seen in Meniere's disease, middle and inner ear surgery; nausea and vomiting (postoperative, malignant neoplasms)	Auditory and visual hallucinations, disorientation, confusion, drowsiness, dry mouth	25–50 mg PO q4h
meclizine	Antivert, *generic*	Same as buclizine	Same as cyclizine	25–100 mg/d PO in divided doses
metoclopramide	Reglan	Prevention of nausea and vomiting associated with chemotherapy for neoplastic disorders; unlabeled use: nausea and vomiting due to a variety of causes	Restlessness, nausea, diarrhea, fatigue, lassitude, transient hypertension	Chemotherapy: 1–2 mg/kg IV; other uses: 5–10 mg PO, 5–20 mg IM, IV
perphenazine	Trilafon	Same as chlorpromazine; see Summary Drug Table 34-1 for other uses	See Summary Drug Table 34-1	8–24 mg/d PO in divided doses, 5 mg IM, IV
prochlorperazine	Compazine, *generic*	Same as chlorpromazine; see Summary Drug Table 34-1 for other uses	See Summary Drug Table 34-1	5–10 mg PO tid or qid, 5–10 mg IM, IV, 25 mg rectally
promethazine hydrochloride	Phenergan, *generic*	Motion sickness and nausea, vomiting asociated with anesthesia and surgery; see Summary Drug Table 34-1 for other uses	See Summary Drug Table 34-1	12.5–25 mg PO, IM, IV
scopolamine, transdermal	Trans-dermscop	Prevention of nausea and vomiting associated with motion sickness; see Summary Drug Table 9-1 for other uses	Dry mouth, drowsiness, transient impairment of eye accommodation	Apply 1 system behind the ear several hours before travel; may be replaced every 3 d

[handwritten annotations: "give c̄ chemo therapy", "intrac. hiccups — Post-op", "drowsiness?", "work good together"]

* The term *generic* indicates that the drug is available in a generic form.

▷ Uses of Antiemetic and Antivertigo Drugs

Antiemetic Drugs

An antiemetic is used for the prevention (prophylaxis) or treatment of nausea and vomiting. An example of prophylactic use is the administration of an antiemetic before surgery to prevent vomiting in the immediate postoperative period when the patient is recovering from anesthesia. Another example is giving an antiemetic before the administration of an antineoplastic drug (see chap 31) when there is a high incidence of vomiting after administration of the drug.

Other causes of nausea and vomiting that may be treated with an antiemetic include the postoperative period, during radiation therapy for a malignancy, bacterial and viral infections, nausea and vomiting due to drugs, Meniere's disease and other ear disorders, and neurological diseases and disorders. Some of these drugs are also of use in the treatment of the nausea and vomiting seen with motion sickness. Examples of antiemetics include cyclizine (Marezine) and chlorpromazine (Thorazine). Cyclizine also is used as an antivertigo agent.

Antivertigo Drugs

An antivertigo drug is used in the treatment of vertigo, which is a feeling of a spinning or rotation-type motion which is usually accompanied by lightheadedness, dizziness, and weakness. The individual often has difficulty walking. Some of the causes of vertigo include a high alcohol consumption over a short time, certain drugs, inner ear disease, and postural hypotension. Motion sickness (sea sickness, car sickness) has similar symptoms but is caused by repetitive motion as may be seen in riding in an airplane, boat, or car. Both vertigo and motion sickness may result in nausea and vomiting.

Antivertigo drugs are essentially antiemetics since many of these preparations, whether used for motion sickness or vertigo, also have direct or indirect antiemetic properties. They prevent the nausea and vomiting that occur because of stimulation of the vestibular apparatus in the ear. Stimulation of this apparatus results in vertigo, which is often followed by nausea and vomiting. Examples of antivertigo drugs include meclizine (Antivert) and dimenhydrinate (Marmine).

▷ Adverse Reactions Associated with the Administration of Antiemetic and Antivertigo Drugs

Varying degrees of drowsiness may be seen with the use of antiemetic and antivertigo drugs. Additional adverse reactions are listed in Summary Drug Table 37-1.

▶ NURSING PROCESS
THE PATIENT RECEIVING AN ANTIEMETIC OR ANTIVERTIGO DRUG

ASSESSMENT

Patients receiving one of these drugs for nausea and vomiting are assessed for signs of fluid and electrolyte imbalances. The number of times the patient has vomited and the approximate amount of fluid lost should be estimated. Before starting therapy, the vital signs should be taken.

NURSING DIAGNOSIS

Depending on the severity of symptoms and the reason for administration, one or more of the following nursing diagnoses may apply to the patient receiving an antiemetic or antivertigo drug:

▶ Anxiety related to nausea, vomiting, other symptoms (vertigo, dizziness, if present)
▶ Fluid volume deficit related to nausea and vomiting
▶ High risk for injury related to adverse drug effects
▶ Knowledge deficit of medication regimen, adverse drug effects, treatment modalities

PLANNING AND IMPLEMENTATION

The major goals of the patient may include a reduction in anxiety, absence of symptoms, a normal fluid and electrolyte balance, absence of injury, and an understanding of the medication regimen.

The major goals of nursing management may include a reduction in the patient's anxiety, correction of a fluid and electrolyte imbalance, prevention of injury, and the development and implementation of an effective teaching plan.

If vomiting is severe, the blood pressure, pulse, and respiratory rate are monitored every 2 to 4 hours or as ordered by the physician. Daily to weekly weights may also be indicated in those with prolonged and repeated episodes of vomiting, for example, those receiving chemotherapy for malignant disease. The intake and output (urine, emesis) is also measured until vomiting ceases and the patient is able to take oral fluids in sufficient quantity. The emesis is described in the patient's chart and the physician is notified if there is blood in the emesis or vomiting suddenly becomes more severe.

ADMINISTRATION. If the patient is unable to retain the oral form of the drug, it needs to be given parenterally or as a rectal suppository (if the prescribed drug is available in these forms). If only the oral form has been ordered and the patient is unable to retain the medication, the physician is contacted regarding an order for a parenteral or suppository form of this or another antiemetic drug.

The patient should be assessed at frequent intervals for the effectiveness of the drug to relieve symptoms (eg, nausea, vomiting, or vertigo). The physician is informed if the drug fails to relieve or diminish symptoms.

FLUID AND ELECTROLYTE IMBALANCE. The patient is observed for signs of dehydration, which include poor skin turgor, dry mucous membranes, decrease or absence of urinary output, concentrated urine, restlessness, irritability, increased respiratory rate, and confusion. The patient is also observed for signs of electrolyte imbalance, particularly sodium and potassium deficits.

If signs of dehydration or electrolyte imbalance are noted, the physician is informed because parenteral administration of fluids or fluids with electrolytes may be necessary. These observations are particularly important in the aged or chronically ill patient in whom severe dehydration may develop in a short time. If the patient is able to take and retain small amounts of oral fluids, water should be offered at frequent intervals.

HIGH RISK FOR INJURY. Administration of these drugs may result in varying degrees of drowsiness. To prevent accidental falls and other injuries, the patient who is allowed out of bed should be assisted with ambulatory activities.

ANXIETY. Nausea, vomiting, vertigo, and dizziness are disagreeable sensations. The patient with one or more of these problems additionally experiences anxiety and concern over these symptoms. It is most important that the patient and the bedding and clothing are changed as needed because the odor of vomitus may only intensify the symptoms. The patient should be provided with an emesis basin, which should be checked and emptied at frequent intervals. The patient should also be pro-

vided with a damp washcloth and a towel to wipe the hands and face as needed. Mouth wash or frequent oral rinses may help in removing the disagreeable taste that accompanies vomiting.

KNOWLEDGE DEFICIT. When one of these drugs is prescribed for outpatient use, the following information may be included in a patient teaching plan:

- ▶ Drowsiness may occur with use. Avoid driving or performing other hazardous tasks when taking this medication.
- ▶ If nausea and vomiting persist or become worse, contact the physician.
- ▶ Use only as directed. Do not increase the dose or frequency of use unless told to do so by the physician.
- ▶ Avoid the use of alcohol and other sedative-type drugs unless use has been approved by the physician.

When one of these drugs is prescribed for the prevention of vomiting during chemotherapy, the patient is told when to take the antiemetic (ie, how to time the taking of the antiemetic with chemotherapy administration). At the time of each chemotherapy treatment, the patient is asked about the effectiveness of the antiemetic.

When these drugs are prescribed for nausea that may accompany motion sickness, instruct the patient to take the medication about 1 hour before travel.

EVALUATION

- ▶ Anxiety is reduced
- ▶ No evidence of a fluid volume deficit or electrolyte imbalance
- ▶ No evidence of injury
- ▶ Verbalizes importance of complying with the prescribed treatment regimen
- ▶ Demonstrates understanding of drug regimen

38

Heavy Metal Compounds and Heavy Metal Antagonists

On completion of this chapter the student will:

- ▶ *List actions, uses, and more common adverse reactions of heavy metal compounds and heavy metal antagonists*
- ▶ *Use the nursing process when administering a gold or a silver compound*
- ▶ *Discuss the reasons for using a heavy metal antagonist*
- ▶ *Use the nursing process when administering a heavy metal antagonist*
- ▶ *Discuss the nursing implications to be considered when administering a heavy metal or heavy metal antagonist*

▶ HEAVY METAL COMPOUNDS

Gold (as compounds) and silver (as silver nitrate, silver protein, and silver sulfadiazine) are two heavy metals used in medicine.

▷ Actions of Heavy Metal Compounds

Gold suppresses or prevents the inflammatory reac-

tions seen with rheumatoid arthritis, but the exact mechanism of its action is not known. Examples of gold compounds include auranofin (Ridaura), gold sodium thiomalate (Myochrysine), and aurothioglucose (Solganal).

Silver acts topically on the cell wall and cell membrane of bacteria, producing a bactericidal effect. Examples of silver compounds include silver nitrate ($AgNO_3$) and silver sulfadiazine (Silvadene).

Summary Drug Table 38-1 lists the various gold and silver preparations.

SUMMARY DRUG TABLE 38–1
Heavy Metal Compounds and Heavy Metal Antagonists

GENERIC NAME	TRADE NAME*	USES	ADVERSE REACTIONS	DOSE RANGES
HEAVY METAL COMPOUNDS				
GOLD COMPOUNDS				
auranofin	Ridaura	Active rheumatoid arthritis	Dermatitis, skin eruptions, ulcers in mouth, nephrotic syndrome, flushing, nausea, vomiting, anorexia fainting, diarrhea	6 mg/d PO in single or divided doses; up to 9 mg/d may be given in 3 divided doses
aurothioglucose	Solganol	Same as auranofin	Same as auranofin	Initial dose: 10 mg IM; dosage increased weekly until a total of 0.8–1 g has been given
gold sodium thiomalate	Myochrysine	Same as auranofin	Same as auranofin	Initial dose: 10 mg IM; dosage increased weekly until a total of 1 g has been given
SILVER COMPOUNDS				
silver nitrate (AgNO₃)	Generic	1% ophthalmic: prevention and treatment of gonorrheal ophthalmia neonatorum; 10%, 25%, 50% solutions: plantar warts, impetigo, pruritus, granulation tissue	Chemical conjunctivitis (ophthalmic use)	Ophthalmic: 2 drops of 1% solution; 25%, 50% solutions: apply as directed by the physician
silver protein, mild	Argyrol	Preoperatively in eye surgery, eye infections	Skin and conjunctiva discoloration with prolonged use	Preoperatively: 2–3 drops in eye(s); eye infections: 1–3 drops q3–4h
silver sulfadiazine	Silvadene, generic	Prevention and treatment of sepsis in 2nd- and 3rd-degree burns	Burning, rash, itching	Apply 1–2 times/d in a thickness of about 1/16 inch or as directed by the physician
HEAVY METAL ANTAGONISTS				
deferoxamine mesylate	Desferal Mesylate	Acute iron intoxication, chronic iron overload	Pain and induration at injection site, urticaria, hypotension, erythema	Acute: 1 g IM, IV then 0.5 g for 4 doses; chronic: 0.5–1 g IM, 1–2 g SC
dimercaprol	BAL in Oil	Gold, arsenic and mercury poisoning, acute lead poisoning (with edetate calcium disodium)	Rise in blood pressure, tachycardia	Gold, arsenic poisoning, mild: 2.5 mg/kg IM qid for 2 d, bid the third day, then daily for 10 d; severe: 3 mg/kg IM q4h for 2 d, qid on the 3rd day, then bid for 10 d; mercury poisoning: 5 mg/kg IM initially, then 2.5 mg/kg 1–2 times/d for 10 d
edetate calcium disodium	Calcium Disodium Versenate	Acute and chronic lead poisoning	Renal tubular necrosis	IM: up to 35 mg/kg bid; IV: 1 ampule diluted in 250–500 mL normal saline or 5% dextrose given over a period of 1 h bid
penicillamine	Cuprimine, Depen	To promote excretion of copper in Wilson's disease; see Summary Drug Table 42-1 for use for rheumatoid arthritis	Pruritus, rash, anorexia, nausea, vomiting, epigastric pain, bone marrow depression, proteinuria, hematuria, tinnitus	Up to 2 g/d PO; see Summary Drug Table 42-1
trientine hydrochloride	Cuprid	Wilson's disease	Heartburn, epigastric pain, thickening and flaking of the skin, anemia	Up to 2 g/d PO in 2, 3, or 4 divided doses

* The term generic indicates that the drug is available in a generic form.

▷ Uses of the Heavy Metal Compounds

Gold Compounds

Gold compounds are used in the management of rheumatoid arthritis in adults and children. The greatest benefits of these drugs appears to occur when they are used in the early active stages of the disease. These drugs do not cure rheumatoid arthritis or reverse the damage caused by the disease. They halt the progression of the disease in some patients.

Silver Compounds

Silver compounds may be used as topical antiseptics. Silver nitrate may be used in the treatment of burns, plantar warts, impetigo, pruritus, and granulation tissue. It may be instilled in the eyes of newborn infants for the prevention and treatment of gonorrheal eye infection. Children born of mothers with active gonorrhea (which may be without symptoms in women) may come in contact with the microorganism during passage through the birth canal. Because the microorganism does not survive on the skin but does survive on mucous membranes, the conjunctiva may become infected. If untreated, blindness may result. In some states, the instillation of silver nitrate or another antibacterial agent in the eyes of all newborns is required by law.

Silver sulfadiazine is used for the prevention and treatment of infection in second- and third-degree burns.

▷ Adverse Reactions Associated with the Administration of Heavy Metal Compounds

Gold Compounds

Adverse reactions to gold compounds may occur any time during treatment, as well as many months after therapy is discontinued. Dermatitis is the most common reaction and *any* skin eruption is considered a drug reaction until proved otherwise. Pruritus often occurs before the skin eruption becomes apparent and is considered a warning sign of a possible impending skin reaction.

Stomatitis is the second most common adverse reaction to this drug. Shallow ulcers on the mucous membranes of the cheek, the tongue, the palate, and the pharynx may be seen. A metallic taste may precede these adverse reactions and is a warning that stomatitis may occur.

Other adverse reactions seen with the administration of these drugs include flushing, fainting, nausea, vomiting, anorexia, diarrhea, and the nephrotic syndrome, which may be evidenced by hematuria and proteinuria.

Gastrointestinal (GI) reactions (nausea, vomiting, diarrhea, abdominal pain or cramps, and anorexia) have been seen. Hematologic reactions may also be seen. Examples of hematologic reactions include thrombocytopenia, leukopenia, aplastic anemia, and granulocytopenia.

Some adverse reactions to gold compounds can be severe and sometimes fatal. Laboratory monitoring of the blood (complete blood count [CBC] and differential, platelet count) and renal function studies are usually performed during and after gold therapy.

Silver Compounds

Silver compounds, which are topical agents, have few adverse reactions. Staining of the skin and permanent discoloration of inanimate objects can occur with silver nitrate. A rash and itching have been seen with the use of silver sulfadiazine.

▶ NURSING PROCESS
THE PATIENT RECEIVING A GOLD COMPOUND

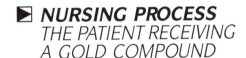

ASSESSMENT

Initial assessment before beginning therapy with a gold compound includes an examination of the areas affected by rheumatoid arthritis and an evaluation of the patient's ability to carry out the activities of daily living [ADL]. These assessments are accurately documented to provide a baseline for comparison during therapy.

NURSING DIAGNOSIS

Depending on the degree of severity of rheumatoid arthritis, one or more of the following nursing diagnoses may apply to the patient receiving a gold compound:

▶ Anxiety related to symptoms of the disorder, other factors

▶ Noncompliance related to failure of the drug to produce immediate results

▶ Knowledge deficit of medication regimen, adverse drug effects, treatment modalities

PLANNING AND IMPLEMENTATION

The major goals of the patient may include a reduction in anxiety and understanding of and compliance to the prescribed treatment regimen.

The major goals of nursing management may include a reduction in the patient's anxiety and the development and implementation of an effective teaching plan.

These drugs are usually given on an outpatient basis. The patient's affected joints are inspected at the time of each office or clinic visit and compared to assessments made before starting therapy. Evaluations are recorded on the patient's chart and aid the physician in evaluating the patient's response to therapy.

ADMINISTRATION. Gold sodium thiomalate should be a pale yellow color. The ampule should not be used if the color has darkened. Aurothioglucose must be shaken thoroughly in a horizontal position in order to suspend all material. Heating the vial to body temperature by immersing it in warm water makes it easier to withdraw the drug from the vial. An 18-gauge, 1½-inch needle is used for withdrawal and administration. When giving gold compounds, the drug is injected deep intramuscularly (IM) and injection sites are rotated.

ADVERSE DRUG REACTIONS. The patient is questioned about or observed for adverse drug reactions to gold compounds, especially dermatitis and stomatitis, as well as the warning signs of these adverse reactions (pruritus, metallic taste). If these or any GI reactions occur, the physician is informed because it may be necessary to temporarily or permanently discontinue the drug. The oral cavity is inspected for signs of ulceration. While the patient is hospitalized, good oral care is important; the patient with rheumatoid arthritis may have difficulty with this activity and require assistance.

ANXIETY. Patients with rheumatoid arthritis have pain and discomfort. Their activities may be limited because of pain or joint deformities. The medication may provide relief for varying time periods, only to be followed by a recurrence of symptoms. Improvement, when it does occur, is often slow and the patient becomes discouraged.

Many of these patients have a great deal of anxiety, not only because of their diagnosis and symptoms, but because treatment may not always be successful. If treatment is successful, the length of time symptoms are controlled may be brief for some. On the other hand, some patients do experience relief with treatment and the progression of the disease may be postponed.

These patients often need emotional support and encouragement. They need time to talk about their problems and encouragement to be as self-sufficient as possible.

NONCOMPLIANCE AND KNOWLEDGE DEFICIT. Response to the gold preparation may be slow; the patient may become discouraged and stop taking the medication or skip doses. It is most important that adherence to the prescribed therapy is stressed and that the patient understands the uninterrupted therapy is necessary to produce the desired results.

The possibility of toxic adverse reactions to these drugs is explained to the patient and family by the physician or nurse, along with the signs and symptoms that may indicate an adverse reaction.

The following points may be included in a patient teaching plan:

▶ Pain in the joints (arthralgia) may occur for a few days after an injection. This usually subsides after the first few injections.

▶ Report any adverse reactions to the physician immediately.

▶ Periodic laboratory tests may be ordered.

▶ Avoid exposure to sunlight because a skin reaction may occur.

▶ Good oral care is essential. Brush the teeth and rinse the mouth well each time food is eaten.

EVALUATION

▶ Anxiety is reduced

▶ Verbalizes an understanding of treatment modalities and importance of continued follow-up care

▶ Patient and family demonstrate understanding of drug regimen

▶ Patient complies with the prescribed drug therapy

▶ Adverse reactions are identified and reported to the physician

▶ NURSING PROCESS
THE PATIENT RECEIVING A SILVER COMPOUND

ASSESSMENT

Initial assessment before beginning therapy with a silver compound includes examining the area to be treated and recording findings in the patient's chart.

NURSING DIAGNOSIS

▶ Anxiety related to pain, other symptoms of the disorder

▶ Knowledge deficit of treatment modality

PLANNING AND IMPLEMENTATION

The major goals of the patient may include a reduction in anxiety and understanding of the prescribed treatment regimen.

The major goals of nursing management may include a reduction in the patient's anxiety and the development and implementation of an effective teaching plan.

ADMINISTRATION. Use, instill, or apply silver compounds as directed by the physician. Silver nitrate imparts a permanent stain on inanimate objects such as clothing, bedding, metal fixtures, jewelry, and so on. The nurse should wear protective clothing when applying the liquid form to large areas of the body. The patient's clothing and other valuables (such as jewelry) must also be protected or removed to prevent a permanent discoloration. Staining of the skin, which usually cannot be prevented, will not wash off with soap or other chemicals but will disappear in time.

Silver sulfadiazine is applied with a sterile gloved hand. The burned area is covered to about 1/16 inch with the cream. Whenever necessary, the cream is reapplied to areas from which it has been removed by the patient's movements so that the burned area remains covered at all times. The physician may order periodic removal and reapplication of the cream. Dressings are normally not required but individual patient requirements may make dressings necessary. This product does not stain the skin or inanimate objects.

Because silver compounds are used to prevent or treat an infection, the area treated is observed for signs of infection or an improvement in the infected tissues.

KNOWLEDGE DEFICIT. Silver compounds are rarely prescribed for outpatient use except for eye infections. The patient is advised to use the product (silver nitrate or silver protein, mild) only as directed and told that the drug can stain the skin and clothing. The patient may also require instructions regarding instillation of the drug in the eye.

When a silver compound is used in the treatment of burns, the application procedure is explained to the patient. The patient is also warned that discomfort may be felt when the drug is applied.

EVALUATION

▶ Anxiety is reduced
▶ Demonstrates understanding of treatment regimen

▶ HEAVY METAL ANTAGONISTS

Poisoning by or excessive blood levels of the heavy metals lead, iron, gold, arsenic, mercury, and copper can be treated with drugs called heavy metal antagonists.

▷ Actions and Uses of Heavy Metal Antagonists

Deferoxamine. Deferoxamine (Desferal) is an iron chelating drug. A chelating agent selectively and chemically binds the ion of a metal to itself, thus aiding in the elimination of the metallic ion from the body. Deferoxamine chelates and then removes excess iron from the body. Excessive iron (or iron overload) may be seen in those who have accidentally or purposely ingested excessive amounts of a drug containing iron, for example, ferrous sulfate. This type of iron overload may be acute or chronic, depending on the amount of drug ingested. Acute iron overload may be seen in persons ingesting large doses of an iron preparation in a short time. Chronic iron overload may be seen in persons taking excessive doses of an iron preparation over a time, as well as in persons receiving multiple blood transfusions.

Dimercaprol. Dimercaprol (BAL in Oil) promotes the excretion of arsenic, gold, and mercury by chelation. It may also be used with edetate calcium disodium (see the following section) to promote the excretion of lead in acute lead poisoning. Arsenic poisoning may occur in persons who have been exposed to certain insecticides and weed killers, as well as those who have been exposed to this chemical in industry. Gold poisoning may be seen in persons receiving gold compounds for arthritis. Mercury poisoning can occur in those eating fish caught in water contaminated with industrial wastes containing mercury. Lead poisoning is discussed next.

Edetate Calcium Disodium. The calcium in edetate calcium disodium (Calcium Disodium Versenate) is displaced by heavy metals, such as lead, to form a stable chemical that is excreted in the urine. This drug is used in the treatment of acute and chronic lead poisoning. Poisoning with this heavy metal may be seen in persons working in industries where lead is used, such as the petroleum industry, as well as in small children ingesting paint fragments containing lead. Federal regulations now require all paint to be lead-free, but lead-based paint may still be seen in older homes on walls and furniture that have not recently been refinished.

Penicillamine and Trientine. Penicillamine (Cuprimine) and trientine (Cuprid) are chelating drugs that remove excess copper in those with Wilson's disease (a degenerative disease of the liver). Penicillamine is also used in the treatment of rheumatoid arthritis (see chap 42) and cystinuria (the presence of cystine, an amino acid, in the urine). Cystinuria is an inherited metabolic disorder that can cause recurrent stones in the urinary tract.

▷ Adverse Reactions Associated with the Administration of Heavy Metal Antagonists

Deferoxamine.   Occasionally, pain and induration at the injection site may occur. Other adverse reactions that may occur during therapy for acute iron intoxication are urticaria, generalized erythema, and hypotension.

Dimercaprol.   One of the most common adverse reactions is a rise in blood pressure accompanied by a rise in pulse rate. Nausea, vomiting, and headache may occur when doses higher than recommended are given.

Edetate Calcium Disodium.   The principal toxic effect of this drug is renal tubular necrosis.

Penicillamine.   This drug has a high incidence of adverse reactions, some of which are potentially fatal, such as bone marrow depression and the nephrotic syndrome. Other adverse reactions include pruritus, skin rash, anorexia, nausea, vomiting, tinnitus, and epigastric pain.

Trientine.   This drug is used when patients experience adverse reactions to penicillamine. Heartburn, epigastric pain and tenderness, thickening and flaking of the skin, and anemia may be seen with the use of this drug.

▶ NURSING PROCESS
THE PATIENT RECEIVING A HEAVY METAL ANTAGONIST

ASSESSMENT

When the patient is diagnosed as having excessive levels of a heavy metal (regardless of the cause), a complete history is obtained with a background of the circumstances surrounding the heavy metal poisoning.

In many instances, it is necessary to question the patient extensively regarding exposure to a heavy metal.

Before starting therapy, the vital signs are taken, the patient is weighed, and the signs and symptoms of the poisoning are documented.

NURSING DIAGNOSIS

Depending on the patient's general physical condition and the reason for use, one or more of the following nursing diagnoses may apply to the patient receiving a heavy metal antagonist:

▶ Anxiety related to diagnosis, severity of symptoms, necessary preventive measures, other factors

▶ Knowledge deficit of treatment regimen, prevention

▶ Noncompliance to preventive measures related to indifference, lack of knowledge, other factors

PLANNING AND IMPLEMENTATION

The major goals of the patient may include a reduction in anxiety, knowledge of preventive measures, and an understanding of and compliance to the prescribed treatment regimen.

The major goals of nursing management may include a reduction in the patient's anxiety and the development and implementation of an effective teaching plan.

The following general points of management are included in a nursing care plan for a patient receiving a heavy metal antagonist:

▶ Depending on the patient's condition, the vital signs are monitored every 1 to 4 hours.

▶ The intake and output are measured and recorded. For the acutely ill patient, it may be necessary to measure the urinary output hourly. As iron is chelated, it is excreted through the kidneys, and the urine becomes a reddish color. Alkalinization of the urine is recommended when dimercaprol or penicillamine are given. The physician may order monitoring of the urinary pH and administration of a urinary alkalinizer, such as sodium bicarbonate or potassium and sodium citrate. Patients with cystinuria who are receiving penicillamine are encouraged to drink copious amounts of fluid, because an excess fluid intake lowers the required drug dosage.

▶ The patient is observed closely for adverse reactions, especially those that may be seen with the administration of penicillamine. All adverse reactions are reported to the physician immediately.

► Therapy may be evaluated by means of laboratory tests, as well as daily assessments of the patient's general condition and a comparison of these symptoms with those recorded during the initial physical assessment. Noticeable improvement may be slow in some cases.

► When the drug is administered IM, the previous injection sites are inspected for signs of induration and inflammation. If these occur, the physician is notified of the problem.

► If dimercaprol is given, a rise in blood pressure and pulse are common responses to therapy. The physician is notified if these vital signs show a significant rise at any time during therapy.

► Some patients may exhibit a marked rise in temperature during therapy with penicillamine. The physician is notified if this occurs because a temporary interruption in therapy may be necessary.

► Additional treatment modalities particular to the type of poisoning and the patient's general condition may also be instituted.

ANXIETY. There can be temporary or permanent serious consequences attached to heavy metal poisoning. The patient or the family may be concerned over the heavy metal poisoning that has occurred, the success or possible failure of therapy, and the possible effects the poisoning may have. They must be allowed time to ask questions about the problems that have occurred because of the heavy metal poisoning, as well as to discuss possible ways to prevent this problem in the future.

Children suffering from chronic lead poisoning may develop mental retardation and other problems. Methods of preventing lead poisoning in children exposed to lead-based paint may require expensive household renovations. Repainting the furniture or walls may not be sufficient because the lead from the lead-based paint that is painted over may still leach through. Some families may be unable to afford the extensive work that may be required because all lead-based paint must first be removed from the surface before lead-free paint is applied. The nurse must spend time with these families and find measures that may help them remove the offending paint from walls and furniture. In some instances, a referral to a social agency for financial assistance may be necessary.

NONCOMPLIANCE AND KNOWLEDGE DEFICIT. Penicillamine and trientine, which are given orally, may be prescribed for outpatient use. The other heavy metal antagonists are given by the parenteral route. However, the patient may be admitted to a short-term unit for parenteral administration of one of these drugs.

Edetate calcium disodium occasionally may be given subcutaneously or IM on an outpatient basis.

To prevent noncompliance, the nurse should emphasize the importance of treatment with a heavy metal antagonist, elimination of those elements that caused the poisoning, and continued and uninterrupted treatment and follow-up care. The patient or family is strongly encouraged to keep all physician or clinic appointments for immediate treatment and for long-term follow-up care (when applicable).

When the cause of poisoning is known, the nurse must work with the patient or family to eliminate those factors (whenever possible) that caused the heavy metal poisoning.

Penicillamine and Trientine

► Take this drug on an empty stomach 1 hour before or 2 hours after a meal. If iron therapy is prescribed, 2 hours must elapse between taking the penicillamine and iron preparation.

► Swallow the capsule form whole; do not chew.

► Notify the physician immediately if fever, skin rash, or other unusual symptoms occur.

► Do not take any nonprescription drug unless use of a specific drug has been approved by the physician.

► Notify the physician if any of the following occurs: skin rash or other types of skin lesions, unusual bruising, sore throat, fever, sores in the mouth, persistent anorexia, nausea, vomiting, diarrhea, unusual fatigue, blood in the urine, or any other unusual symptoms that were not present before therapy was started.

► Patients with cystinuria receiving penicillamine—Drink 4000 mL or more of water or other fluids per day; this is about 16 to 17 large glasses of fluid.

► Follow the diet outlined by the physician; this is an important part of therapy.

EVALUATION

► Anxiety is reduced

► Patient or family verbalize an understanding of treatment modalities and importance of continued follow-up care

► Patient or family member demonstrates understanding of drug regimen

► Verbalizes importance of complying with the prescribed treatment regimen, recommended preventive measures

► Discusses preventive measures and actively seeks assistance with preventive measures

39

Vitamins; Drugs Used in the Treatment of Anemias

On completion of this chapter the student will:

▶ *Name the water- and fat-soluble vitamins*

▶ *Discuss the actions, uses, and adverse reactions of the water- and fat-soluble vitamins*

▶ *Use the nursing process when administering a water- or fat-soluble vitamin*

▶ *Discuss the nursing implications to be considered when administering a water- or fat-soluble vitamin*

▶ *List the drugs used in the treatment of anemia*

▶ *Discuss the actions, uses, and adverse reactions of the drugs used to treat anemia*

▶ *Use the nursing process when administering a drug used for the treatment of anemia*

▶ *Discuss the nursing implications to be considered when administering a drug used for the treatment of anemia*

▶ VITAMINS

A vitamin is a substance needed for normal growth and nutrition. The exact role of some vitamins in human nutrition remains unclear. Most vitamins are obtained from outside sources, namely food, because they cannot be manufactured by the body. The vitamins manufactured by the body are vitamin D, which is produced upon exposure of the skin to sunlight, and vitamin K, which is synthesized by bacteria normally residing in the intestine.

Vitamins are divided into two main groups: the **water-soluble vitamins** and the **fat-soluble vitamins.** Recommended dietary allowances of vitamins for adults are given in Table 39-1.

TABLE 39–1
Recommended Dietary Allowances of
Vitamins for Adults*

WATER-SOLUBLE VITAMINS
Vitamin C (ascorbic acid): 60 mg
Vitamin B_1 (thiamine): men, 1.4 mg; women, 1 mg
Vitamin B_2 (riboflavin); men, 1.6 mg; women, 1.2 mg
Vitamin B_5 (pantothenic acid): approximately 10 mg
Vitamin B_6 (pyridoxine): men, 2.2 mg; women, 2 mg
Niacin (nicotinic acid): men, 18 mg; women, 13 mg

FAT-SOLUBLE VITAMINS

Vitamin A: men, 5000 IU; women, 4000 IU
Vitamin D: 400 IU
Vitamin E: men, 15 IU; women, 12 IU
Vitamin K: minimum daily requirement estimated to be
    0.03 mcg/kg

DRUGS USED TO TREAT ANEMIAS

Iron: men, 10 mg; women, 18 mg (higher during pregnancy and
    lactation)
Folic acid: 500 mcg
Vitamin B_{12}: 3 mcg

* Other references may vary slightly from the RDAs given here.

▶ THE WATER-SOLUBLE VITAMINS

The water soluble vitamins are vitamin C (ascorbic acid) and the B-complex vitamins: vitamins B_1 (thiamine), B_2 (riboflavin), B_5 (pantothenic acid), B_6 (pyridoxine), niacin (vitamin B_3, nicotinic acid), and vitamin B_{12} (cyanocobalamin).

▷ Actions of the Water-Soluble Vitamins

Vitamin C (Ascorbic Acid)

Vitamin C is necessary for the development of teeth, bone, blood vessels, and collagen and is also involved with carbohydrate metabolism. This vitamin also appears to aid in wound healing, which is why it may be given during the postoperative period.

Vitamin C or ascorbic acid is found in citrus fruits and some vegetables. A deficiency of this vitamin results in scurvy, a condition characterized by swollen, red, bleeding gums, a loosening of the teeth, fatigue, pallor, anemia, and hemorrhage of the skin, joints, and muscles due to capillary fragility. In most instances, a normal diet provides sufficient amounts of this vitamin. Examples of situations that may require additional vitamin C are a decreased or inadequate food intake, pregnancy, patients having major surgery, and infants and growing children.

Vitamin B_1 (Thiamine)

Vitamin B_1 plays an important role in carbohydrate metabolism. When the diet is high in carbohydrates, there is an increased need for vitamin B_1. This vitamin is found in many foods. Large amounts of this vitamin are found in wheat germ, whole grains, pork, and enriched grain products. Smaller amounts of the vitamin may be found in milk and milk products.

A deficiency of vitamin B_1 results in beriberi, a disease characterized by neurological, gastrointestinal (GI), and cardiovascular symptoms. Symptoms that may be seen with beriberi are muscle weakness, anorexia, peripheral neuritis, cardiac dysrhythmias, and edema of the lower extremities. In most instances, a normal diet provides the recommended daily requirement of this vitamin. Situations that may require administration of vitamin B_1 include a limited dietary intake of the foods containing this vitamin, the chronically ill patient, the postoperative patient, the chronic alcoholic, and the elderly. This vitamin may be given alone, but very often it is given in combination with other B vitamins under the name *vitamin B complex*.

Vitamin B_2 (Riboflavin)

Vitamin B_2 plays a vital role in numerous tissue respiration systems. This vitamin is found in small amounts in almost all foods. Larger amounts of the vitamin are found in milk and milk products, organ meats, and green leafy vegetables.

A deficiency of vitamin B_2 is characterized by changes in the cornea of the eye, cheilosis, glossitis, seborrheic dermatitis (especially in the skin folds), roughness of the eyelids, blepharospasm, and photophobia. Riboflavin deficiency rarely occurs alone and is often seen with deficiency of other B vitamins and protein.

Vitamin B_5 (Pantothenic Acid)

Vitamin B_5 is an essential element in cellular metabolism. A true deficiency of this vitamin rarely occurs in those eating a normal diet because this vitamin is found in a wide variety of foods.

Vitamin B₆ (Pyridoxine)

Vitamin B₆ is involved with the metabolism of protein, carbohydrates, and fats. This vitamin is found in wheat germ, pork, organ and muscle meats, bananas, and whole grain cereals.

A deficiency of vitamin B₆ is rare and is most likely accompanied by other vitamin B deficiencies. When there is a deficiency of vitamin B₆, nausea, depression, anemia, and dermatitis may be seen.

Vitamin B₁₂ (Cyanocobalamin).

Vitamin B₁₂ is discussed in the section on drugs used to treat anemia.

Niacin (Vitamin B₃, Nicotinic Acid).

Niacin is converted by the body to nicotinamide, which is involved with the metabolism of fats, carbohydrates, and proteins. Niacin is found in meat, poultry, fish, enriched bread and bread products, and peanut butter.

A deficiency of niacin results in pellagra, a disease characterized by dermatitis, diarrhea, inflammation of the mouth, tongue, and intestinal lining, and mental changes.

▷ Uses of the Water-Soluble Vitamins

The water-soluble vitamins are not stored in the body to any great extent. One or more of the water-soluble vitamins may be administered to prevent or treat a deficiency of one or more of these vitamins. Examples of situations or diseases that may result in a deficiency of one or more water-soluble vitamins include the following:

▷ Diseases or disorders of the GI tract, such as prolonged episodes of vomiting or diarrhea, or an inability of the body to absorb vitamins from the GI tract

▷ Emotional or psychotic disorders, such as bulimia, anorexia nervosa, and severe depression, when food intake is limited

▷ Fad diets, starvation diets

▷ Poor eating habits or the inability to purchase food for proper nutrition

▷ Prolonged periods without food, such as the time after surgery

▷ Use of niacin (nicotinic acid) to lower the blood cholesterol

The specific uses of each water-soluble vitamin are given in Summary Drug Table 39-1.

▷ Adverse Reactions Associated with the Administration of Water-Soluble Vitamins

Vitamin C.   Large doses of vitamin C may result in diarrhea. Burning on urination may also occur. Soreness may be noted at the intramuscular (IM) injection site, and rapid intravenous (IV) administration may result in temporary faintness and dizziness.

Vitamin B₁.   A feeling of warmth, pruritus, urticaria, sweating, nausea, restlessness, tightness in the chest, angioneurotic edema, cyanosis, and pulmonary edema may be seen with the administration of vitamin B₁. Serious sensitivity reactions can occur and death has been reported with IV use. When taken orally in a multivitamin preparation, adverse reactions are rare unless the recommended dose is exceeded.

Vitamins B₂ and B₅.   No adverse reactions are seen with the administration of these vitamins.

Vitamin B₆.   Paresthesia, somnolence, and low serum folic acid levels may be seen with the administration of vitamin B₆.

Niacin.   Administration of niacin (nicotinic acid, vitamin B₃) may result in nausea, vomiting, abdominal pain, diarrhea, severe generalized flushing of the skin, and a sensation of warmth. Flushing of the skin may also be accompanied by severe itching or tingling, especially when large doses are administered.

▶ *NURSING PROCESS*
THE PATIENT RECEIVING A WATER-SOLUBLE VITAMIN

ASSESSMENT

The history and physical assessment depend on the reason for the administration of any one or a combination of water-soluble vitamins. When the individual has an actual vitamin deficiency due to any cause, the history and assessment include vital signs, looking for signs of the deficiency, a record of the patient's dietary intake, and looking for possible causes of an impaired nutritional state.

SUMMARY DRUG TABLE 39–1
Vitamins

GENERIC NAME	TRADE NAME*	USES	ADVERSE REACTIONS	DOSE RANGES
VITAMIN A PREPARATIONS				
vitamin A	Aquasol A, *generic*	Vitamin A deficiency	None unless overdosage occurs	5000–500,000 IU/d PO, up to 100,000 IU/d IM depending on degree of deficiency
isotretinoin	Accutane	Severe cystic acne	Cheilitis, conjunctivitis, eye irritation, dry skin, fetal abnormalities, pruritus, epistaxis	0.5–2 mg/kg/d PO in 2 divided doses
tretinoin	Retin-A	Same as isotretinoin	Redness, blistering, swelling of the skin	Apply daily hs
VITAMIN B PREPARATIONS				
vitamin B$_1$ (thiamine hydrochloride)	*Generic*	Prevention and treatment of thiamine deficiency	Feeling of warmth, sweating, nausea, tightness in the chest, cyanosis, pulmonary edema, angioneurotic edema, urticaria, restlessness	5–30 mg/d PO, up to 30 mg IV, 10–20 mg IM
vitamin B$_2$ (riboflavin)	*Generic*	Prevention and treatment of riboflavin deficiency	None	5–10 mg or more per day PO
vitamin B$_5$ (calcium pantothenate, pantothenic acid)	*Generic*	Supplement when diet is low in this vitamin	None	10–100 mg PO
vitamin B$_6$ (pyridoxine hydrochloride)	*Generic*	Prevention and treatment of pyridoxine deficiency	Paresthesia, somnolence	10–50 mg/d PO; higher doses may be used under certain conditions
niacin (nicotinic acid, vitamin B$_3$)	Nicobid, Nicolar, *generic*	Prophylaxis and treatment of pellagra, hyperlipidemia, niacin deficiency	Nausea, vomiting, diarrhea, abdominal pain, severe generalized flushing of the skin with severe itching, or tingling and sensation of warmth	Pellagra: up to 500 mg/d PO; hyperlipidemia: 1–2 g PO tid; niacin deficiency: 10–20 mg/d PO; drug may also be given IM, IV, SC
VITAMIN C PREPARATIONS				
ascorbic acid	Cevalin, *generic*	Prevention and treatment of ascorbic acid deficiency	Large doses: diarrhea, burning on urination	50 mg or more per day PO; 100 mg–2 g IM, SC, IV
VITAMIN D PREPARATIONS				
calcifediol	Calderol	Metabolic bone disease, hypocalcemia in those on chronic renal dialysis	Weakness, headache, vomiting, dry mouth, constipation, muscle and bone pain, metallic taste, nausea	300–350 mcg/wk PO in divided doses given qd or every other day
calcitriol	Rocaltrol	Hypocalcemia in those on chronic renal dialysis	Same as calcifediol	0.25–1 mcg/d PO
dihydrotachysterol (DHT)	Hytakerol, *generic*	Acute, chronic, and latent tetany (postoperative, idiopathic) and hypoparathyroidism	Same as calcifediol	0.25–2.4 mg/d PO
ergocalciferol	Calciferol, *generic*	Rickets, familial hypophosphatemia, hypoparathyroidism	Same as calcifediol	Up to 500,000 IU/d PO (dose may be as low as 400 IU/d)

(continued)

SUMMARY DRUG TABLE 39—1
(continued)

GENERIC NAME	TRADE NAME*	USES	ADVERSE REACTIONS	DOSE RANGES
VITAMIN E PREPARATIONS				
vitamin E	Aquasol E, generic	Treatment and prevention of vitamin E deficiency (only established use)	None	12–15 IU/d PO is recommended daily allowance; higher doses may be used
VITAMIN K PREPARATIONS				
menadiol sodium diphosphate (K₄)	Synkayvite	Hypoprothrombinemia due to antibacterial or salicylate therapy, obstructive jaundice, biliary fistulas	Nausea, vomiting, pain at injection site, headache	5–10 mg/d PO, 5–15 mg IM, IV, SC
phytonadione (K₁)	Mephyton, Konakion, AquaMEPHYTON	Anticoagulant-induced prothrombin deficiency (oral anticoagulants), prophylaxis and treatment of hemorrhagic disease of the newborn	Same as menadiol plus severe reactions during and after IV administration	1–25 mg IM, SC, IV, PO; newborn: 0.5–1 mg SC, IM

* The term generic indicates that the drug is available in a generic form.

NURSING DIAGNOSIS

▶ Knowledge deficit of treatment regimen, reason for administration

PLANNING AND IMPLEMENTATION

The major goal of the patient may be an understanding of the treatment regimen and reason for use.

The major goal of nursing management may include the development and implementation of an effective teaching plan.

In those eating poorly or with a severe nutritional problem, an evaluation is made of the patient's nutritional intake. The physician is contacted if the patient fails to eat the prescribed diet.

When niacin (nicotinic acid) is given for treatment of elevated blood cholesterol, the patient is told that a feeling of warmth, flushing, and itching may occur. Often, high doses are necessary for the treatment of an elevated blood cholesterol and these adverse reactions may be severe. The physician is informed immediately of a severe adverse reaction to this vitamin.

KNOWLEDGE DEFICIT. When the patient has a vitamin deficiency, it is necessary to emphasize the importance of improving or correcting eating habits. The first step in developing a teaching plan is to determine the reason for the inadequate dietary intake. This is followed by determining what steps are necessary to improve the patient's nutritional intake. For example, an elderly patient with a history of poor nutrition may have a problem shopping for food or may not have the financial means to eat a well-balanced diet. This problem may require contacting the hospital's social service department. After an interview, the social service worker may refer the patient to those persons or private or government agencies that may provide the funds and means for obtaining the types of food required for a well-balanced diet.

Some nutritional problems are difficult to solve, such as the nutritional deficiencies of the chronic alcoholic refusing treatment for his or her alcoholism or the young woman with anorexia nervosa. Many times, the family may be able to help the patient improve his or her nutritional status, but there are other times when an attempt to improve nutrition fails.

The hospital dietitian is a resource person who can assist the *willing* patient with meal planning and selecting foods that are high in the vitamins required to correct the deficiency. When contacting the dietitian, the nurse gives a full history of the patient's problems, the disease that may be causing a nutritional deficit (when applicable), the diet recommended by the physician, and a list of medications (including vitamin supplements) the patient will be taking at home. The nurse must emphasize the importance of good nutrition and of following the diet prescribed by the physician and outlined by the dietitian.

The nurse also has the responsibility to inform the general public about the adverse effects associated with high vitamin dosages, as well as to give correct information regarding the role of vitamin therapy. Water-soluble vitamins cannot be stored in the body for any appreciable length of time and what the body doesn't need is excreted, sometimes in a few hours. Unless prescribed by the physician, massive doses of these vitamins are of no value.

When applicable, the adverse reactions that may be seen with these drugs are explained to the patient. Patients taking niacin (nicotinic acid) are advised to contact their physician if intense flushing and itching occur.

EVALUATION

▶ Patient and family demonstrate understanding of drug regimen

▶ Verbalizes importance of complying with the prescribed treatment regimen

▶ THE FAT-SOLUBLE VITAMINS

The fat-soluble vitamins are A, D, E, and K. These vitamins are stored in the body and used as needed.

▷ Actions of the Fat-Soluble Vitamins

Vitamin A

Vitamin A is necessary for the eye to adapt to night vision. Vitamin A also prevents retardation of growth and preserves the integrity of epithelial cells. Some of the foods containing vitamin A include kidney, liver, whole milk, eggs, butter, and leafy yellow and green vegetables. Some foods such as skim milk and margarine are fortified with this vitamin. Because vitamin A is a fat-soluble vitamin, absorption of this vitamin requires the presence of bile salts, pancreatic lipase (a pancreatic digestive enzyme), and dietary fat. Vitamin A is stored in the liver.

A deficiency of vitamin A results in night blindness or the inability to see in the dark. Drying of the skin, a lowered resistance to infection, changes in the cornea of the eye, growth retardation, and fetal malformations may occur when a vitamin A deficiency exists.

Vitamin D

Vitamin D is necessary for the metabolism of calcium. It also promotes the absorption of calcium and phosphorus in the intestine, and increases the rate of accretion (accumulation) and resorption of minerals from the bone. Absorption of vitamin D from the intestine depends on an adequate amount of bile. Vitamin D is stored in the liver but is also found in fat, muscle, the skin, brain, spleen, and bones.

Several vitamin D preparations are available for replacement therapy (see Summary Drug Table 39-1). The physician's choice of a vitamin D preparation is based on the problem being treated and the pharmacologic activity of the product selected. Sources of this vitamin are mainly foods fortified with vitamin D. Milk is the main fortified source of this vitamin. Sunlight is also a major source of vitamin D because the skin converts dehydrocholesterol in the skin to vitamin D_3.

A deficiency of vitamin D results in rickets, which is a malformation of the long bones (arms, legs) of the body in children. In adults, a deficiency leads to osteomalacia, which is a loss of calcium from the bones, resulting in a weakening of the bones and an increased tendency toward bone fractures.

Vitamin E

Vitamin E is considered an essential element in human nutrition but its exact function in the body is unclear. A deficiency of this vitamin is rare because it is found in a great many foods and the daily requirement for the vitamin appears to be small. This vitamin requires the presence of bile salts for absorption, and it is stored in the liver and muscle.

Vitamin K

Vitamin K is needed by the liver to manufacture prothrombin and the other factors involved in the blood-clotting mechanism. This vitamin is found in cabbage, liver, egg yolks, cauliflower, and other leafy vegetables. Intestinal bacteria also synthesize vitamin K. This is probably the greatest source of the vitamin.

A deficiency of vitamin K is rare when the individual eats a normal diet and there is an adequate number of vitamin K–producing bacteria in the intestine. A deficiency may exist when drugs, such as the antibiotics, decrease the number of intestinal bacteria responsible for the manufacture of this vitamin. When a deficiency does occur, it is seen as an inability of the blood to clot within a normal time period.

▷ Uses of the Fat-Soluble Vitamins

Vitamin A. Vitamin A is given when a deficiency exists. Conditions that may cause a vitamin A deficiency include biliary tract or pancreatic disease, sprue, colitis, hepatic cirrhosis, celiac disease, regional enteritis, and a poor nutritional intake of foods containing this vitamin.

Isotretinoin (Accutane) and tretinoin (Retin-A) are products chemically related to vitamin A and are used in the treatment of acne. Isotretinoin is an isomer of retinoic acid. (An isomer is a chemical substance that has the same chemical formula but different chemical properties as its related substance). Isotretinoin is taken orally, whereas tretinoin is applied topically.

Vitamin D. Vitamin D, along with the parathyroid hormone, regulates calcium metabolism. Therefore, it may be used in persons with a certain type of calcium deficiency, such as the calcium deficiency seen in those patients on prolonged renal dialysis. Vitamin D is also used in the treatment of rickets in children. Although this condition is relatively rare in the United States, it may be seen in persons living in areas where exposure to sunlight is limited and whose diet is deficient in this vitamin.

Vitamin E. The only established use of vitamin E is in the prevention or treatment of a vitamin E deficiency, which is rare. An unlabeled use of this vitamin is the administration to premature infants receiving oxygen to reduce the incidence of eye damage (retrolental fibroplasia) and lung damage (bronchopulmonary dysplasia) due to oxygen administration. There are also other unlabeled conditions or disorders for which this vitamin has been used.

Vitamin K. Vitamin K is used to correct a vitamin K deficiency. Menadiol sodium diphosphate (Synkayvite) is used in the treatment of hypoprothrombinemia due to antibacterial or salicylate therapy, obstructive jaundice, and biliary fistulas. Phytonadione (Mephyton, AquaMEPHYTON) is an oral anticoagulant antagonist and may be given to patients receiving anticoagulant therapy when an elevated prothrombin time results in bleeding or hemorrhage (see Summary Drug Table 15-1).

▷ Adverse Reactions Associated with the Administration of Fat-Soluble Vitamins

Vitamin A. The adverse effects seen with vitamin A administration are related to overdosage (hypervitaminosis A). Signs of overdosage include fatigue, malaise, headache, abdominal discomfort, anorexia, vomiting, arthralgia, fissures of the lips, drying and cracking of the skin, alopecia, bone pain, and vertigo. Treatment of hypervitaminosis A is immediate withdrawal of the drug along with supportive treatment.

Adverse reactions associated with the administration of isotretinoin for acne include conjunctivitis, dry skin and mucous membranes, rash, brittle nails, and dry mouth. Women who are pregnant or may become pregnant must not use this drug because of a high risk of fetal deformities. Adverse reactions seen with the administration of tretinoin include redness, blistering, and swelling of the skin.

Vitamin D. Administration of vitamin D in normal doses may result in weakness, headache, somnolence, nausea, vomiting, dry mouth, constipation, muscle and bone pain, and a metallic taste. Overdosage of this vitamin may produce hypercalcemia (see chap 17) and the loss of calcium from bone in adults. Severe hypercalcemia can result in a loss of renal function and cardiovascular failure. Deaths have been reported with vitamin D overdosage.

Vitamin E. There appear to be no adverse reactions associated with the administration of this vitamin, nor have there been any adverse reactions seen with overdosage.

Vitamin K. Oral administration of vitamin K may result in nausea, vomiting, and headache. Parenteral administration may cause pain at the injection site. Anaphylactoid reactions have been reported with the IV administration of Aquamephyton.

▶ NURSING PROCESS
THE PATIENT RECEIVING A FAT-SOLUBLE VITAMIN

ASSESSMENT

When a patient is receiving a fat-soluble vitamin for a vitamin deficiency, the signs of the deficiency are recorded in the patient's chart. If a decreased nutritional intake is the cause of the deficiency, the patient is weighed and vital signs are taken.

If isotretinoin is prescribed for acne, the physician discusses with the patient the dangers associated with pregnancy while on this drug. The nurse may be responsible for evaluating the patient's understanding of the precautions to be observed while taking isotretinoin.

NURSING DIAGNOSIS

▶ Knowledge deficit of treatment regimen, reason for administration

PLANNING AND IMPLEMENTATION

The major goal of the patient may be an understanding of the treatment regimen and reason for use.

The major goal of nursing management may include the development and implementation of an effective teaching plan.

When a vitamin deficiency exists, the patient's food intake is monitored. Each meal tray is checked and the physician is informed if the food intake is below normal.

If bleeding has occurred and vitamin K therapy is instituted, the patient is closely observed for a continued bleeding tendency. When parenteral phytonadione is given, the effect on the bleeding time is noted within 1 to 2 hours and hemorrhage, when present, is usually controlled within 3 to 6 hours.

KNOWLEDGE DEFICIT. If the vitamin deficiency is due to a decreased dietary intake, the information included under the water-soluble vitamins is applicable. The following information may also be included in a teaching plan:

Vitamin Preparations

▶ Take this drug as prescribed. Do not increase or decrease the dose unless told to do so by the physician.

▶ Eat the foods recommended by the physician. If there is difficulty in purchasing these foods, discuss this with the physician or a social service worker.

▶ Avoid the use of mineral oil, which can prevent the absorption of these (fat-soluble) vitamins. If a laxative is needed, ask the physician for the type of laxative that will not interfere with vitamin and food absorption.

▶ Do not use multivitamin preparations unless their use is approved by the physician.

Isotretinoin

▶ Take this drug with meals. Do not crush the capsules but swallow whole.

▶ Follow the physician's recommendations regarding contraceptive measures before, during, and after therapy. If pregnancy is suspected, stop taking the drug and immediately notify the physician.

▶ Avoid prolonged exposure to sunlight because a photosensitivity reaction may occur.

Tretinoin

▶ Avoid prolonged exposure to sunlight because a photosensitivity reaction may occur.

▶ Apply the drug as directed. Keep the drug away from the eyes, mouth, and mucous membranes.

EVALUATION

▶ Patient and family demonstrate understanding of drug regimen

▶ Verbalizes importance of complying with the prescribed treatment regimen

▶ Demonstrates understanding of the dangers associated with pregnancy (isotretinoin)

▶ DRUGS USED IN THE TREATMENT OF ANEMIA

Anemia is a decrease in the number of red blood cells, a decrease in the amount of hemoglobin in red blood cells, or *both* a decrease in the number of red blood cells and hemoglobin. There are various types and causes of anemia. Once the type and cause have been identified, the physician selects a method of treatment. Drugs used in treatment of anemia are summarized in Summary Drug Table 39-2.

▷ Actions and Uses of Drugs Used in the Treatment of Anemia

Iron

Iron is a component of hemoglobin, which is in red blood cells. It is the iron in the hemoglobin of red blood cells that picks up oxygen from the lungs and carries it to all body tissues. Iron is stored in the body and is found mainly in the reticuloendothelial cells of the liver, spleen, and bone marrow. Iron salts, for example, ferrous sulfate or ferrous gluconate, are used in the treatment of iron-deficiency anemia, which occurs when there is a loss of iron that is greater than the available iron stored in the body. Iron is found in foods such as meats, fruits, eggs, fish, poultry, grains, and dairy products. Iron dextran is a parenteral iron that is also used for the treatment of iron-deficiency anemia. It is primarily used when the patient cannot take oral drugs or when the patient experiences GI intolerance to oral iron administration.

Folic Acid

Folic acid is required for the manufacture of red blood cells in the bone marrow. Folic acid is found in

SUMMARY DRUG TABLE 39–2
Drugs Used in Treatment of Anemia

GENERIC NAME	TRADE NAME*	USES	ADVERSE REACTIONS	DOSE RANGES
ferrous fumarate (33% elemental iron)	Feostat, *generic*	Prevention and treatment of iron-deficiency anemia	GI irritation, nausea, vomiting, constipation, diarrhea, allergic reactions	15–200 mg PO of elemental iron qd
ferrous gluconate (11.6% elemental iron)	Fergon, *generic*	Same as ferrous fumarate	Same as ferrous fumarate	Same as ferrous fumarate
ferrous sulfate (20% elemental iron)	Feosol, *generic*	Same as ferrous fumarate	Same as ferrous fumarate	Same as ferrous fumarate
folic acid	Folvite, *generic*	Megaloblastic anemias due to deficiency of folic acid	Allergic sensitization	Up to 1 mg/d PO, IM, IV, SC
iron dextran	Imferon, Hematran, *generic*	Iron deficiency anemia	Anaphylactoid reactions, soreness and inflammation at injection site, hypersensitivity reactions	Dosage based on body weight and grams percent (g/dL) of hemoglobin
leucovorin calcium	*Generic*	Megaloblastic anemias, to counteract effect of overdosage of folic acid antagonists	Allergic sensitization	Megaloblastic anemias: up to 1 mg/d IM; overdosage of folic acid antagonists: up to 100 mg/m² dose PO, IM, IV infusion
vitamin B₁₂ (cyanocobalamin)	Rubramin PC, *generic*	B₁₂ deficiency as seen in pernicious anemia, GI pathology; also used when requirements for the vitamin are increased; Schilling test	Mild diarrhea, itching	Up to 1000 mcg/d PO; up to 200 or more mcg/d IM, SC; Schilling test: flushing dose is 100 mcg IM

* The term generic *indicates that the drug is available in a generic form.*

leafy green vegetables, fish, meat, poultry, and whole grains. A deficiency of folic acid results in megaloblastic anemia. Folic acid deficiency may be seen in sprue, anemias of nutritional origin, pregnancy, infancy, and childhood. Folic acid is used in the treatment of megaloblastic anemias that are due to a deficiency of folic acid.

Leucovorin

Leucovorin is a derivative of and an active reduced form of folic acid. The oral and parenteral form of this drug is used in the treatment of megaloblastic anemia. Leucovorin may also be used to diminish the toxicity and counteract the effect of (intentional) massive doses of methotrexate, a drug used in the treatment of certain types of cancers (see chap 31). This technique of administering leucovorin after a large dose of methotrexate is called *folinic acid rescue* or *leucovorin rescue*. Occasionally, high doses of methotrexate are administered to select patients.

Leucovorin is then used either at the time methotrexate is administered or a specific number of hours after the methotrexate has been given. Leucovorin may be ordered to be given IV or by the oral route.

Vitamin B₁₂ (Cyanocobalamin)

Vitamin B₁₂ is essential to growth, cell reproduction, the manufacture of myelin (which surrounds some nerve fibers), and blood cell manufacture. The *intrinsic factor*, which is produced by cells in the stomach, is necessary for the absorption of vitamin B₁₂ in the intestine. A deficiency of vitamin B₁₂ results in megaloblastic anemia and pernicious anemia.

A deficiency of this vitamin due to a low dietary intake of vitamin B₁₂ is rare because it is found in meats, milk, eggs, and cheese. The body is also able to store this vitamin; a deficiency, for any reason, will not occur for 5 to 6 years. A vitamin B₁₂ deficiency may be seen in persons who (1) are strict vegetarians; (2) have had a total gastrectomy or subtotal gastric resection (when the cells producing the intrinsic factor are totally or partially removed); (3) have intestinal diseases such as ulcerative colitis or sprue; (4) have gastric carcinoma; or (5) have a congenital decrease in the number of gastric cells secreting the intrinsic factor.

Vitamin B_{12} is also used to perform the Schilling test, which is used to diagnose pernicious anemia.

▷ Adverse Reactions Associated with the Administration of Drugs Used in the Treatment of Anemia

Iron Salts. Iron salts occasionally cause GI irritation, nausea, vomiting, constipation, diarrhea, and allergic reactions. The stools usually appear darker in color.

Iron dextran is given by the parenteral route. Hypersensitivity reactions, including fatal anaphylactic reactions, have been reported with the use of this form of iron. Additional adverse reactions include soreness, inflammation, and sterile abscesses at the IM injection site. Intravenous administration may result in phlebitis at the injection site.

Folic Acid and Leucovorin. Administration of these drugs may result in allergic sensitization.

Vitamin B_{12}. Mild diarrhea and itching have been reported with the administration of vitamin B_{12}. Other adverse reactions that may be seen include a marked increase in red blood cell production, acne, peripheral vascular thrombosis, congestive heart failure, and pulmonary edema.

▶ NURSING PROCESS
THE PATIENT RECEIVING A DRUG USED IN THE TREATMENT OF ANEMIA

ASSESSMENT

A general health history and the symptoms of the anemia are obtained. The physician orders laboratory tests to determine the type, severity, and possible cause of the anemia. At times, it may be easy to identify the cause of the anemia, but there are also instances where the cause of the anemia is obscure.

If iron dextran is to be given, an allergy history is necessary because this drug is given with caution to those with significant allergies or asthma. The patient's weight may be required for calculating the dosage.

The vital signs are taken to provide a baseline during therapy. Other physical assessments may include the patient's general appearance and, in the severely anemic patient, an evaluation of the patient's ability to carry out the activities of daily living.

NURSING DIAGNOSIS

Depending on the drug, dose, and reason for administration, one or more of the following nursing diagnoses may apply to a person receiving a drug used in the treatment of anemia:

▶ Anxiety related to diagnosis, other factors
▶ Noncompliance related to indifference, lack of knowledge, other factors
▶ Knowledge deficit of medication regimen, adverse drug effects, treatment modalities

PLANNING AND IMPLEMENTATION

The major goals of the patient may include a reduction in anxiety and an understanding of and compliance to the prescribed treatment regimen.

The major goals of nursing management may include a reduction in the patient's anxiety and the development and implementation of an effective teaching plan.

ADMINISTRATION. Iron dextran is given IM or IV. When given IM, the Z-track technique is used (see chap 2). Iron salts are preferably given between meals with water but can be given with food or meals if GI upset occurs. If the patient is receiving other medications, check with the hospital pharmacist regarding the simultaneous administration of iron salts with other drugs. When a liquid iron salt preparation is ordered, the dose is mixed with 2 to 4 ounces of water to prevent staining of the teeth.

When leucovorin is administered after a large dose of methotrexate, the timing of the administration is outlined by the physician. It is essential that the leucovorin be given at the *exact* time ordered because the purpose of folinic acid rescue is to allow a high dose of a toxic drug to remain in the body for only a limited time.

OBSERVATIONS AND NURSING MANAGEMENT. The following assessments, evaluations, and nursing tasks may be included in the nursing care plan:

▶ The vital signs are taken daily; more frequent monitoring may be needed if the patient is moderately to acutely ill.

► The patient is observed for adverse reactions. Any occurrence of adverse reactions is reported to the physician before the next dose is due. Severe adverse reactions are reported immediately.

► Iron salt therapy—The patient is informed that the color of the stool will change. If diarrhea or constipation occurs, the physician should be informed of this problem.

► Iron dextran—The patient should be informed that soreness at the injection site may occur. Injection sites are checked daily for signs of inflammation, swelling, or abscess formation.

► A special diet (eg, foods high in iron or foods high in folic acid) may be prescribed. If the diet is taken poorly, this is noted on the patient's chart and the problem is discussed with the physician.

► The patient is observed for relief of the symptoms of anemia. Some patients may note a relief of symptoms after a few days of therapy.

► Periodic laboratory tests are necessary to monitor the results of therapy.

ANXIETY. Some patients may have varying degrees of anxiety because of their diagnosis or the necessity of treatment. The nurse should explain the purpose of treatment and allow the patient time to ask questions.

NONCOMPLIANCE AND KNOWLEDGE DEFICIT. It is most important that the medical regimen be explained to the patient and family. The importance of following the prescribed treatment regimen is emphasized.

The following points may be included in a patient and family teaching plan:

Iron Salts

► Take this drug on an empty stomach with water. If GI upset occurs, take the drug with food or meals.

► Do not take other drugs (prescription or nonprescription) at the same time or 2 hours before or after taking iron without first checking with the physician.

► This drug may cause a darkening of the stools, constipation, or diarrhea. If constipation or diarrhea becomes severe, contact the physician.

► Avoid the indiscriminate use of advertised iron products. If a true iron deficiency occurs, the cause must be determined and therapy should be under the care of a physician.

Folic Acid

► Avoid the use of multivitamin preparations unless use has been approved by the physician.

► Follow the diet recommended by the physician because diet and medication are necessary to correct a folic acid deficiency.

Leucovorin

► Megaloblastic anemia—Adhere to the diet prescribed by the physician. If the purchase of foods high in protein (which can be expensive) becomes a problem, discuss this with the physician.

► Folinic acid rescue—Take this drug at the exact prescribed intervals. If nausea and vomiting occur, contact the physician *immediately.*

Vitamin B$_{12}$

► Nutritional deficiency of vitamin B$_{12}$—Eat a well-balanced diet including seafood, eggs, meats, and dairy products.

► Pernicious anemia—Lifetime therapy is necessary. Eat a well-balanced diet including seafood, eggs, meats, and dairy products. Avoid contact with infections and report any signs of infection to the physician immediately because an increase in dosage may be necessary.

Note: Therapy for pernicious anemia almost always requires parenteral administration of the drug at periodic intervals (usually monthly). The importance of receiving the monthly injection must be emphasized. In some instances, the physician may allow the patient or a family member to give the drug, and instruction in administration is necessary.

EVALUATION

► Anxiety is reduced
► Patient and family demonstrate understanding of drug regimen
► Verbalizes importance of complying with the prescribed treatment regimen

40

Immunologic Agents

On completion of this chapter the student will:

▶ *Define the terms used in immunology*

▶ *Distinguish between and define the three different types of immunity*

▶ *Discuss the positive and negative aspects of an immunization program*

▶ *Discuss the nursing implications to be considered when administering an immunologic agent*

▷ Terminology

An **antigen** is a foreign protein substance that invades the body. Two examples of antigens are the virus causing chickenpox and the bacteria causing tuberculosis. When a virus, bacteria, or other foreign protein (or antigen) enters the body, antibodies against this invading foreign substance are formed. An **antibody** is also a protein that is manufactured by lymphoid tissue and the reticuloendothelial system. *Specific* antibodies are formed for a *specific* antigen, that is, chickenpox antibodies are formed when the person is exposed to the chickenpox virus (the antigen). This is called an *antigen–antibody response*. Once manufactured, antibodies circulate in the bloodstream, sometimes for only a short time and at other times, for the life of the person. When an antigen enters the body, specific antibodies neutralize the specific invading antigen. This is called *immunity*. Thus, the individual with *specific* circulating antibodies is immune (or has immunity) to a *specific* antigen.

Antibody-producing tissues cannot distinguish between an antigen that is capable of causing disease (a live antigen) or an attenuated (weakened) antigen or a killed antigen. Because of this phenomenon, **vaccines,** which contain either an attenuated or killed antigen, have been developed to create immunity to certain diseases. The live antigens are either killed or weakened during the manufacturing process. Vaccines containing specific attenuated or killed antigens are used to create immunity to specific diseases.

A **toxin** is a substance produced by some bacteria, such as the *Clostridium tetani*, the bacteria that causes tetanus. A toxin is capable of stimulating the lymphoid tissues and the reticuloendothelial system to produce **antitoxins,** which are substances that act in the same manner as antibodies. Toxins are powerful substances and like other antigens, they can be attenuated. When a toxin is attenuated (or weakened), it is called a **toxoid.** Like toxins, toxoids also stimulate the formation of antibodies because the body cannot distinguish between a toxin or a toxoid.

Globulins are proteins present in blood serum or plasma and contain antibodies. **Immune globulins** are given for passive immunity against disease because they contain antibodies.

▷ Active and Passive Immunity

When a person is exposed to certain infectious microorganisms (antigens), the body begins to form antibodies (or build an immunity) to the invading microorganism. There are three types of immunity: naturally acquired active immunity, artificially acquired active immunity, and passive immunity.

Figure 40-1 shows the sequence of active and passive immunity.

Naturally Acquired Active Immunity

Naturally acquired active immunity occurs when the person is exposed to a disease and develops the disease, and the body manufactures antibodies to provide future immunity to the disease. Naturally acquired immunity is immunity that occurs after the individual has a disease caused by an invading antigen. It is called *active* immunity because the antibodies that provide the immunity were produced by the person who had the disease.

An example of naturally acquired active immunity is when the individual is exposed to chickenpox for the *first* time and has no immunity to the disease. The body immediately begins to manufacture antibodies against the chickenpox virus. However, the production of a sufficient quantity of antibodies takes time, and the individual gets the disease. At the time of exposure and while the individual still has chickenpox, the body continues to manufacture antibodies. These antibodies circulate in the individual's bloodstream for life. In the future, any exposure to the chickenpox virus results in the antibodies' destroying the invading antigen.

Artificially Acquired Active Immunity

Artificially acquired active immunity occurs when an individual is given a killed or weakened antigen, which stimulates the formation of antibodies against the antigen. Because the antigen is either killed or weakened, it does not cause the disease but the individual will still manufacture specific antibodies against the disease. When a vaccine containing an attenuated antigen is given, the individual *may* develop a few minor symptoms of the disease or even a mild form of the disease but the symptoms

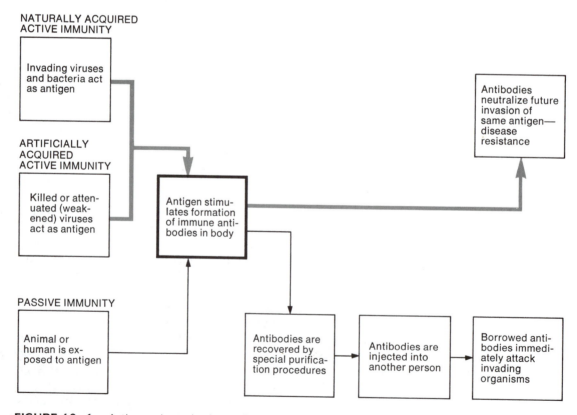

FIGURE 40–1. Active and passive immunity.

are almost always milder and usually last for a shorter time.

The decision to use an attenuated or a killed virus for a vaccine is based on research, which shows the results of the administration of either an attenuated or a killed antigen. Some antigens, when killed, show a poor antibody response, whereas when the antigen is merely weakened, a good antibody response occurs. This is why some vaccines contain a killed antigen and others contain an attenuated antigen.

An example of artificially acquired active immunity is the administration of the measles vaccine to an individual who has not had measles. The measles (rubeola) vaccine contains the live, attenuated measles virus. The individual receiving the vaccine develops a *mild or modified* measles infection, which then produces lifetime immunity against the rubeola virus.

Artificially acquired immunity against some diseases may require periodic *booster* injections to keep an adequate antibody level (or antibody *titer*). A booster injection may be necessary because the life of some antibodies is relatively short. The immunization schedules for children are given in Table 40-1.

Passive Immunity

Passive immunity provides the individual with antibodies made by another human or by an animal. Passive immunity provides *immediate* immunity to the invading antigen, but this type of immunity lasts for only a short time.

An example of passive immunity is the administration of diphtheria antitoxin. Diphtheria antitoxin would be given if the individual (1) has never had diphtheria (which would have provided naturally acquired active immunity); (2) has never received the diphtheria vaccine (which would have provided artificially acquired active immunity); or (3) was exposed to or began to develop the disease. Because diphtheria is extremely serious and may even be fatal, it is necessary to provide the individual with *immediate* immunity by the administration of diphtheria antitoxin. The antitoxin that is given was produced by an animal (a horse) injected with the live diphtheria virus. The animal produces an antitoxin identical to the antitoxin that can be manufactured by a human. The individual exposed to diphtheria would also produce his or her own antitoxin, but this may take days or even weeks. Because immediate immunity is required in this instance, passive immunity is the chosen method of providing temporary immunity to this disease.

Another example of passive immunity is the administration of immune globulins (Summary Drug Table 40-1) such as hepatitis B immune globulin. Administration of this vaccine is an attempt to prevent hepatitis B *after* the individual has been exposed to the virus.

▷ Nursing Implications

Immunization is an important method of controlling some of the infectious diseases that are capable of causing serious and sometimes fatal consequences. An example of this is the poliovirus vaccine. Before the development of this vaccine, many children and adults were afflicted with this disease each year. Some years produced an epidemic of poliomyelitis (polio). Many persons were admitted to the hospital daily and often required weeks and even months of hospitalization. Many of these victims were permanently paralyzed. For some, the paralysis affected one or both arms or legs. Others developed a form of the disease that affected the respira-

TABLE 40–1
Recommended Immunization Schedules

	2 MONTHS	4 MONTHS	6 MONTHS	15 MONTHS	4–6 YEARS
Diphtheria toxoid	•	•	•	•	•
Tetanus toxoid	•	•	•	•	•
Pertussis vaccine	•	•	•	•	•
Trivalent oral polio vaccine	•	•	•	•	•
Measles vaccine				•	
Rubella vaccine				•	
Mumps vaccine				•	

SUMMARY DRUG TABLE 40–1
Immunologic Agents

GENERIC NAME	TRADE NAME*	USES	ADVERSE REACTIONS	DOSE RANGES
AGENTS FOR ACTIVE IMMUNIZATION				
BCG vaccine	*Generic*	Those with negative tuberculin skin tests exposed to sputum-positive cases of tuberculosis	Incidence is low	0.1 mL intradermally
cholera vaccine	*Generic*	Travel to areas requiring cholera vaccination	Transitory local reactions, malaise, fever, headache	2 doses of 0.5 mL SC, IM 1 wk to 1 mo apart
diphtheria and tetanus toxoids, combined (labeled for pediatric or adult use)	*Generic*	Pediatric form used until age 6; adult form for children age 7 or over and adults	Local reactions, drowsiness, anorexia, vomiting, fever, malaise, generalized aches and pains	Pediatric: 2–3 doses (depending on age) of 0.5 mL IM 4 wk apart, then 0.5 mL in 6–12 mo and a booster of 0.5 mL when starting school; adults: 2 doses of 0.5 mL IM 4–8 wk apart, reinforcing dose of 0.5 mL 6–12 mo later; booster dose of 0.5 mL every 10 y
diphtheria and tetanus toxoids and pertussis vaccine adsorbed (DTP)	Tri-Immunol, *generic*	Immunization of infants and children through age 6	Local reactions, fever, chills, irritability	3 doses of 0.5 mL IM at 4–8-wk intervals; booster: 0.5 mL when child is 4–8 y old
hemophilus b conjugate vaccine	HibTITER, ProHIBIT, PedavaxHIB	Immunization for children 24 mo to 6 y against diseases caused by *Haemophilus influenzae* b	Redness at injection site, fever	0.5 mL SC
hepatitis B vaccine	Heptavax-B, Recombivax-HB, Engerix-B	Immunization against all known subtypes of hepatitis B virus	Local reactions, malaise, fatigue, headache, nausea, myalgia	See package insert of specific trade name for amount and dosage schedule
influenza virus vaccine	Fluogen, Fluzone, *generic*	Annual vaccination of those at increased risk of consequences from infections of lower respiratory tract, older persons, those providing essential community services	Local reactions, fever, malaise, myalgia	See package insert for recommended dosage schedule; vaccine prepared for use during a specific year
measles (rubeola) virus vaccine, live, attenuated	Attenuvax	Given before or immediately after exposure to natural measles; immunization for children 15 mo or older	Fever, rash (between 5th and 12th days after administration)	1 ampule SC
measles (rubeola) and rubella virus vaccine	M-R-Vax II	Immunization for children 15 mo to puberty	Same as measles (rubeola) virus vaccine, live, attenuated and rubella virus vaccine, live	1 ampule SC
measles, mumps, and rubella virus vaccine	M-M-R II	Immunization for children 15 mo to puberty, and adults	Same as measles (rubeola) virus vaccine, live, attenuated and rubella and mumps virus vaccines, live	1 ampule SC
meningococcal polysaccharide vaccine, groups A, C, Y, and W-135	Menomune-A/C/Y/W-135	Immunization for medical and laboratory personnel, travelers to endemic areas, household travelers to endemic areas, household contacts of meningococcal disease	Headache, malaise, fever, chills; tenderness, pain, and redness at injection site	0.5 mL SC

(continued)

SUMMARY DRUG TABLE 40–1

(continued)

GENERIC NAME	TRADE NAME*	USES	ADVERSE REACTIONS	DOSE RANGES
mumps virus vaccine, live	Mumpsvax	Immunization for children 15 mos or older and adults	Fever, parotitis	1 ampule SC
plague vaccine	*Generic*	Those at high risk for exposure	Malaise, headache, local erythema, sensitivity reactions	First dose 1 mL IM; 2nd dose: 0.2 mL IM 1–3 mo after 1st dose
pneumococcal vaccine, polyvalent	Pneumovax 23, Pnu-Immune 23	Immunization against pneumococcal pneumonia and bacteremia	Erythema and soreness at injection site, fever, myalgia	0.5 mL SC, IM
poliovirus vaccine, inactivated (Salk, IPV)	*Generic*	Immunization against poliomyelitis (adults at risk, infants)	Allergic reactions, erythema and tenderness at injection site, fever	Primary immunization: 3 doses of 1 mL each SC at 4–8-wk intervals then 4th dose of 1 mL 6–12 mo after the 3rd dose; booster: 1 mL SC every 2–3 y
poliovirus vaccine live, oral, trivalent (Sabin, TOPV)	Orimune	Prevention of poliomyelitis in infants, children up to 18 y	Vaccine-associated paralysis (rare)	Primary series: 3 doses of 0.5 mL PO started at 6–12 wk of age, 2nd dose 6–8 wk later, 3rd dose 8–12 months after 2nd dose; booster: on entering school
rabies vaccine, human diploid cell cultures (HDCV)	Imovax Rabies Vaccine	Preexposure and postexposure immunization	Local reactions, nausea, headache, muscle aches, abdominal pain	See package insert for dosage recommendations and suggested schedules
rabies vaccines, human diploid cell cultures (for intradermal use)	Imovax Rabies I.D. Vaccine	Preexposure immunization for those at risk	Same as for rabies vaccine, human diploid cell cultures	3 doses of 0.1 mL given intradermally; 2nd dose given 7 d after 1st dose, 3rd dose in 21 or 28 d after the 1st dose
rubella virus vaccine, live	Meruvax II	Immunization for children age 1 y to puberty, adolescent and adult males, nonpregnant adolescent and adult females	Fever, joint pain, rash, malaise, sore throat, lymphadenopathy, headache	1 vial SC
rubella and mumps virus vaccine, live	Biavax-II	Immunization for children aged 1 mo to puberty	Same as rubella virus vaccine, live and mumps virus vaccine, live	1 ampule SC
tetanus toxoid, fluid and tetanus toxoid, adsorbed	*Generic*	Immunization in adults and children	Local reactions, fever, chills, malaise, myalgia	Tetanus toxoid adsorbed: 2 doses of 0.5 mL IM given 4–8 wk apart; booster—every 10 y; tetanus toxoid, fluid: 3 doses of 0.5 mL IM, SC at 4–8-wk intervals and 4th dose 6–12 mo after 3rd dose; booster—every 10 y
typhoid vaccine	*Generic*	Intimate exposure to known carrier, travel to area where typhoid is endemic	Local reactions, malaise, myalgia, fever	Primary immunization: 2 doses of 0.5 mL SC at intervals of ≥4 wk; children under 10—each dose is 0.25 mL; booster: 0.5 mL SC or 0.1 mL intradermal every 3 y; children under 10—each dose is 0.25 mL SC or 0.1 mL intradermal

(continued)

SUMMARY DRUG TABLE 40–1
(continued)

GENERIC NAME	TRADE NAME*	USES	ADVERSE REACTIONS	DOSE RANGES
AGENTS FOR PASSIVE IMMUNIZATION				
antirabies serum, equine origin (ARS)	*Generic*	Suspected exposure to rabies	Serum sickness, local pain, erythema, urticara	See package insert for schedule and dilution
diphtheria antitoxin	*Generic*	Prevention or treatment of diphtheria	Anaphylaxis, pain and redness at injection site	Therapeutic: 20,000–120,000 U IM, IV; prophylaxis: 10,000 U IM
hepatitis B immune globulin (HBIG)	H-BIG, HyperHep, Hep-B-Gammagee	Postexposure prophylaxis	Local reactions, fever, urticaria	0.06 mg/kg IM as soon as possible after exposure and repeated 28–30 d after exposure; see package insert for additional dosage and schedules
immune globulin intramuscular	Gamastan, Gammar	Hepatitis A (before or soon after exposure), rubeola (prevention and modification in those exposed < 6 d previously), immunoglobulin deficiency, passive immunization for varicella in immunosuppressed patients	Same as hepatitis B immune globulin	0.02–1.3 mL/kg IM depending on reason for use
immune globulin, intravenous (IGIV)	Gamimune N, Sandoglobulin, Gammagard, Venoglobulin-I	Immunodeficiency syndrome	Hypersensitivity reactions	See package insert of specific product (by trade name) for dosage
rabies immune globulin, human (RIG)	Imogam	Immunization for those suspected of exposure	Fever, soreness at injection site	20 IU/kg IM; 1/2 the dose may be used to infiltrate the wound
RH₀(D) immune globulin	Gamulin Rh, RhoGAM	Prevention of sensitization to Rh0 (D) factor and of hemolytic disease in the newborn in a subsequent pregnancy; transfusion accidents (Rh0-[D] negative patient transfused with Rh₀-[D] positive blood)	Same as hepatitis B immune globulin	≥1 vial IM depending on reason for use
tetanus immune globulin	Hyper-Tet	Passive immunization	Tenderness, pain, muscle stiffness	Adults: 250 U IM; children: dose based on weight (4 U/kg)
tetanus antitoxin	*Generic*	Tetanus; prevention of tetanus when tetanus immune globulin not available	Tenderness, pain at injection site	Prophylactic: 1500–5000 U IM, SC; treatment: 50,000–100,000 U IM *and* IV (part of dose given IV and remainder IM)
varicella-zoster immune globulin (human)	*Generic*	Passive immunization of immune deficient individuals in those meeting required criteria (see package insert)	Tenderness, pain at injection site	Dosage based on weight (125 U/10 kg; maximum dose: 625 U

* The term generic *indicates that the drug is available in a generic form.*

tory center, resulting in permanent respiratory paralysis requiring lifetime use of artificial ventilation because they would never be able to breathe on their own. Today, poliomyelitis is rare because administration of the poliovirus vaccine has provided immunity to a large number of the population.

History

Before the administration of any vaccine, an allergy history is obtained. If the individual is known or thought to have allergies of any kind, this is told to the physician before the vaccine is given. Some passive immunization vaccines contain antibodies obtained from animals, such as the horse, whereas other vaccines may contain proteins or preservatives to which the individual may be allergic. A highly allergic person may have an allergic reaction (which could be serious and even fatal) if he or she is allergic to these substances. If the patient has an allergy history, the physician may decide to skin test him for allergy to one or more of the components or proteins in the vaccine.

Administration

If a vaccine is not in liquid form and must be reconstituted, the nurse must read the directions enclosed with the vaccine. It is important to follow the enclosed directions carefully. Package inserts also contain information regarding dosage, adverse reactions, method of administration, administration sites (when appropriate), and, when needed, recommended booster schedules. The various types of vaccines for immunization are given in Summary Drug Table 40-1.

Patient and Family Teaching

Because of the effectiveness of various types of vaccines in the prevention of disease, nurses must inform the public about the advantages of immunization. Parents should be encouraged to have infants and young children receive the immunizations suggested by the physician.

Those traveling to a foreign country are advised to contact their physician or local health department well in advance of their departure date for information about the immunizations that will be needed. Immunizations should be given well in advance of departure because it may take several weeks to produce adequate immunity.

When an adult or child is receiving a vaccine for immunization, the patient or a family member is made aware of the possible reactions that may occur, for example, soreness at the injection site, fever, and so on.

There have been fatalities, as well as serious viral infections of the central nervous system, associated with the use of vaccines. Although the number of these incidents is small, a risk factor still remains when some vaccines are given. However, a risk is also associated with *not* receiving immunization against some infectious diseases, and that risk may be higher and just as serious as the risk associated with the use of vaccines. It must also be remembered that when a large segment of the population is immunized, the small number of those not immunized are less likely to be exposed to and be infected with the disease-producing microorganism. But when large numbers of the population are *not* immunized, there is a great increase in the chances of exposure to the infectious disease and a significant increase in the probability that the individual will develop the disease.

41

Anesthetic Agents

On completion of this chapter the student will:

▶ *Discuss the uses of local and general anesthetics*

▶ *Discuss the four stages of general anesthesia*

▶ *List and discuss the nursing responsibilities when a local or general anesthetic is given*

There are two types of anesthetic agents: **general anesthetics** and **local anesthetics.** When a general anesthetic is given, the patient loses consciousness and feels no pain. Reflexes, such as the swallowing and gag reflexes, are lost during deep general anesthesia. When a local anesthetic is given, the patient is fully awake but does not feel pain in the area that has been anesthetized. Some procedures done under local anesthesia may require the patient to be sedated, and although not fully awake, the patient may hear what is going on around him.

▶ LOCAL ANESTHESIA

▷ Preparing the Patient for Local Anesthesia

Depending on the procedure performed, preparation for local anesthesia may or may not be similar to preparing the patient for general anesthesia. For example, the administration of a local anesthetic for

dental surgery or the suturing of a small wound may require an explanation of how the anesthetic will be administered, an allergy history, and, when applicable, preparation of the area (cleaning the area with an antiseptic, shaving the area, and so forth). Other local anesthetic procedures may require the patient to be in a fasting state because a sedative may also be administered. Intravenous diazepam (Valium), a tranquilizer (see chap 34), may be used as a sedative during some local anesthetic procedures, such as cataract surgery.

▷ Administration of Local Anesthetics

A local injectable anesthetic is administered by a physician or dentist. Table 41-1 lists the more commonly used local anesthetics. Topical anesthetics may, in some instances, be administered by the nurse.

TABLE 41–1
Local Anesthetics

GENERIC NAME	TRADE NAME*
bupivacaine hydrochloride	Marcaine HCl, *generic*
chloroprocaine hydrochloride	Nesacaine
lidocaine hydrochloride	Dilocaine, L-Caine, Xylocaine, *generic*
mepivacaine hydrochloride	Carbocaine, Isocaine
prilocaine hydrochloride	Citanest HCl
tetracaine hydrochloride	Pontocaine HCl

* The term generic *indicates that the drug is available in a generic form.*

▷ Nursing Management After Administration of a Local Anesthetic

When applicable, the nurse may be responsible for applying a dressing to the area. Depending on the reason for using a local anesthetic, the nurse may also be responsible for observing the area for bleeding, oozing, and signs of infection during the period after the administration of a local anesthetic.

▶ GENERAL ANESTHESIA

Before general anesthesia is administered, a *preanesthetic* agent may be given. Preanesthetic agents may be omitted in those 60 years or older because some preanesthetic agents are contraindicated in certain disorders. For example, atropine, which can be used to decrease secretions of the upper respiratory tract, is contraindicated in certain medical disorders, for example, prostatic hypertrophy, glaucoma, and myocardial ischemia. Many of the medical disorders for which atropine is contraindicated are seen in older individuals. Other preanesthetic agents that depress the central nervous system (CNS), such as narcotics, barbiturates, tranquilizers with antiemetic properties, may be contraindicated in the older individual.

The preanesthetic agent may consist of one drug or a combination of drugs. The general purpose of the preanesthetic agent is to prepare the patient for anesthesia. The more specific purposes of these agents are the following:

▷ To decrease anxiety and apprehension immediately before surgery. The patient who is calm and relaxed can be anesthetized more quickly, usually requires a smaller dose of an induction agent, may require less anesthesia during surgery, and may have a smoother anesthesia recovery period (wakening from anesthesia).

▷ To decrease secretions of the upper respiratory tract. Some anesthetic gases and volatile liquids are irritating to the lining of the respiratory tract and thereby increase mucus secretions. The cough and swallowing reflexes are lost during general anesthesia and excessive secretions can pool in the lungs, resulting in pneumonia or atelectasis during the postoperative period. The administration of an agent such as glycopyrrolate (a cholinergic blocking drug) dries up secretions of the upper respiratory tract and lessens the possibility of excessive mucus production.

▷ To lessen the incidence of nausea and vomiting during the immediate postoperative recovery period.

The preanesthetic agent is usually selected by the anesthesiologist and may consist of one or more drugs (Table 41-2). A *narcotic* or *barbiturate* may be given to relax (or sedate) the patient. Barbiturates are used only occasionally; narcotics are usually preferred for sedation. A *cholinergic blocking* drug is given to dry secretions in the upper respiratory tract. Scopolamine and glycopyrrolate also have

TABLE 41–2
Preanesthetic Drugs

GENERIC NAME	TRADE NAME*
NARCOTICS	
meperidine	Demerol, *generic*
morphine	*Generic*
fentanyl	Sublimaze, *generic*
BARBITURATES	
pentobarbital	Nembutal Sodium, *generic*
secobarbital	*Generic*
CHOLINERGIC BLOCKING DRUGS	
atropine	*Generic*
glycopyrrolate	Robinul, *generic*
scopolamine	*Generic*
TRANQUILIZERS WITH ANTIEMETIC PROPERTIES	
hydroxyzine	Vistaril, *generic*
perphenazine	Trilafon
prochlorperazine	Compazine, *generic*
promethazine	Phenergan, *generic*

* The term generic *indicates that the drug is available in a generic form.*

mild sedative properties and atropine may or may not produce some sedation. *Tranquilizers* with antiemetic properties may also be given. The tranquilizers also have sedative action; when combined with a narcotic, they allow for a lowering of the narcotic dosage because they also have the ability to potentiate the sedative action of the narcotic.

In most hospitals, the anesthesiologist examines the patient the day or evening before surgery, although this may not be possible in emergency situations. The patient's physical status is evaluated and an explanation of the anesthesia is given. Proper explanation of anesthesia, the surgery itself, and the events that may occur in preparation for and after surgery require a team approach. The nurse's responsibility is as follows:

▷ Describing or explaining the preparations for surgery ordered by the physician. Examples of preoperative preparations include fasting from midnight (or the time specified by the physician), enemas, shaving, a hypnotic for sleep the night before, and the preoperative injection approximately 30 minutes before going to surgery.

▷ Describing or explaining immediate postoperative care, such as the recovery room or a special postoperative surgical unit and the activities of the physicians and nurses during this period. The patient should know that his or her vital signs will be monitored frequently, and that other equipment, such as intravenous (IV) and monitors, may be used.

▷ Describing, explaining, and demonstrating postoperative patient activities such as deep breathing, coughing, and leg exercises.

The preoperative explanations given by the nurse are tailored to fit the type of surgery scheduled. Not all of the above teaching points may be included in every explanation.

▷ Agents Used for General Anesthesia

The administration of an anesthetic requires the use of one or more agents. The choice of anesthetic agents depends on many factors including the following:

▷ The general physical condition of the patient
▷ The area, organ, or system being operated on
▷ The anticipated length of the surgical procedure

The anesthesiologist selects the anesthetic agent that will produce safe anesthesia, analgesia, and, in some surgeries, effective skeletal muscle relaxation. The agents used for general anesthesia are discussed below.

Methohexital, Thiamylal, and Thiopental. Methohexital (Brevital), thiamylal (Surital), and thiopental (Pentothal), which are short-acting barbiturates, are used for the following: induction of anesthesia, short surgical procedures with minimal painful stimuli, and in conjunction with or as a supplement to other anesthetics. Thiopental may also be used for the control of convulsive states. These agents have a rapid onset and a short duration of action. They depress the CNS to produce hypnosis and anesthesia but do not produce analgesia. Recovery after a small dose is rapid.

Etomidate. Etomidate (Amidate), a nonbarbiturate, is used for induction of anesthesia. Etomidate may also be used to supplement other anesthetics, such as nitrous oxide, for short surgical procedures. It is a hypnotic without analgesic activity.

Propofol. Propofol (Diprivan) is used for induction and maintenance of anesthesia.

Midazolam. Midazolam (Versed), a short-acting benzodiazepine CNS depressant, is used for induction of anesthesia, for conscious sedation before minor procedures, such as endoscopic procedures, and to supplement nitrous oxide and oxygen for short surgical procedures. When used for induction anesthesia, the patient gradually loses consciousness over 1 to 2 minutes.

Ketamine. Ketamine (Ketalar) is a rapid-acting general anesthetic. It produces an anesthetic state characterized by profound analgesia, cardiovascular and respiratory stimulation, normal or enhanced skeletal muscle tone, and occasionally mild respiratory depression. Ketamine is used for diagnostic and surgical procedures that do not require relaxation of skeletal muscles, for induction of anesthesia before the administration of other anesthetic agents, and as a supplement to other anesthetic agents.

Cyclopropane. An anesthetic gas, cyclopropane has a rapid onset of action and may be used for induction and maintenance of anesthesia. Skeletal muscle relaxation is produced with full anesthetic doses. Cyclopropane is supplied in orange cylinders. Disadvantages of cyclopropane are difficulty in detecting the planes of anesthesia, occasionally laryngospasm, cardiac dysrhythmias, and postanesthesia nausea, vomiting, and headache. Cyclopropane and oxygen mixtures are explosive, which limits the use of this gas anesthetic.

Ethylene. Ethylene is an anesthetic gas with a rapid onset of action and a rapid recovery from its anesthetic effects. It provides adequate analgesia but has poor muscle-relaxant properties. The advantages of ethylene include minimal bronchospasm, laryngospasm, and postanesthesia vomiting. A disadvantage of ethylene is hypoxia. This gas is supplied in red cylinders. Mixtures of ethylene and oxygen are flammable and explosive.

Nitrous Oxide. Nitrous oxide is a commonly used anesthetic gas. It is a weak anesthetic and is usually used in combination with other anesthetic agents. It does not cause skeletal muscle relaxation. The chief danger in the use of nitrous oxide is hypoxemia. Nitrous oxide is nonexplosive and is supplied in blue cylinders.

Enflurane. Enflurane (Ethrane) is a volatile liquid (a liquid that evaporates on exposure to air) anesthetic that is delivered by inhalation. Induction and recovery from anesthesia are rapid. Muscle relaxation for abdominal surgery is adequate, but greater relaxation may be necessary and may require the use of a skeletal muscle relaxant. Enflurane may produce mild stimulation of respiratory and bronchial secretions when used alone. Hypotension may occur when anesthesia deepens.

Halothane. Halothane (Fluothane) is a volatile liquid given by inhalation for induction and maintenance of anesthesia. Induction and recovery from anesthesia are rapid and the depth of anesthesia can be rapidly altered. Halothane does not irritate the respiratory tract and an increase in tracheobronchial secretions usually does not occur. Halothane produces moderate muscle relaxation, but skeletal muscle relaxants may be used in certain types of surgeries. This anesthetic may be given with a mixture of nitrous oxide and oxygen.

Isoflurane. Isoflurane (Forane) is a volatile liquid given by inhalation. It is used for induction and maintenance of anesthesia.

Methoxyflurane. Methoxyflurane (Penthrane), a volatile liquid, provides analgesia and anesthesia. It is usually used in combination with nitrous oxide but may also be used alone. It does not produce good muscle relaxation and a skeletal muscle relaxant may be required.

Fentanyl and Droperidol. The narcotic analgesic fentanyl (Sublimaze) and the neuroleptic (major tranquilizer) droperidol (Inapsine) may be used to-

gether as a single agent called Innovar. The combination of these two drugs results in *neuroleptanalgesia*, which is characterized by general quietness, reduced motor activity, and profound analgesia. Complete loss of consciousness may not occur unless other anesthetic agents are used. A fentanyl and droperidol combination may be used to produce tranquilization and analgesia for surgical and diagnostic procedures. It may also be used as a preanesthetic medication for the induction of anesthesia and in the maintenance of general anesthesia.

Droperidol may be used as a single agent to produce tranquilization, to reduce nausea and vomiting during the immediate postanesthesia period, as an induction agent, and as an adjunct to general anesthesia. Fentanyl may be used alone as a supplement to general or regional anesthesia. It may also be administered as a single agent or with other agents as a preoperative medication and as an analgesic in the immediate postoperative (recovery room) period.

Skeletal Muscle Relaxants. The various skeletal muscle relaxants that may be used during general anesthesia are listed in Table 41-3. These drugs are administered to produce relaxation of the skeletal muscles during certain types of surgeries, such as those involving the chest or abdomen. They may also be used to facilitate the insertion of an endotracheal tube. Their onset of action is usually rapid (45 seconds to a few minutes) and the duration of action is 30 minutes or more.

▷ The Stages of General Anesthesia

General surgical anesthesia is divided into the following stages:

Stage I—the stage of analgesia
Stage II—the stage of delirium
Stage III—the stage of surgical analgesia
Stage IV—the stage of respiratory paralysis

With newer drugs and techniques, the stages of anesthesia may not be as prominent as described above. In addition, movement through the first two stages is usually very rapid.

Stage I

Induction is a part of stage I anesthesia. It begins with the administration of an anesthetic agent and lasts until consciousness is lost. With some induc-

TABLE 41–3
Muscle Relaxants Used During General Anesthesia

GENERIC NAME	TRADE NAME*
atracurium besylate	Tracrium
gallamine triethiodide	Flaxedil
metocurine iodide	Metubine Iodide
pancuronium bromide	Pavulon
pipecuronium bromide	Arduan
succinylcholine chloride	Anectine
tubocurarine chloride	*Generic*
vecuronium bromide	Norcuron

* The term generic *indicates that the drug is available in a generic form.*

tion agents, such as the short-acting barbiturates, this stage may last only 5 to 10 seconds.

Stage II

Stage II is the stage of delirium and is also brief. During this stage, the patient may move about and mumble incoherently. The muscles are somewhat rigid and the patient is unconscious and cannot feel pain. If surgery were attempted at this stage, there would be a physical reaction to painful stimuli, yet the patient would not remember sensing pain.

Stage III

Stage III is the stage of surgical analgesia and is divided into four parts, planes, or substages. The anesthesiologist differentiates these planes by the character of the respirations, eye movements, certain reflexes, pupil size, and so on. At plane 2 or 3, the patient is usually ready for the surgical procedure.

Stage IV

Stage IV is the stage of respiratory paralysis and is a rare and dangerous stage of anesthesia. At this stage, respiratory arrest and cessation of all vital signs may occur.

Anesthesia begins with a loss of consciousness. This is part of the induction stage (stage I). Often, the short-acting barbiturates are used to produce an almost immediate loss of consciousness. The patient is now relaxed and can no longer see or hear what is going on around him or her. After consciousness is lost, additional anesthetic agents are administered. Some of these agents are also used as part of the induction phase, as well as for deepening anesthesia. Depending on the type of surgery, an endotracheal

tube may also be inserted into the trachea to provide an adequate airway and to assist in the administration of oxygen and other anesthetic agents. The endotracheal tube is removed during the postanesthesia period once the gag and swallowing reflexes have returned. If an IV line was not inserted before the patient's arrival in surgery, it is inserted by the anesthesiologist before the administration of an induction agent.

▷ Nursing Implications

Preanesthesia

Before surgery, the nurse has the following responsibilities:

▷ Performing the required tasks and procedures as prescribed by the physician and hospital policy the day, evening, or morning before surgery. These tasks may include administration of a hypnotic the night before surgery, shaving, taking vital signs, seeing that the operative consent is signed, checking to see if all jewelry or metal objects are removed, administering enemas, inserting a catheter, inserting a nasogastric tube, preoperative teaching, and so on. All tasks are recorded on the patient's chart.

▷ Checking the chart for any recent, abnormal laboratory tests. If a recent, abnormal laboratory test was attached to the patient's chart shortly before surgery, the surgeon and the anesthesiologist must be made aware of the abnormality. A note can be attached to the front of the chart and the surgeon or anesthesiologist can be contacted by telephone.

▷ Placing a list of known or suspected drug allergies or idiosyncrasies on the front of the chart

▷ Administering preanesthetic (preoperative) medication. These medications must be given *on time* to produce their intended effects.

▷ Instructing the patient to remain in bed and placing the side rails up once the preanesthetic medication is administered

After surgery the nurse has the following responsibilities, which vary according to where the nurse first sees the postoperative patient.

Postanesthesia Recovery Room

▷ Admitting the patient to the unit according to hospital procedure or policy

▷ Checking the airway for patency, assessing the respiratory status, and giving oxygen as needed

▷ Positioning the patient to prevent aspiration of vomitus and secretions

▷ Checking the following: blood pressure, pulse, IV lines, catheters, drainage tubes, surgical dressings, casts, and so forth

▷ Reviewing the patient's surgical and anesthesia records

▷ Monitoring the blood pressure, pulse, and respiratory rate every 5 to 15 minutes until the patient is discharged from the area

▷ Checking the patient for emergence from anesthesia every 5 to 15 minutes

▷ Providing suction as needed

▷ Exercising caution in administering narcotics. The respiratory rate, blood pressure, and pulse must be checked before these drugs are given and 20 to 30 minutes after administration (see chap 10). The physician is contacted if the respiratory rate is below 10 before the drug is given, and if the respirations fall below 10 after the drug is given.

▷ Discharging the patient from the area to his or her room or other specified area. All drugs administered and nursing tasks performed must be recorded before the patient leaves the recovery room.

42

Drugs Used in the Management of Musculoskeletal Disorders

On completion of this chapter the student will:

▶ *Discuss the actions and uses of drugs used in the treatment of musculoskeletal disorders*

▶ *List and discuss the adverse reactions of drugs used in the treatment of musculoskeletal disorders*

▶ *Use the nursing process when administering drugs used in the treatment of musculoskeletal disorders*

▶ *Discuss the nursing implications to be considered when administering drugs used in the treatment of musculoskeletal disorders*

A variety of drugs are used in the treatment of musculoskeletal disorders. The drug selected is based on the musculoskeletal disorder being treated and the severity of the disorder. For example, early cases of rheumatoid arthritis may respond well to the salicylates, whereas advanced rheumatoid arthritis not responding to other drug therapies may require the use of one of the gold salts. The physician may base the selection of a drug for treatment of a chronic musculoskeletal disorder on the patient's positive or negative response to past therapy. Administration of some of these drugs may result in serious adverse effects, which may require dosage adjustments or a change in drug therapy.

▷ Actions of the Drugs Used in the Treatment of Musculoskeletal Disorders

The Salicylates

Aspirin (acetylsalicylic acid) has greater antiinflammatory activity than the other salicylates, and therefore is preferred for the treatment of arthritic disorders. The antiinflammatory activity of aspirin is thought to be due to its ability to inhibit the synthesis of prostaglandins (see chap 11), a substance thought to increase the sensitivity of peripheral pain receptors to painful stimuli. When inflammation is reduced, pain is also relieved. In addition to an antiinflammatory action, the salicylates also relieve mild pain.

Gold Salts

Gold salts, for example, gold sodium thiomalate (Myochrysine) and auranofin (Ridaura), may be used to suppress or prevent the inflammatory reactions seen with rheumatoid arthritis. The exact mechanism of their action is unknown.

Nonsteroidal Antiinflammatory Drugs

The nonsteroidal antiinflammatory drugs (NSAIDs) are so called because they do not belong to the steroid group of drugs, do not possess the adverse reactions associated with the steroids (or corticosteroids) and yet have antiinflammatory activity. Their exact mechanism of action is unknown. In addition to their antiinflammatory activity, they possess analgesic and antipyretic actions. Examples of these drugs include fenoprofen (Nalfon) and ibuprofen (Advil).

Drugs Used for Gout

The deposit or collection of urate crystals in the joints causes the symptoms of gout. Allopurinol (Zyloprim) reduces the production of uric acid, thus decreasing serum uric acid levels and the deposit of urate crystals in joints.

The exact mechanism of action of colchicine is unknown, but it does reduce the inflammation associated with the deposit of urate crystals in the joints. This probably accounts for its ability to relieve the severe pain of acute gout. Colchicine has no effect on uric acid metabolism.

Sulfinpyrazone (Anturane) increases the excretion of uric acid by the kidneys, which lowers serum uric acid levels and consequently retards the deposit of urate crystals in the joints. Probenecid (Benemid) works in the same manner and may be given alone or with colchicine (Colabid) as combination therapy when there are frequent, recurrent attacks of gout. Probenecid also has been used to prolong the plasma levels of the penicillins and cephalosporins.

Skeletal Muscle Relaxants

The mode of action of carisoprodol (Soma), chlorphenesin (Maolate), and chlorzoxazone (Paraflex), is not clearly understood. These drugs do not relax skeletal muscles but their ability to relieve acute painful musculoskeletal conditions may be due to their sedative action.

Cyclobenzaprine (Flexeril) appears to have an effect on muscle tone, thus reducing muscle spasm.

The exact mode of action of diazepam (Valium), a tranquilizer (see chap 34), in the relief of painful musculoskeletal conditions is unknown. The drug does have a sedative action, which may account for some of its ability to relieve muscle spasm and pain.

The Corticosteroids

The potent antiinflammatory action of the corticosteroids make these drugs useful in the treatment of many types of musculoskeletal disorders. The corticosteroids are also discussed in chapter 26.

Miscellaneous Drugs

Phenylbutazone (Butazolidin) and oxyphenbutazone are chemically related. These drugs have antiinflammatory, as well as antipyretic and analgesic, activity. The exact mode of their antiinflammatory action is not well understood. These drugs may inhibit prostaglandin synthesis, which may partially account for their antiinflammatory activity. The mechanism of action of penicillamine (Cuprimine) in the treatment of rheumatoid arthritis is unknown. This drug is also discussed in chapter 38.

▷ Uses of the Drugs Used in the Treatment of Musculoskeletal Disorders

The specific uses of the drugs used in the treatment of musculoskeletal disorders are given in Summary Drug Table 42-1.

SUMMARY DRUG TABLE 42–1
Drugs Used in the Management of Musculoskeletal Disorders

GENERIC NAME	TRADE NAME*	USES	ADVERSE REACTIONS	DOSE RANGES
THE SALICYLATES				
aspirin (acetyl-salicylic acid)	Bayer, Ecotrin, Bufferin, *generic*	Rheumatoid arthritis, osteoarthritis; see Summary Drug Table 11-1	See Summary Drug Table 11-1	Arthritis, other rheumatic conditions 3.6–5.4 g/d PO in divided doses
GOLD SALTS				
See Summary Drug Table 38-1				
NONSTEROIDAL ANTIINFLAMMATORY DRUGS				
diclofenac sodium	Voltaren	Signs and symptoms of rheumatoid arthritis and osteoarthritis, ankylosing spondylitis	Nausea, vomiting, diarrhea, constipation, abdominal discomfort, gastric or duodenal ulcer formation, GI bleeding, hematologic changes	Osteoarthritis: 100–150 mg/d PO in divided doses; rheumatoid arthritis: 150–200 mg/d PO in divided doses; ankylosing spondylitis: 100–125 mg/d PO in divided doses
fenoprofen calcium	Nalfon	Signs and symptoms of rheumatoid arthritis and osteoarthritis, long-term management of mild to moderate pain	Same as diclofenac sodium	Rheumatoid and osteoarthritis: 300–600 mg PO tid, qid; pain: 200 mg PO q4–6h
flurbiprofen	Ansaid	Signs and symptoms of rheumatoid arthritis and osteoarthritis	Same as diclofenac sodium	Up to 300 mg/d PO in divided doses
ibuprofen	Advil, Motrin, Nuprin, *generic*	Same as fenoprofen plus painful dysmenorrhea	Same as diclofenac sodium	Rheumatoid arthritis and osteoarthritis: 1.2–3.2 g/d PO in divided doses; pain: 400 mg PO q4–6h; dysmenorrhea: 400 mg PO q4h
indomethacin	Indocin	Rheumatoid arthritis, ankylosing spondylitis, moderate to severe osteoarthritis, acute painful shoulder, acute gouty arthritis	Same as diclofenac sodium; hematologic changes may be more serious	Rheumatoid arthritis and osteoarthritis, ankylosing spondylitis: 25 mg PO bid, tid and up to 200 mg/d in divided doses; acute shoulder: 75–150 mg/d PO in 3–4 divided doses; gouty arthritis: 50 mg PO tid until pain is tolerated, then dosage is reduced
ketoprofen	Orudis	Same as ibuprofen	Same as diclofenac sodium	Up to 300 mg/d PO in divided doses
meclofenamate sodium	Meclomen, *generic*	Rheumatoid arthritis, osteoarthritis, mild to moderate pain	Same as diclofenac sodium; GI side effects may be severe	Rheumatoid arthritis and osteoarthritis: 200–400 mg/d PO in divided doses; pain: 50–100 mg PO q4–6h
naproxen	Naprosyn	Same as indomethacin, dysmenorrhea	Same as diclofenac	Rheumatoid arthritis, osteoarthritis, ankylosing spondylitis: 250–500 mg PO bid; gout: initially 750 mg PO then 250 mg PO q6–8h; pain, dysmenorrhea, painful shoulder: 500 mg PO then 250 mg q6–8h
piroxicam	Feldene	Same as flurbiprofen	Same as diclofenac sodium	20 mg/d PO as a single dose

(continued)

SUMMARY DRUG TABLE 42–1
(continued)

GENERIC NAME	TRADE NAME*	USES	ADVERSE REACTIONS	DOSE RANGES
sulindac	Clinoril	Same as indomethacin	Same as diclofenac sodium	Rheumatoid arthritis and osteoarthritis, ankylosing spondylitis: initially 150 mg PO bid; acute painful shoulder, acute gouty arthritis: initially 200 mg PO bid; dosages reduced after satisfactory respone
tolmetin sodium	Tolectin	Same as flurbiprofen	Same as diclofenac sodium	Up to 1800 mg/d PO in divided doses
DRUGS USED FOR GOUT				
allopurinol	Zyloprim, *generic*	Gout, uric acid stone formation, prophylactic treatment to prevent urate deposits	Rash, nausea, vomiting, diarrhea, hematologic changes, abdominal pain	100–800 mg/d PO in single or divided doses
colchicine	*Generic*	Gout	Vomiting, diarrhea, abdominal pain, nausea, bone marrow depression	Acute gouty arthritis: 1–1.2 mg PO followed by 0.5–1.2 mg q1–2h until pain relieved; 2 mg IV followed by 0.5 mg IV q6h until pain relieved; prophylaxis: 0.5–1.8 mg/d PO
probenecid	Benemid, *generic*	Hyperuricemia associated with gout and gouty arthritis, prolongation of plasma levels of the penicillins and cephalosporins	Headache, GI symptoms urinary frequency, hypersensitivity reactions	Gout: 0.25–0.5 g PO bid; penicillin, cephalosporin therapy: 2 g/d PO in divided doses
probenecid and colchicine	ColBenemid, Colabid, *generic*	Gouty arthritis	Same as benemid and colchicine	1 tablet PO 1–2 times/d
sulfinpyrazone	Anturane, *generic*	Chronic or intermittent gouty arthritis	Upper GI disturbances	Initial dose: 200 mg/d PO in 2 divided doses; maintenance dose: 400–800 mg/d PO in 2 divided doses
SKELETAL MUSCLE RELAXANTS				
carisoprodol	Rela, Soma, *generic*	Discomfort associated with acute, painful musculoskeletal conditions	Dizziness, drowsiness, ataxia, nausea, vomiting, hiccups, tachycardia, vertigo	350 mg PO tid, qid
chlorphenesin carbamate	Maolate	Same as carisoprodol	Drowsiness, dizziness, confusion, epigastric distress	400 mg PO qid to 800 mg PO tid
chlorzoxazone	Paraflex, *generic*	Same as carisoprodol	GI disturbances, dizziness, rash, drowsiness	250–750 mm PO tid, qid
cyclobenzaprine hydrochloride	Flexeril	Same as carisoprodol	Drowsiness, dry mouth, dizziness, fatigue, blurred vision, headache	20–60 mg/d PO in divided doses
diazepam	Valium	Skeletal muscle spasm; see Summary Drug Table 34-1	See Summary Drug Table 34-1	2–10 mg PO tid, qid; 2–10 mg IM, IV
methocarbamol	Robaxin, *generic*	Acute, painful musculoskeletal conditions	Syncope, hypotension, dizziness, lightheadedness, blurred vision, vertigo, headache, rash	1.5 g PO initially, maintenance: up to 8 g/d PO in divided doses; 1–3 g IM; up to 1 vial IV

(continued)

SUMMARY DRUG TABLE 42–1
(continued)

GENERIC NAME	TRADE NAME*	USES	ADVERSE REACTIONS	DOSE RANGES
CORTICOSTEROID DRUGS				
See Summary Drug Table 27-2				
GOLD COMPOUNDS				
See Summary Drug Table 38-1				
MISCELLANEOUS DRUGS				
hydroxy-chloroquine sulfate	Plaquenil Sulfate	Chronic discoid and systemic lupus erythematosus, acute or chronic rheumatoid arthritis; see chap 25 for additional uses	Irritability, nervousness, skeletal muscle weakness, bleaching of hair, alopecia, anorexia, nausea, vomiting	Rheumatoid arthritis: 200–600 mg/d PO; lupus erythematosus: 400–800 mg/d PO; see Summary Drug Table 25-1
oxyphenbutazone	*Generic*	Acute gouty arthritis, rheumatoid arthritis, ankylosing spondylitis, degenerative joint disease of hips and knees, painful shoulder	Abnominal discomfort, nausea, dyspepsia, rash, edema	Rheumatoid arthritis, ankylosing spondylitis, painful shoulder, degenerative joint disease: 100–600 mg/d PO in divided doses; gouty arthritis: initially 400 mg PO, then 100 mg q4h
penicillamine	Cuprimine, Depen	Rheumatoid arthritis; see Summary Drug Table 38-1 for use in WIlson's disease	Pruritus, rash, anorexia, nausea, vomiting, epigastric pain, bone marrow depression, proteinuria, hematuria, tinnitus	125–250 mg/d PO as a single dose and increased at 1–3-mo intervals
phenylbutazone	Azolild, Butazolidin, *generic*	Same as oxyphenbutazone	Same as oxyphenbutazone	Same as oxyphenbutazone

* The term generic *indicates that the drug is available in a generic form.*

▷ Adverse Reactions Associated with the Administration of Drugs Used in the Treatment of Musculoskeletal Disorders

The Salicylates.   The adverse reactions associated with the administration of the salicylates are listed in Summary Drug Table 11-1. Because relatively high doses of these drugs may be required for some arthritic disorders, such as rheumatoid arthritis, common adverse reactions seen with high doses are tinnitus, gastrointestinal (GI) distress, and GI bleeding. At times, adverse reactions are severe and the dosage may need to be decreased or the drug discontinued.

Gold Salts.   Adverse reactions to gold salts may occur any time during therapy, as well as many months after therapy has been discontinued. Dermatitis and stomatitis are the most common adverse reactions seen. Pruritus often occurs before the skin eruption becomes apparent. The gold salts are also discussed in chapter 38.

Nonsteroidal Antiinflammatory Drugs.   GI symptoms are the most common adverse reactions seen with nonsteroidal antiinflammatory drugs. These reactions may include nausea, vomiting, abdominal discomfort, diarrhea, constipation, gastric or duodenal ulcer formation, and GI bleeding, which can be potentially serious. Hematologic changes can occur, and in some instances are serious. Other adverse reactions that may be seen include jaundice, toxic hepatitis, visual disturbances, rash, dermatitis, and hypersensitivity reactions.

Drugs Used for Gout.   One adverse reaction associated with allopurinol is skin rash, which in some cases has been followed by serious hypersensitivity reactions such as exfoliative dermatitis and the

Stevens-Johnson syndrome. Other adverse reactions include nausea, vomiting, diarrhea, abdominal pain, and hematologic changes.

Colchicine administration may result in nausea, vomiting, diarrhea, abdominal pain, and bone marrow depression. When this drug is given to patients with an acute attack of gout, the physician may order the drug given at frequent intervals until GI symptoms occur. Probenecid administration may cause headache, GI symptoms, urinary frequency, and hypersensitivity reactions. Upper GI disturbances may be seen with the administration of sulfinpyrazone. Even when the drug is given with food, milk, or antacids, GI distress may persist and the drug may need to be discontinued.

The adverse reactions seen with other agents used in the treatment of gout are listed in Summary Drug Table 42-1.

Skeletal Muscle Relaxants. Drowsiness is the most common reaction seen with the use of skeletal muscle relaxants. Additional adverse reactions are given in Summary Drug Table 42-1. The adverse reactions seen with the administration of diazepam are listed in Summary Drug Table 34-1.

The Corticosteroids. Corticosteroids may be given in high doses for some arthritic disorders. There are many adverse reactions associated with high dose and long-term therapy. A list of these adverse reactions may be found in Table 27-2.

Miscellaneous Drugs. Phenylbutazone and oxyphenbutazone have the same adverse reactions, which include abdominal discomfort, edema, nausea, rash, indigestion, and heartburn. Less common adverse reactions include vomiting, constipation, diarrhea, and epigastric pain. The adverse reactions seen with penicillamine include pruritus, rash, anorexia, nausea, vomiting, epigastric pain, bone marrow depression, proteinuria, hematuria, increased skin friability, and tinnitus. Penicillamine is capable of causing severe toxic reactions.

▶ NURSING PROCESS
THE PATIENT RECEIVING A DRUG FOR A MUSCULOSKELETAL DISORDER

ASSESSMENT

The patient with a musculoskeletal disorder may be in acute pain or have longstanding mild to moderate pain, which can be just as difficult to tolerate as severe pain.

Along with pain, there may be skeletal deformities, for example, the joint deformities seen with advanced rheumatoid arthritis. For many musculoskeletal conditions, drug therapy is a major treatment modality. Therapy with these drugs may keep the disorder under control (eg, therapy for gout), improve the patient's ability to carry out the activities of daily living (ADL), or make the pain and discomfort tolerable.

The patient history should include a summary of the disorder including onset, symptoms, and current treatment or therapy. In some instances, it may be necessary to question the patient regarding his or her ability to carry out ADL, including employment, when applicable.

The physical assessment includes a general appraisal of the patient's physical condition and limitations. If the patient has arthritis (any type), the affected joints in the extremities are examined for appearance of the skin over the joint, evidence of joint deformity, and mobility of the affected joint. The vital signs and weight are taken to provide a baseline for comparison during therapy. If the patient has gout, the affected joints are examined and the appearance of the skin over the joints and any joint enlargement are noted.

NURSING DIAGNOSIS

Depending on the drug, dose, and reason for administration, one or more of the following nursing diagnoses may apply to a person receiving a drug for a musculoskeletal disorder:

▶ Anxiety related to symptoms of disorder, other factors

▶ Noncompliance related to indifference, lack of knowledge, other factors

▶ Knowledge deficit of medication regimen, adverse drug effects, treatment modalities

PLANNING AND IMPLEMENTATION

The major goals of the patient may include a reduction in anxiety and an understanding of and compliance to the prescribed treatment regimen.

The major goals of nursing management may include a reduction in the patient's anxiety, a reduction in or relief of pain and discomfort, recognition of adverse drug reactions, and the development and implementation of an effective teaching plan.

ADMINISTRATION. Some of the drugs prescribed for a musculoskeletal disorder have specific administration requirements.

SALICYLATES. These drugs may be given with food or milk or a full glass of water. The physician may prescribe an antacid to be given with the drug to minimize GI distress.

GOLD SALTS. Aurothioglucose and gold sodium thiomalate are given intramuscularly (IM), preferably in the upper outer quadrant of the gluteus muscle. Auranofin is given orally.

NONSTEROIDAL ANTIINFLAMMATORY DRUGS. Indomethacin (Indocin) is given with an antacid (when prescribed by the physician), food, or milk. Sulindac (Clinoril) is given with food. The other nonsteroidal antiinflammatory agents may be given with food or milk if GI upset occurs.

DRUGS USED FOR GOUT. Allopurinol, probenemid, and sulfinpyrazone are given with or immediately after meals to minimize GI distress. Colchicine usually can be given with food or milk. When this drug is used for the treatment of an acute gout attack, it may be given every 1 to 2 hours until the pain is relieved or the patient develops vomiting or diarrhea. The physician writes specific orders for administration of the drug and when the drug is to be stopped. The patient is carefully evaluated for relief of pain or the occurrence of nausea, vomiting, or diarrhea. After this evaluation, the nurse makes the decision to administer or withhold the drug. Colchicine may be given with food or milk when it is given as a prophylaxis for gout. The nurse should check with the physician regarding administration with food when the drug is given at 1- to 2-hour intervals. Colchicine may be given IV for severe gout.

SKELETAL MUSCLE RELAXANTS. These drugs may be given with food to minimize GI distress.

CORTICOSTEROIDS. When the patient is receiving one of these drugs on alternate days (alternate-day therapy), the drug *must be given before 9 AM.* It is extremely important that these drugs not be omitted or suddenly discontinued. When the drug is discontinued, the dosage is tapered gradually over several days. If high dosages have been given, it may take a week or more to taper the dosage. These drugs are also discussed in chapter 27.

PHENYLBUTAZONE AND OXYPHENBUTAZONE. These drugs *must* be given with food or milk to minimize GI distress.

PENICILLAMINE. This drug *must* be given on an empty stomach, 1 hour before or 2 hours after a meal.

OBSERVATIONS AND NURSING MANAGEMENT. Periodic evaluation is an important part of therapy for musculoskeletal disorders. With some disorders such as acute gout, the patient can be expected to respond to therapy in hours. Therefore, the joints involved are inspected every 1 to 2 hours to identify immediately a

response or nonresponse to therapy. At this time, the patient is also questioned regarding the relief of pain, as well as adverse drug reactions. In other disorders, response is gradual and may take days, weeks, and even months of treatment. Depending on the drug administered and the disorder being treated, evaluation of therapy may be daily or weekly. These evaluations help the physician plan present and future therapy including dosage changes, changes in the drug administered, institution of physical therapy, and so on.

Patients on complete bed rest require position changes and good skin care every 2 hours. The patient with an arthritic disorder may experience much pain or discomfort and require assistance with activities such as ambulating, eating, and grooming.

Nursing assessments and management for specific drugs are the following:

The Salicylates
▶ The patient is observed closely for signs of salicylate toxicity: tinnitus, impaired hearing, nausea, vomiting, flushing, sweating, rapid deep breathing, thirst, headache, tachycardia, diarrhea, and drowsiness. Any one or more of these symptoms should be considered signs of salicylate toxicity and the physician should be notified before the next dose is due.

▶ Periodic monitoring of plasma salicylate acid levels may be ordered. Therapeutic levels are between 100 and 300 mcg/mL.

▶ The color of the stools is checked. Black or dark stools or bright red blood in the stool may indicate GI bleeding. Any change in the color of the stool is reported to the physician.

Gold Salts
▶ The patient is observed closely for evidence of dermatitis. Itching may occur before a skin reaction and is reported to the physician immediately.

▶ The mouth of the patient is inspected daily for evidence of ulceration of the mucous membranes. A metallic taste may be noted before stomatitis becomes evident. The patient is advised to inform the nurse if a metallic taste occurs.

▶ Good oral care is necessary. The teeth should be brushed after each meal and the mouth rinsed with plain water to remove food particles. Mouthwash may also be used but excessive use may result in oral infections due to the destruction of the normal bacteria present in the mouth.

Nonsteroidal Antiinflammatory Drugs
▶ GI reactions may occur with the use of these drugs and can be severe and even fatal, especially in patients with a history of upper GI disease such as stomach ulcers. Withhold the next dose and notify

the physician if diarrhea, nausea, vomiting, tarry stools, or abdominal pain occurs.

▶ The patient should be advised that the drug may take several days to produce an effect (relief of pain and tenderness).

▶ Diabetic patient: the insulin dosage may require adjustment when these drugs are given. The urine is tested four times per day or as ordered and the physician is informed of any change in urine testing results.

Drugs Used for Gout

▶ When these drugs are given, a liberal fluid intake is encouraged and the intake and output are measured. The daily urine output should be at least 2 L. An increase in urinary output is necessary to excrete the urates (uric acid) and prevent urate acid stone formation in the genitourinary tract.

▶ Adequate fluids are made available and the patient is frequently reminded of the importance of increasing his or her fluid intake. If the patient fails to increase his or her oral intake, the physician is informed. In some instances, it may be necessary to administer IV fluids to supplement the oral intake when the patient fails to drink about 3000 mL of fluid per day.

Skeletal Muscle Relaxants

▶ In addition to drug therapy, rest, physical therapy, and other measures may be part of treatment.

▶ These drugs may cause drowsiness. The patient should be carefully evaluated before being allowed to ambulate alone. If drowsiness does occur, assistance with ambulatory activities is necessary. If drowsiness is severe, the physician is notified before the next dose is due.

Corticosteroids

▶ See chapter 27 for the nursing management of the patient receiving a corticosteroid.

Phenylbutazone and Oxyphenbutazone

▶ If drowsiness occurs, the patient requires assistance with ambulatory activities.

▶ Once a therapeutic response is obtained, the dosage may be reduced or the drug discontinued.

▶ These drugs may depress the bone marrow. The next dose is withheld and the physician is notified if any of the following occur: sore throat, fever, soreness of the mouth, stomatitis, unusual bleeding or bruising, or tarry stools.

Penicillamine

▶ Administration of this drug has been associated with many adverse reactions, some of which are potentially serious and even fatal. Any complaint or comment made by the patient is carefully evaluated and reported to the physician.

▶ Increased skin friability may occur, which may result in easy breakdown of the skin at pressure sites such as the hips, elbows, and shoulders. The patient who is unable to ambulate must have his or her position changed and pressure sites inspected for skin breakdown every 2 hours.

ADVERSE DRUG REACTIONS. Some of these drugs are toxic and the patient is carefully observed for the development of adverse reactions. Should any one or more adverse reactions occur, the physician is notified before the next dose is due. Serious adverse reactions require notifying the physician immediately.

ANXIETY. Patients with a musculoskeletal disorder often have anxiety related to the symptoms and the chronicity of their disorder. In addition to physical care, these patients often require emotional support, especially when a disorder is disabling and chronic. Therapy with some drugs may take weeks or longer before any benefit is noted. When this is explained before therapy is started, the patient is less likely to become discouraged over the results of drug therapy.

NONCOMPLIANCE AND KNOWLEDGE DEFICIT. The points included in a patient and family teaching plan depend on the type and severity of the musculoskeletal disorder being treated. Drug therapy, as well as other medical management, such as diet, exercise, limitations or nonlimitations of activity, periodic physical therapy treatments, and so on, are carefully explained.

The patient must also understand the importance of complying with the prescribed treatment regimen and taking the drug exactly as directed to obtain the best results from therapy. The patient is also told not to take any nonprescription drugs unless their use has been approved by the physician.

The following points for specific drugs may be included in the patient teaching plan. Information included for the patient taking a corticosteroid is covered in chapter 27.

Salicylates
▶ Take with food or milk to minimize GI distress.
▶ Notify the physician if nausea, vomiting, abdominal pain, easy bruising or bleeding, tinnitus, impaired hearing, sweating, thirst, diarrhea, or black tarry stools occur.

Gold Salts
▶ *Note:* The possibility of toxic reactions must be explained before therapy is started on an outpatient basis. This is usually the responsibility of the physician. Give the patient a list of the adverse

reactions that require notifying the physician of their occurrence as soon as possible.

► Inform the patient that arthralgia (pain in the joints) may be noted for 1 or 2 days after the parenteral form is given.

► Avoid exposure to sunlight because a photosensitivity reaction may occur.

Nonsteroidal Antiinflammatory Drugs

► Do not take aspirin during therapy with this drug; aspirin may interfere with the drug's action.

► Take this drug with food or milk to prevent GI upset. Take indomethacin with food or milk; sulindac is taken with food.

► Notify the physician if skin rash, itching, visual disturbances, weight gain, diarrhea, black stools, nausea, vomiting, or persistent headache occurs.

► Diabetic patient—Test urine daily or as recommended by the physician. Notify the physician if there is an increased amount of glucose in the urine because an adjustment in insulin dosage may be needed.

Drugs Used for Gout

► Drink at least 10 glasses of water a day until the acute attack has subsided. Then water intake can be lessened.

► Take this drug with food to minimize GI upset.

► If drowsiness occurs, avoid driving or performing other hazardous tasks.

► Acute gout—Notify the physician if pain is not relieved in a few days.

► Colchicine for acute gout: take at the intervals prescribed by the physician. Stop taking the medication when the pain is relieved or when diarrhea or vomiting occurs. If the pain is not relieved in about 12 hours, notify the physician.

► Allopurinol—Notify the physician if a skin rash occurs.

► Colchicine—Notify the physician if skin rash, sore throat, fever, unusual bleeding or bruising, unusual fatigue, or weakness occurs.

Skeletal Muscle Relaxants

► This drug may cause drowsiness. Do not drive or perform other hazardous tasks if drowsiness occurs during use of the drug.

Penicillamine

► *Note:* The toxic effects associated with this drug must be explained before therapy is started. This is usually done by the physician. The patient must know which toxic reactions require contacting the physician immediately.

► Take this drug on an empty stomach 1 hour before or 2 hours after a meal.

► If other drugs are prescribed, penicillamine is taken 1 hour apart from any other drug.

► Observe skin areas over the elbows, shoulders, and buttocks for evidence of bruising, bleeding, or break in the skin. If these occur, do not self-treat the problem but notify the physician immediately.

Phenylbutazone and Oxyphenbutazone

► Take this drug with food or milk to prevent GI upset.

► Notify the physician immediately if any of the following occur: sore throat, sores in the mouth, unusual bleeding or bruising, fever, blurred vision, black tarry stools, or skin rash.

EVALUATION

► Anxiety is reduced

► Adverse reactions are identified and reported to the physician

► Verbalizes importance of complying with the prescribed treatment regimen

► Patient and family demonstrate understanding of drug regimen

Abstract Abbreviations

AC	before meals	—	**KVO**	keep vein open
ADL	activities of daily living		**mEq**	milliequivalent
AIDS	acquired immunodeficiency syndrome		**mL**	milliliter
ARC	AIDS-related complex		**mm**	millimeter
BUN	blood urea nitrogen		**ng**	nanogram
CBC	complete blood count		**NPO**	nothing by mouth
CHF	congestive heart failure		**OTC**	over-the-counter (nonprescription) drugs
CNS	central nervous system		**PC**	after meals
CVP	central venous pressure		**PO**	orally, by mouth
d	day		**prn**	whenever necessary, when needed
dL	decaliter		**PVCs**	premature ventricular contractions
ECG	electrocardiogram		**qh**	every hour (q2h, q3h, q4h, q6h, etc—every 2, 3, 4, 6 hours and so on)
GI	gastrointestinal			
GU	genitourinary		**RBC**	red blood cell
h	hour	—	**REM**	rapid eye movement
HS	hour of sleep		**SC**	subcutaneous
IM	intramuscular		**URI**	upper respiratory infection
IU	international units		**UTI**	urinary tract infection
IV	intravenous		**WBC**	white blood cell

Handwritten annotations:

BC p̄ meals

Dig Level

g day

as - L
OD - R eye

Ung - ointment
3 - dram
3 - oz ounce
kg - kilogram

OD - once a day
h - hour
aa - of each
Caps - capsule
Tabs - tablet
CC - Cubic Centimeters
(Cough Syrup) - Elix - Elixir
gr - grain
GM - gram

gtt - drop
L - liter
ML - milliliter
O - pint
OD = Rt eye
OS - lt eye
OU = Both eyes
QOD - every other day
Rx - take
SP - frumenti = whiskey
SS - half
Stat - immediately

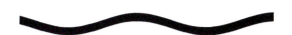

Glossary

acidosis a disturbance of the acid–base balance of the body with a shift toward the acid state

agranulocytosis a decrease in or absence of agranulocytes (a type of white blood cell)

alkalosis a disturbance of the acid–base balance of the body with an accumulation of alkali

alopecia loss of hair

analeptic a drug that stimulates respiration

analgesia relief of pain

analgesic a drug capable of relieving pain

anaphylactic reaction a sudden, severe reaction whose symptoms progress rapidly and may result in death if not treated

angioneurotic edema localized wheals or swellings occurring in subcutaneous tissue or mucous membrane probably as an allergic response to a drug or substance

anorexia loss of appetite

antibacterial against bacteria

antibiotic a drug that destroys or slows the multiplication rate of organisms

antiemetic a drug given to relieve or prevent nausea and vomiting

antimicrobial a drug that prevents the multiplication of microorganisms

antipyretic a drug capable of reducing an elevated body temperature (fever)

aplastic anemia a blood disorder caused by damage to the bone marrow resulting in a marked reduction in the number of red blood cells and some white cells

arterioles small arteries

ataxia muscular incoordination

auscultation the act of listening

bactericidal a drug or agent that destroys bacteria

bacteriostatic a drug or agent that slows or retards the multiplication of bacteria

bigeminy an irregular pulse rate consisting of two beats followed by a pause before the next two paired beats

blepharospasm a twitching or spasm of the eyelid

bradycardia slow pulse rate, usually below 60/min

bronchospasm spasm or constriction of the bronchi resulting in difficulty in breating

carcinoma cancer

cheilosis cracking at the edges of the lips

chemotherapy treatment with a drug, often used when referring to treatment with an antineoplastic drug

crystalluria crystals in the urine

cyclopegia paralysis of the ciliary muscle of the eye resulting in an inability to focus the eye

decaliter 10 liters or 10,000 mL

diluent a fluid that dilutes

diplopia double vision

diuresis production and passage of abnormally large amounts of urine

diuretic an agent that promotes the excretion of water and electrolytes

dyscrasia abnormal or disease

edema the retention of excess fluid in body tissues

endogenous produced by the body

exogenous originating outside of an organ or part; originating outside of the body

extravasation the escape of fluid into surrounding tissue

febrile   related to fever

glossitis   inflammation of the tongue

glucosuria   glucose (sugar) in the urine

granulocytopenia   a reducion or decrease in the number of granulocytes (a type of white blood cell)

hematologic   pertaining to blood cells or the blood

hematopoietic   pertaining to the production and development of blood cells

hematuria   blood in the urine

hyperglycemia   elevated blood glucose

hyperkalemia   an excessive amount of potassium in the blood

hypernatremia   an excessive amount of sodium in the blood

hypersensitive   allergic

hypersensitivity reaction   an allergic reaction

hyperuricemia   elevated serum uric acid levels

hypocalcemia   low blood calcium

hypoglycemia   low blood glucose

hyokalemia   low blood potassium

hyponatremia   low blood sodium

hypoproteinemia   a deficiency of protein in the blood

hypoprothrombinemia   a decrease in the amount of prothrombin in the blood

hypotension, orthostatic   a decrease in blood pressure occurring after standing in one place for an extended period

hypotension, postural   a decrease in blood pressure following a sudden change in body position

hypovolemia   a decrease in the circulating blood volume (*adj.,* hypovolemic)

ketonuria   ketones in the urine

laryngospasm   spasm of the laryngeal muscles resulting in dyspnea and noisy respirations

latent   not active; hidden

leukopenia   a decrease in the number of white blood cells

lipodystrophy   atrophy of subcutaneous fat

lumen   opening; the space within a blood vessel

miosis   pinpoint pupils; constriction of the pupils

mydriasis   dilatation of the pupil of the eye

myocardium   the muscle layer of the heart (*adj.,* myocardial)

necrosis   death of tissue

neoplastic   new abnormal tissue growth, usually referring to malignant tumors

nephrotoxic   harmful to the kidney

nonsteroidal   not a steroid

nystagmus   an involuntary and constant movement of the eyeball

oliguria   a decrease in urinary output (*adj.,* oliguric)

osmotic pressure   the pressure developing when two solutions of different concentrations are separated by a semipermeable membrane; a pressure necessary for osmosis

osteomalacia   a softening of the bones

osteoporosis   a loss of calcium from the bones, resulting in a decrease in bone density

ototoxic   harmful to the ear

overt   not hidden; clearly evident

parenteral   administration of a substance, such as a drug, by any route other than the oral route

paresthesia   an abnormal sensation such as numbness, tingling, prickling, or heightened sensitivity

pathogenic   capable of causing disease

phlebitis   inflammation of a vein

photophobia   an aversion to or intolerance of light

photosensitivity   sensitivity to light

photosensitivity reaction   an exaggerated sunburn reaction when the skin is exposed to sunlight

polydipsia   excessive thirst

polyphagia   eating large amounts of food

polyuria   excessive production and voiding of urine

postpartum   after childbirth

postural hypotension   *see* hypotension, postural

prepubertal   before puberty

prophylaxis   prevention

pruritus   itching

resorption   the act of removing something by absorption

rhinitis; vasomotor rhinitis   inflammation of the nasal passages resulting in increased nasal secretions

serum sickness   symptoms of chills, fever, edema, joint and muscle pain, malaise

stomatitis   inflammation of the mouth

sublingual   under the tongue

superinfection   a new infection caused by a microorganism different from that which caused the original infection

sympathomimetic   acting like the sympathetic nervous system

thrombocytopenia   a decrease in the number of platelets

thrombosis   development of a thrombus

thrombus   a blood clot (*pl.,* thrombi)

tinnitus   ringing in the ears

trigeminy   an irregular pulse rate consisting of three beats followed by a pause before the next three beats

urticaria   hives

vasodilation   dilation of a vessel

vasopressor   a constriction of the blood vessels, which when widespread results in a rise in blood pressure

venous   pertaining to the veins

venules   small veins

vertigo   a sensation of moving or objects moving usually accompanied by difficulty in walking and maintaining balance

vestibular   pertaining to the structures of the inner ear

Metric – Apothecary Equivalents and Conversions

Liquid Measurements

METRIC	APPROXIMATE APOTHECARY EQUIVALENTS	APPROXIMATE HOUSEHOLD EQUIVALENTS
1000 mL*	32 fluid ounces (1 quart)	1 quart
500 mL	16 fluid ounces (1 pint)	1 pint
250 mL	8 fluid ounces	1 measuring cup
30 mL	1 fluid ounce	2 tablespoonfuls
15 mL	4 fluid drams	1 tablespoonful
4 or 5 mL	1 fluid dram	1 teaspoonful
1 mL	15 or 16 minims	
0.06 mL	1 minim	1 drop

* 1 milliliter (mL) is the approximate equivalent of 1 cubic centimeter (cc).

Weights

METRIC	APPROXIMATE APOTHECARY EQUIVALENTS
30 g	1 ounce
15 g	4 drams
4 g	60 grains (1 dram)
1 g	15 or 16 grains
300 mg	5 grains
60 mg	1 grain
30 mg	1/2 grain
10 mg	1/6 grain
6 mg	1/10 grain
1 mg	1/60 grain
0.6 mg	1/100 grain
0.5 mg	1/120 grain
0.4 mg	1/150 grain
0.3 mg	1/200 grain
0.2 mg	1/300 grain
0.1 mg	1/600 grain

Other Equivalents and Conversions

METRIC

1 kg = 1000 g
1 g = 1000 mg
1 mg = 0.001 g
1 mcg = 0.001 mg
1 liter = 1000 mL

WEIGHT

1 kg = 2.2 pounds (lb)
1 lb = 453.6 g (0.454 kg)

LENGTH

1 cm = 0.39 inch
1 inch = 2.54 cm

Celsius (Centigrade) and Fahrenheit Temperatures

CELSIUS (CENTRIGRADE) 0	FARENHEIT 32
36.0	96.8
36.5	97.7
37.0	98.6
37.5	99.5
38.0	100.4
38.5	101.3
39.0	102.2
39.5	103.1
40.0	104.0
40.5	104.9
41.0	105.8
41.5	106.7
42.0	107.6

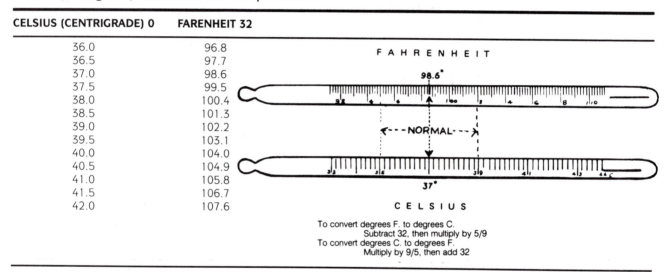

To convert degrees F. to degrees C.
Subtract 32, then multiply by 5/9
To convert degrees C. to degrees F.
Multiply by 9/5, then add 32

Comparative Scales of Measures, Weights, and Temperatures

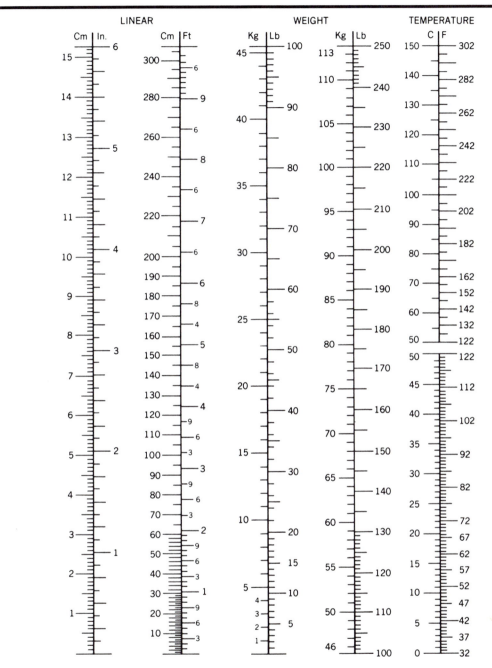

LINEAR   WEIGHT   TEMPERATURE

* 2.5 cm. = 1 inch   1 kg. = 2.2 lb.

Body Surface Area Nomograms

Nomogram for Estimating Body Surface Area of Infants and Young Children

HEIGHT		SURFACE AREA	WEIGHT	
feet	centimeters	in square meters	pounds	kilograms

HEIGHT (feet):
- 3′
- 34″
- 32″
- 30″
- 28″
- 26″
- 2′
- 22″
- 20″
- 18″
- 16″
- 14″
- 1′
- 10″
- 9″
- 8″

HEIGHT (centimeters):
- 95
- 90
- 85
- 80
- 75
- 70
- 65
- 60
- 55
- 50
- 45
- 40
- 35
- 30
- 25
- 20

SURFACE AREA (in square meters):
- .8
- .7
- .6
- .5
- .4
- .3
- .2
- .1

WEIGHT (pounds):
- 65
- 60
- 55
- 50
- 45
- 40
- 35
- 30
- 25
- 20
- 15
- 10
- 5
- 4
- 3

WEIGHT (kilograms):
- 30
- 25
- 20
- 15
- 10
- 5
- 4
- 3
- 2
- 1

To determine the surface area of the patient, draw a straight line between the point representing his height on the left vertical scale to the point representing his weight on the right vertical scale. The point at which this line intersects the middle vertical scale represents the patient's surface area in square meters. (Courtesy of Abbott Laboratories)

Nomogram for Estimating Body Surface Area of Older Children and Adults

HEIGHT		SURFACE AREA	WEIGHT	
feet	centimeters	in square meters	pounds	kilograms

HEIGHT (feet): 7', 10", 8", 6", 4", 2", 6', 10", 8", 6", 4", 2", 5', 10", 8", 6", 4", 2", 4', 10", 8", 6", 4", 2", 3', 10", 8", 6"

HEIGHT (centimeters): 220, 215, 210, 205, 200, 195, 190, 185, 180, 175, 170, 165, 160, 155, 150, 145, 140, 135, 130, 125, 120, 115, 110, 105, 100, 95, 90, 85, 80, 75

SURFACE AREA (square meters): 3.00, 2.90, 2.80, 2.70, 2.60, 2.50, 2.40, 2.30, 2.20, 2.10, 2.00, 1.95, 1.90, 1.85, 1.80, 1.75, 1.70, 1.65, 1.60, 1.55, 1.50, 1.45, 1.40, 1.35, 1.30, 1.25, 1.20, 1.15, 1.10, 1.05, 1.00, .95, .90, .85, .80, .75, .70, .65, .60

WEIGHT (pounds): 440, 420, 400, 380, 360, 340, 320, 300, 290, 280, 270, 260, 250, 240, 230, 220, 210, 200, 190, 180, 170, 160, 150, 140, 130, 120, 110, 100, 90, 80, 70, 60, 50

WEIGHT (kilograms): 200, 190, 180, 170, 160, 150, 140, 130, 120, 110, 100, 95, 90, 85, 80, 75, 70, 65, 60, 55, 50, 45, 40, 35, 30, 25, 20

(Courtesy, Abbott Laboratories.)

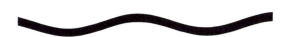

Index

Drugs are indexed under their generic names. Page numbers followed by *f* indicate illustrations; *t* following a page number indicates tabular material; *g* following a page number indicates a glossary entry.

A

AA (Alcoholics Anonymous), 86
Abbokinase (urokinase), 98*t*, 103
Abbreviations, 323
Abnormal behavior syndrome (attention deficit disorder), CNS stimulants for, 135
  nursing management with, 136
  patient teaching with, 137
Abortifacient(s), 225*t*, 228–230
Abstinence syndrome, defined, 81
Accutane. *See* Isotretinoin
Acebutolol hydrochloride (Sectral), 43*t*, 130*t*
Acetaminophen (Anacin-3, Tylenol), 72*t*
  actions of, 71
  adverse reactions to, 72
  uses of, 71
Acetazolamide (Diamox), 122*t*, 123*t*
Acetohexamide (Dymelor), 145*t*
  administration of, 146
Acetylcholine (ACh), 49
Acetylcholinesterase (AChE), 49
Acetylcysteine (Mucomyst), 269*t*
  administration of, 269–270
  patient teaching with, 270
Acetylsalicylic acid. *See* Aspirin
ACh (acetylcholine), 49

AChE (acetylcholinesterase), 49
Acidosis, 324*g*
Acquired immunodeficiency syndrome (AIDS)
  antiviral agents used in, 186
  Pneumocystis carinii pneumonia treatment in, 189–190
  transmission of, through needle sharing, 82
  tuberculosis prophylaxis in, 173
ACTH (adrenocorticotropic hormone), 198*f*, 199*t*, 201–202
Acthar (adrenocorticotropic hormone), 199*t*, 201–202
Actigall (ursodiol), 273*t*, 274
Activase (alteplase), 98*t*
Acyclovir (Zovirax), 187*t*
  actions of, 185
  administration of, 186
  uses of, 186
Adapin (doxepin hydrochloride), 254*t*
Addiction. *See also* Drug dependency; Substance abuse
  defined, 81–82
Adenohypophysis, 197
  hormones produced by, 197–202, 198*f*, 199*t*
ADH (vasopressin), 198*f*, 199*t*, 202–204

Adphen (phendimetrazine tartrate), 134*t*
Adrenalin. *See* Epinephrine
Adrenalin Chloride. *See* Epinephrine hydrochloride
Adrenergic blocking agent(s), 42–48, 43–44*t*
  actions of, 42–43
  adverse reactions to, 45
  as antihypertensive drugs, 46, 47–48, 128, 129–130*t*
  nursing process with, 45–48
  uses of, 43–45
Adrenergic drug(s), 36–41, 39*t*
  actions of, 37
  adverse reactions to, 37
  as bronchodilators, 263, 264*t*
    administration of, 266
    adverse reactions to, 263, 266
  nursing process with, 37–41
  uses of, 37
Adrenocortical hormone(s), 204–208, 204*t*, 206*t*
  actions of, 205
  adverse reactions to, 205, 206*t*
  nursing process with, 205–208
  uses of, 205, 206*t*
Adrenocorticotropic hormone (ACTH, corticotropin, Acthar), 198*f*, 199*t*, 201–202